Publicly Funded Healthcare
Comprehensive Reference Guide & Citation Source

Contents

Chapter 1

Introduction & Overview

1.1 Publicly funded health care

Publicly funded healthcare is a form of health care financing designed to meet the cost of all or most healthcare needs from a publicly managed fund. Usually this is under some form of democratic accountability, the right of access to which are set down in rules applying to the whole population contributing to the fund or receiving benefits from it.

The fund may be a not-for-profit trust that pays out for healthcare according to common rules established by the members or by some other democratic form. In some countries, the fund is controlled directly by the government or by an agency of the government for the benefit of the entire population. That distinguishes it from other forms of private medical insurance, the rights of access to which are subject to contractual obligations between an insurer (or his sponsor) and an insurance company, which seeks to make a profit by managing the flow of funds between funders and providers of health care services.

When taxation is the primary means of financing health care and sometimes with compulsory insurance, all eligible people receive the same level of cover regardless of their financial circumstances or risk factors.[1]

1.1.1 Varieties of public systems

Main article: Health care system

Most developed countries have partially or fully publicly funded health systems. Most western industrial countries have a system of social insurance based on the principle of social solidarity that covers eligible people from bearing the direct burden of most health care expenditure, funded by taxation during their working life.

Among countries with significant public funding of healthcare there are many different approaches to the funding and provision of medical services. Systems may be funded from general government revenues (as in Canada) or through a government social security system (as in Australia, France, Belgium, Japan and Germany) with a separate budget and hypothecated taxes or contributions. The proportion of the cost of care covered also differs: in Canada, all hospital care is paid for by the government, while in Japan, patients must pay 10 to 30% of the cost of a hospital stay. Services provided by public systems vary. For example, the Belgian government pays the bulk of the fees for dental and eye care, while the Australian government covers eye care but not dental care.

Publicly funded medicine may be administered and provided by the government, as in the Nordic countries, Portugal, Spain, and Italy; in some systems, though, medicine is publicly funded but most hospital providers are private entities, as in Canada. The organization providing public health insurance is not necessarily a public administration, and its budget may be isolated from the main state budget. Some systems do not provide universal healthcare or restrict coverage to public health facilities. Some countries, such as Germany, have multiple public insurance organizations linked by a common legal framework. Some, such as the Netherlands, allow private for-profit insurers to participate.

Two-tier healthcare

Main article: Two-tier healthcare

Almost every major country that has a publicly funded healthcare system also has a parallel private system for patients who hold private medical insurance or themselves pay for treatment.[2] In those states, those able to pay have access to treatment and comforts that may not be available to those dependent upon the state system.

From the inception of the NHS model (1948), public hospitals in the United Kingdom have included "amenity beds" which would typically be siderooms fitted more comfortably, and private wards in some hospitals where for a fee more amenities are provided. Patients using these beds are

1

in an NHS hospital for surgical treatment, and operations are generally carried out in the same operating theatres as NHS work and by the same personnel but the hospital and the physician receive funding from an insurance company or the patient. These amenity beds do not exist in all publicly funded systems, such as in Spain. The NHS also pays for private hospitals to take on surgical cases under contract.

1.1.2 Policy discussion

Main articles: Health system and Health care reform

Many countries are seeking the right balance of public and private insurance, public subsidies, and out-of-pocket payments.

Many OECD countries have implemented reforms to achieve policy goals of ensuring access to health care, improving the quality of health care and health outcomes, allocating an appropriate level of public sector other resources to healthcare but at the same time ensuring that services are provided in a cost-efficient and cost-effective manner (microeconomic efficiency). A range of measures, such as better payment methods, have improved the microeconomic incentives facing providers. However, introducing improved incentives through a more competitive environment among providers and insurers has proved difficult.[3]

A 2009 Harvard study published in the American Journal of Public Health found more than 44,800 excess deaths annually in the United States because of Americans' lacking health insurance, equivalent to one excess death every 12 min.[4][5] More broadly, the total number of people in the United States, whether insured or uninsured, who die because of lack of medical care was estimated in a 1997 analysis to be nearly 100,000 per year.[6]

1.1.3 See also

- Health care compared for varying degrees of public funding

- National health insurance

- Public opinion on health care reform in the United States

- Single-payer health care

- Socialized medicine

- Social insurance

- Universal health care

- National Health Service of the United Kingdom

1.1.4 References

[1] Claude Blanchette, Erin Tolley. "PUBLIC- AND PRIVATE-SECTOR INVOLVEMENT IN HEALTHCARE SYSTEMS: A COMPARISON OF OECD COUNTRIES." May 1997. Retrieved September 12, 2006.

[2] http://scc.lexum.umontreal.ca/en/2005/2005scc35/2005scc35.html Canadian Supreme Court, after expert testimony, found that all OECD countries and four of the ten Canadian provinces allow private medical insurance alongside the state system

[3] Elizabeth Docteur; Howard Oxley (2003). "Health-Care Systems: Lessons from the Reform Experience" (PDF). OECD.

[4] Wilper AP, Woolhandler S, Lasser KE, McCormick D, Bor DH, Himmelstein DU (December 2009). "Health Insurance and Mortality in US Adults" (PDF). American Journal of Public Health. 99 (12): 2289–2295. doi:10.2105/ajph.2008.157685. PMC 2775760. PMID 19762659. Retrieved 10 September 2014.

[5] State-by-state breakout of excess deaths from lack of insurance

[6] A 1997 study carried out by Professors David Himmelstein and Steffie Woolhandler (New England Journal of Medicine 336, no. 11 [1997]) "concluded that almost 100,000 people died in the United States each year because of lack of needed care—three times the number of people who died of AIDs." The Inhuman State of U.S. Health Care, Monthly Review, Vicente Navarro, September 2003. Retrieved 2009-09-10

1.1.5 Further reading

- Devereaux PJ, Choi PT, Lacchetti C, et al. (May 2002). "A systematic review and meta-analysis of studies comparing mortality rates of private for-profit and private not-for-profit hospitals". CMAJ. 166 (11): 1399–406. PMC 111211. PMID 12054406.

- Devereaux PJ, Heels-Ansdell D, Lacchetti C, et al. (June 2004). "Payments for care at private for-profit and private not-for-profit hospitals: a systematic review and meta-analysis". CMAJ. 170 (12): 1817–24. doi:10.1503/cmaj.1040722. PMC 419772. PMID 15184339.

- Doctors support universal health care: survey, Reuters, March 31, 2008 (first reported in Annals of Internal Medicine).

- Krauss, C. As Canada's Slow-Motion Public Health System Falters, Private Medical Care is Surging, New York Times, February 26, 2006.

- Woolhandler S, Himmelstein DU (August 1999). "When money is the mission—the high costs of investor-owned care". *N. Engl. J. Med.* **341** (6): 444–6. doi:10.1056/NEJM199908053410611. PMID 10432332.

1.2 Single-payer healthcare

Single-payer healthcare is a system in which the state, rather than private insurers, pays for all healthcare costs.[1] Single-payer systems may contract for healthcare services from private organizations (as is the case in Canada) or may own and employ healthcare resources and personnel (as is the case in the United Kingdom).

The term "single-payer" thus describes the funding mechanism, referring to healthcare financed by a single public body from a single fund, not the type of delivery or for whom physicians work. The British system is technically not single payer, as it consists of a number of financially and legally autonomous trusts and private health insurance options are also allowed. Only Canada and Taiwan have true single-payer systems.[2]

The actual funding of a "single payer" system comes from all or a portion of the covered population. Although the fund holder is usually the state, some forms of single-payer use a mixed public-private system.

1.2.1 Description

Single-payer health insurance collects all medical fees and then pays for all services, by a single government (or government-related) source.[3] In wealthy nations, that kind of publicly managed insurance is typically extended to all citizens and legal residents. Examples include the United Kingdom's National Health Service, Australia's Medicare, Canada's Medicare, and Taiwan's National Health Insurance.

The standard usage of the term "single-payer healthcare" refers to health insurance, as opposed to healthcare delivery, operating as a public service and offered to citizens and legal residents towards providing nearly universal or universal healthcare. The fund can be managed by the government directly or as a publicly owned and regulated agency.[3] Some writers describe publicly administered systems as "single-payer plans". Some writers have described any system of healthcare which intends to cover the entire population, such as voucher plans, as "single-payer plans",[4] but that is uncommon.

1.2.2 Countries with single payer systems

Main article: Health care system § International comparisons

Many nations worldwide have single-payer health insurance programs. These programs generally provide some form of universal healthcare, which are implemented in a variety of ways. In some cases doctors are employed, and hospitals run by, the government such as in the United Kingdom[5] or Spain.[6] Alternatively the government may purchase healthcare services from outside organizations, such as the approach taken in Canada.

Canada

Main article: Health care in Canada
See also: Canadian and American health care systems compared and Medicare (Canada)

Healthcare in Canada is delivered through a publicly funded healthcare system, which is mostly free at the point of use and has most services provided by private entities.[7] It is guided by the provisions of the Canada Health Act of 1984.[8] The government assures the quality of care through federal standards. The government does not participate in day-to-day care or collect any information about an individual's health, which remains confidential between a person and his or her physician. Canada's provincially based Medicare systems are cost-effective partly because of their administrative simplicity. In each province each doctor handles the insurance claim against the provincial insurer. There is no need for the person who accesses healthcare to be involved in billing and reclaim. Private insurance represents a minimal part of the overall system.

Competitive practices such as advertising are kept to a minimum, thus maximizing the percentage of revenues that go directly towards care. In general, costs are paid through funding from income taxes, except in British Columbia, the only province to impose a fixed monthly premium which is waived or reduced for those on low incomes.[9] There are no deductibles on basic health care and co-pays are extremely low or non-existent (supplemental insurance such as Fair Pharmacare may have deductibles, depending on income). A health card is issued by the Provincial Ministry of Health to each individual who enrolls for the program and everyone receives the same level of care.[10] There is no need for a variety of plans because virtually all essential basic care is covered, including maternity and infertility problems. Depending on the province, dental and vision care may not be covered but are often insured by employers through private companies. In some provinces, private supplemental plans are available for those who desire private rooms if they are hospitalized. Cosmetic surgery and some forms of elective surgery are not considered essential care and are generally not covered. These can be paid out-of-pocket or through private insurers. Health coverage is not affected by loss or change of jobs, as long as premiums are up to date, and there are no lifetime limits or exclusions for pre-existing conditions.

Pharmaceutical medications are covered by public funds for the elderly or indigent,[11] or through employment-based private insurance. Drug prices are negotiated with suppliers by the federal government to control costs. Family physicians (often known as general practitioners or GPs in Canada) are chosen by individuals. If a patient wishes to see a specialist or is counseled to see a specialist, a referral can be made by a GP. Canadians do wait for some treatments and diagnostic services. Survey data shows that the median wait time to see a special physician is a little over four weeks with 89.5% waiting less than three months. The median wait time for diagnostic services such as MRI and CAT scans[12] is two weeks, with 86.4% waiting less than three months.[13] The median wait time for surgery is four weeks, with 82.2% waiting less than three months.[14]

While physician income initially boomed after the implementation of a single-payer program, a reduction in physician salaries followed, which many feared would be a long-term result of government-run healthcare. However, by the beginning of the 21st century, medical professionals were again among Canada's top earners.[15]

Taiwan

Main article: Healthcare in Taiwan

Healthcare in Taiwan is administrated by the Department of Health of the Executive Yuan. As with other developed economies, Taiwanese people are well-nourished but face such health problems as chronic obesity and heart disease.[16] In 2002 Taiwan had nearly 1.6 physicians and 5.9 hospital beds per 1,000 population.[16] In 2002, there were a total of 36 hospitals and 2,601 clinics in the country. Per capita health expenditures totaled US$752 in 2000.[16] Health expenditures constituted 5.8 percent of the gross domestic product (GDP) in 2001 (or $951 US in 2009[17]); 64.9 percent of the expenditures were from public funds.[16] Overall life expectancy in 2009 was 78 years.[18] Despite the initial shock on Taiwan's economy from increased costs of expanded healthcare coverage, the single-payer system has provided protection from greater financial risks and has made healthcare more financially accessible for the population, resulting in a steady 70% public satisfaction rating.[19]

The current healthcare system in Taiwan, known as National Health Insurance (NHI), was instituted in 1995. NHI is a single-payer compulsory social insurance plan which centralizes the disbursement of health care funds. The system promises equal access to health care for all citizens, and the population coverage had reached 99% by the end of 2004.[20] NHI is mainly financed through premiums, which are based on the payroll tax, and is supplemented with out-of-pocket payments and direct government funding. In the initial stage, fee-for-service predominated for both public and private providers. Most health providers operate in the private sector and form a competitive market on the health delivery side. However, many healthcare providers took advantage of the system by offering unnecessary services to a larger number of patients and then billing the government. In the face of increasing loss and the need for cost containment, NHI changed the payment system from fee-for-service to a global budget, a kind of prospective payment system, in 2002. Taiwan's success with a single-payer health insurance program is owed, in part, to the country's human resources and the government's organizational skills, allowing for the effective and efficient management of government-run health insurance program.[19]

1.2.3 Countries with hybrid single-payer/private insurance systems

Australia

Main article: Health care in Australia

Healthcare in Australia is provided by both private and government institutions. Medicare is the publicly funded universal health care venture in Australia. It was instituted in 1984 and coexists with a private health system. Medicare is funded partly by a 2% income tax levy[21] (with exceptions for low-income earners), but mostly out of general revenue. An additional levy of 1% is imposed on high-income earners without private health insurance. As well as Medicare, there is a separate Pharmaceutical Benefits Scheme that considerably subsidises a range of prescription medications. The Minister for Health administers national health policy, elements of which (such as the operation of hospitals) are overseen by individual states.

France

Main article: Health care in France

Everyone is covered by the French national health insurance scheme, known as "Assurance Maladie", but more than 90% of its residents have private, supplemental insurance, known as "complémentaire santé", which is either provided by their employer or purchased on the market.[22]

Spain

Building upon less structured foundations, in 1963 the existence of a single-payer healthcare system in Spain was established by the Spanish government.[23] The system was sustained by contributions from workers, and covered them and their dependents.[24] The universality of the system was established later in 1986. At the same time, management of public healthcare was delegated to the different autonomous communities in the country.[25]

While previously this was not the case, in 1997 it was established that public authorities can delegate management of publicly funded healthcare to private companies.[26] Additionally, in parallel to the single-payer healthcare system there are private insurers, which provide coverage for some private doctors and hospitals. Employers will sometimes offer private health insurance as a benefit,[27] with 14.8% of the Spanish population being covered under private health insurance in 2013.[28]

In 2000, the Spanish healthcare system was rated by the World Health Organization as the 7th best in the world.

United Kingdom

Main article: Healthcare in the United Kingdom

Healthcare in the United Kingdom is a devolved matter, meaning England, Northern Ireland, Scotland and Wales each have their own systems of private and publicly funded healthcare, generally referred to as the National Health Service (NHS). Each country having different policies and priorities has resulted in a variety of differences existing between the systems.[29][30] That said, each country provides public healthcare to all UK permanent residents that is free at the point of use, being paid for from general taxation. In addition, each also has a private sector which is considerably smaller than its public equivalent, with provision of private healthcare acquired by means of private health insurance, funded as part of an employer funded healthcare scheme or paid directly by the customer, though provision can be restricted for those with conditions such as AIDS/HIV.[31][32]

The individual systems are:

- England: National Health Service

- Northern Ireland: Health and Social Care in Northern Ireland (HSCNI)

- Scotland: NHS Scotland

- Wales: NHS Wales

In England, funding from general taxation is channeled through NHS England, which is responsible for commissioning mainly specialist services and primary care, and Clinical Commissioning Groups (CCGs), which hold 60% of the budget and are responsible for commissioning health services for their local populations.[33] These commissioning bodies do not provide services themselves directly, but procure these from NHS Trusts and Foundation Trusts, as well as private, voluntary and social enterprise sector providers.[34]

United States

Main article: Health care in the United States

A number of proposals have been made for a universal single-payer healthcare system in the United States, most recently the United States National Health Care Act, (popularly known as H.R. 676 or "Medicare for All") but none has achieved more than 20% congressional co-sponsorship.

Advocates argue that preventive healthcare expenditures can save several hundreds of billions of dollars per year because publicly funded universal healthcare would benefit employers and consumers, that employers would benefit from a bigger pool of potential customers and that employers would likely pay less, would be spared administrative costs, and inequities between employers would be reduced. Advocates also argue that single payer could benefit from a more fluid economy with increasing economic growth, aggregate demand, corporate profit, and quality of life.[35][36][37] Also, for example, cancer patients are more likely to be diagnosed at Stage I where curative treatment is typically a few outpatient visits, instead of at Stage III or later in an emergency room where treatment can involve years of hospitalization and is often terminal.[38][39] Others have estimated a long-term savings amounting to 40% of all national health expenditures due to preventive health care,[40] although estimates from the Congressional Budget Office and *The New England Journal of Medicine* have found that preventive care is more expensive due to increased utilization.[41]

Any national system would be paid for in part through taxes replacing insurance premiums, but advocates also believe savings would be realized through preventive care and the elimination of insurance company overhead and hospital billing costs.[42] An analysis of a single-payer bill by Physicians for a National Health Program estimated the immediate savings at $350 billion per year.[43] The Commonwealth Fund believes that, if the United States adopted a universal health care system, the mortality rate would improve and the country would save approximately $570 billion a year.[44]

Recent enactments of single-payer systems within individual states, such as in Vermont in 2011, are seen as possible routes to enacting single-payer on the federal level.[45][46] In December 2014, Vermont cancelled its plan for single payer healthcare.[47]

National policies and proposals Medicare in the United States is a single-payer healthcare system, but is restricted to only senior citizens over the age of 65, people under 65 who have specific disabilities, and anyone with End-Stage Renal Disease.[48] Government is increasingly involved in U.S. health care spending, paying about 45% of the $2.2 trillion the nation spent on individuals' medical care in 2004.[49] However, studies have shown that the publicly administered share of health spending in the U.S. may be closer to 60% as of 2002.[50]

According to Princeton University health economist Uwe Reinhardt, U.S. Medicare, Medicaid, and State Children's Health Insurance Program (SCHIP) represent "forms of 'social insurance' coupled with a largely private healthcare delivery system" rather than forms of "socialized medicine." In contrast, he describes the Veterans Administration healthcare system as a pure form of socialized medicine because it is "owned, operated and financed by government."[51]

In a peer-reviewed paper published in the *Annals of Internal Medicine*, researchers of the RAND Corporation reported that the quality of care received by Veterans Administration patients scored significantly higher overall than did comparable metrics for patients currently using United States Medicare.[52]

The United States National Health Care Act, is a perennial piece of legislation introduced in the United States House of Representatives by Representative John Conyers (D-MI) every year since 2002.[53] The act would establish a universal single-payer health care system in the United States, the rough equivalent of Canada's Medicare, the United Kingdom's National Health Service, and Taiwan's Bureau of National Health Insurance, among other examples. Under a single payer system, all medical care would be paid for by the Government of the United States, ending the need for private health insurance and premiums, and probably recasting private insurance companies as providing purely supplemental coverage, to be used when non-essential care is sought. The bill was first introduced in 2002,[53] and has been reintroduced in each Congress since. During the 2009 health care debates over the bill that became the Patient Protection and Affordable Care Act, H.R. 676 was expected to be debated and voted upon by the House in September 2009,[54] but was never debated.[55]

The Congressional Budget Office and related government agencies scored the cost of a single payer health care system several times since 1991. The General Accounting Office published a report in 1991 noting that "[I]f the US were to shift to a system of universal coverage and a single payer, as in Canada, the savings in administrative costs [10 percent of health spending] would be more than enough to offset the expense of universal coverage."[56] The CBO scored the cost in 1991, noting that "the population that is currently uninsured could be covered without dramatically increasing national spending on health" and that "all US residents might be covered by health insurance for roughly the current level of spending or even somewhat less, because of savings in administrative costs and lower payment rates for services used by the privately insured.[57] A CBO report in 1993 stated that "[t]he net cost of achieving universal insurance coverage under this single payer system would be negative" in part because "consumer payments for health would fall by $1,118 per capita, but taxes would have to increase by $1,261 per capita" in order to pay for the plan.[58] A July 1993 scoring also resulted in positive outcomes, with the CBO stating that, "[a]s the program was phased in, the administrative savings from switching to a single-payer system would offset much of the increased demand for health care services. Later, the cap on the growth of the national health budget would hold the rate of growth of spending below the baseline."[59] The CBO also scored Sen. Paul Wellstone's American Health and Security Act of 1993 in December 1993, finding that "by year five (and in subsequent years) the new system would cost less than baseline."[60] A 2014 study published in the journal BMC Medical Services Research by James Kahn, etal, found that the actual administrative burden of health care in the United States was 27.4% of all national health expenditures. The study examined both direct costs charged by insurers for profit, administration and marketing but also the indirect burden placed on health care providers like hospitals, nursing homes and doctors for costs they incurred in working with private health insurers including contract negotiations, financial and clinical record-keeping (variable and idiosyncratic for each payer). Kahn, et al. estimate that the added cost for the private insurer health system in the US was about $471 billion in 2012 compared to a single payer system like Canada's. This represents just over 20% of the total national healthcare expenditure in 2012. Kahn asserts that this excess administrative cost will increase under the Affordable Care Act with its reliance on the provision of health coverage through a multi-payer system.[61]

State proposals Several single-payer state referendums and bills from state legislatures have been proposed, but, with the exception of Vermont,[62] all have failed. In December 2014, Vermont canceled its plan for single payer health care.[47]

California California attempted passage of a single-payer bill as early as 1994,[63] and the first successful passages of legislation through the California State Legislature, SB 840 or "The California Universal Healthcare Act" (authored by Sheila Kuehl), occurred in 2006 and again in 2008.[64] Both times, Governor Arnold Schwarzenegger vetoed the bill.[65] State Senator Mark Leno has reintroduced the bill in each legislative session since.[66]

Colorado Main article: ColoradoCare

The Colorado State Health Care System Initiative, Amendment 69, was a citizen-initiated constitutional amendment proposal in November 2016 to vote on a single payer healthcare system funded by a 10% payroll tax split 2:1 between employers and employees. This would have replaced the private health insurance premiums currently paid by employees and companies.[67] The ballot was rejected by 79% of the electorate.[68]

Hawaii In 2009, the Hawaii state legislature passed a single-payer healthcare bill that was vetoed by Republican Governor Linda Lingle. While the veto was overridden by the legislature, the bill was not implemented.[69]

Illinois In 2007, the Health Care for All Illinois Act was introduced and the Illinois House of Representatives' Health Availability Access Committee passed the single-payer bill favorably out of committee by an 8–4 vote. The legislation was eventually referred back to the House rules committee and not taken up again during that session.[70]

Massachusetts Massachusetts had passed a universal healthcare program in 1986, but budget constraints and partisan control of the legislature resulted in its repeal before the legislation could be enacted.[71] Question 4, a nonbinding referendum, was on the ballot in 14 state districts in November 2010, asking voters, "[S]hall the representative from this district be instructed to support legislation that would establish healthcare as a human right regardless of age, state of health or employment status, by creating a single payer health insurance system like Medicare that is comprehensive, cost effective, and publicly provided to all residents of Massachusetts?" The ballot question passed in all 14 districts that offered the question.[72][73]

Minnesota The Minnesota Health Act, which would establish a statewide single payer health plan, has been presented to the Minnesota legislature regularly since 2009. The bill was passed out of both the Senate Health Housing and Family Security Committee[74] and the Senate Commerce and Consumer Protection Committee[75] in 2009, but the House version was ultimately tabled.[76] In 2010, the bill passed the Senate Judiciary Committee on a voice vote[77] as well as the House Health Care & Human Services Policy and Oversight Committee.[78] In 2011, the bill was introduced as a two-year bill in both the Senate[79] and House,[80] but did not progress. It has been introduced again in the 2013 session in both chambers.[81][82]

Montana In September 2011, Governor Brian Schweitzer announced his intention to seek a waiver from the federal government allowing Montana to set up a single payer healthcare system.[83] Governor Schweitzer was unable to implement single-payer health care in Montana, but did make moves to open government-run clinics[84] and, in his final budget as governor, increased coverage for lower-income Montana residents.[85]

New York New York State has been attempting passage of the New York Health Act, which would establish a statewide single-payer health plan, since 1992. The New York Health Act has passed the Assembly twice, once in 1992 and again in 2015, but has failed to advance through the Senate after referrals to the Health Committee. On both occasions, the legislation passed the Assembly by an almost two-to-one ratio of support.[86]

Oregon The state of Oregon attempted to pass single payer healthcare via Oregon Ballot Measure 23 in 2002, and the measure was rejected by a significant majority.[87] Previous bills, including the Affordable Health Care for All Oregon Act, have been introduced in the legislature but have never left committee. The Affordable Health Care Act may be reintroduced in the 2013 session.[88]

Pennsylvania The Family Business and Healthcare Security Act has been introduced in the Pennsylvania legislature numerous times, but has never been able to pass.[89][90][91]

Vermont Main article: Vermont health care reform

In December 2014, Vermont canceled its plan for single payer healthcare.[47] Vermont passed legislation in 2011 creating Green Mountain Care.[92] When Governor Peter Shumlin signed the bill into law, Vermont became the first state to functionally have a single payer health care system.[93] While the bill is considered a single-payer bill, private insurers can continue to operate in the state indefinitely, meaning it does not fit the strict definition of single-payer. Representative Mark Larson, the initial sponsor of the bill, has described Green Mountain Care's provisions "as close as we can get [to single-payer] at the state level."[94][95]

Vermont abandoned the plan in 2014, citing costs and tax increases as too high to implement.[96]

Public opinion   Advocates for single payer point to support in polls, although the polling is mixed depending on how the question is asked.[97] Polls from Harvard University in 1988,[98] the Los Angeles Times in 1990,[99] and the Wall Street Journal in 1991[100] all showed strong support for a health care system comparable to the system in Canada. More recently, however, polling support has declined.[97][101] A 2007 Yahoo/AP poll showed a majority of respondents considered themselves supporters of "single-payer health care,"[102] and a plurality of respondents in a 2009 poll for Time Magazine showed support for "a national single-payer plan similar to Medicare for all."[103] Polls by Rasmussen Reports in 2011[104] and 2012[105] showed pluralities opposed to single payer health care.

A 2001 article in the public health journal *Health Affairs* studied fifty years of American public opinion of various health care plans and concluded that, while there appears to be general support of a "national health care plan," poll respondents "remain satisfied with their current medical arrangements, do not trust the federal government to do what is right, and do not favor a single-payer type of national health plan."[101] Politifact rated a statement by Michael Moore "false" when he stated that "[t]he majority actually want single-payer health care." According to Politifact, responses on these polls largely depend on the wording. For example, people respond more favorably when they are asked if they want a system "like Medicare."[97]

Advocacy groups   Physicians for a National Health Program[106] the American Medical Student Association,[107] Healthcare-NOW! and the California Nurses Association[108] are among advocacy groups that have called for the introduction of a single payer healthcare program in the United States. A 2007 study published in the *Annals of Internal Medicine* found that 59% of physicians "supported legislation to establish national health insurance" while 9% were neutral on the topic, and 32% opposed it.[109]

1.2.4   Criticisms of single-payer healthcare

Criticisms of a single-payer healthcare system include:

- Public mistrust and reluctance to expand the size of government.

- Fears that set wages will reduce incentives for the development of new medicines and technology, concerns that easier access to medicine will reinforce drug addiction.

- The unwillingness of individuals to pay for a service (via increased taxes) that may not benefit them personally.

- The belief that state-funded healthcare will create a free-rider problem where individuals abuse government services, creating longer wait-times for the critically ill.[110]

Criticisms from physicians include fears that government-run healthcare will limit their discretion when treating patients, decrease physician salaries, and leave less money to cover more services, potentially reducing the quality of treatment.[111]

1.2.5   See also

- Health care reform debate in the United States

- International comparisons of health care systems – tabular comparisons of the US, Canada, and other countries not shown above.

- The Kucinich Amendment, an amendment to the America's Affordable Health Choices Act of 2009 which would have empowered the Secretary of Health and Human Services to waive the federal law that preempts state law on employee-related health care.

- National health insurance

- Public health insurance option ("the public option")

- All payer healthcare

1.2.6   References

[1] single-payer, Merriam Webster Dictionary

[2] Julie Rovner (January 22, 2016). "Debate Sharpens Over Single-Payer Health Care, But What Is It Exactly?". NPR.

[3] Medical Subject Headings thesaurus, National Library of Medicine."Single-Payer System" Year introduced: 1996, (From Slee and Slee, Health Care Reform Terms, 1993, p106)

[4] Frank, Robert H. (2007-02-15). A Health Care Plan So Simple, Even Stephen Colbert Couldn't Simplify It, By ROBERT H. FRANK. New York Times, February 15, 2007. Retrieved from http://www.nytimes.com/2007/02/15/business/15scene.html.

[5] Aguirre, Jessica Camille (August 6, 2012). "In British Emergency Room, 'There's No Card To Show; There Are No Bills'". *NPR*. Retrieved August 9, 2012.

[6] Socolovsky, Jerome. "What Makes Spain's Health Care System The Best?". *NPR*. Retrieved 21 September 2014.

[7] Public vs. private health care *CBC*, December 1, 2006.

[8] "Overview of the Canada Health Act".

[9] "Ministry of Health - Redirect".

[10] "Provincial/Territorial Role in Health".

[11] CIHI p. 91

[12] Diagnostic tests defined as the following: non-emergency magnetic resonance imaging (MRI) devices; computed tomography (CT or CAT) scans; and angiographies that use X-rays to examine the inner opening of blood-filled structures such as veins and arteries.

[13] Section from Healthy Canadians: A Federal report on Comparable Health Indicators Archived June 4, 2008, at the Wayback Machine.

[14] , *Canadian Medical Association Journal*

[15] Duffin, Jacalyn (2016-11-17). "The Impact of Single-Payer Health Care on Physician Income in Canada, 1850–2005". *American Journal of Public Health*. **101** (7): 1198–1208. doi:10.2105/AJPH.2010.300093. ISSN 0090-0036. PMC 3110239Ⓒ. PMID 21566029.

[16] "Taiwan country profile" (PDF). Library of Congress Federal Research Division. March 2005. Retrieved 2008-05-04. *This article incorporates text from this source, which is in the public domain.*

[17] GDP data refer to the year 2009. World Economic Outlook Database-April 2010, International Monetary Fund. Accessed on April 24, 2010.

[18] List by the CIA World Factbook (2009 estimates)

[19] Lu, Jui-Fen Rachel; Hsiao, William C. (2003-05-01). "Does Universal Health Insurance Make Health Care Unaffordable? Lessons From Taiwan". *Health Affairs*. **22** (3): 77–88. doi:10.1377/hlthaff.22.3.77. ISSN 0278-2715. PMID 12757274.

[20] Fanchiang, Cecilia."New IC health insurance card expected to offer many benefits", *Taiwan Journal, January 2nd, 2004* Accessed March 28, 2008

[21] "Medicare levy increase to fund DisabilityCare Australia". *www.ato.gov.au*. Retrieved 28 February 2015.

[22] Maggie Mahar (February 25, 2014). "Single-Payer Health Care: Is That What Makes France So Different?". HealthBeat.

[23] "Seguridad Social:Conócenos".

[24] "Historia de la Sanidad Pública española. Revisión bibliográfica - Revista Médica Electrónica PortalesMedicos.com". November 23, 2013.

[25] La protección de la salud en España

[26] "BOE.es - Documento BOE-A-1997-9021".

[27] González, Alejandro Nieto (September 22, 2014). "Muface y la sanidad privada, ¿de verdad tiene sentido?".

[28] Informe IDIS, Análisis de situación 2013

[29] 'Huge contrasts' in devolved NHS BBC News, 28 August 2008

[30] NHS now four different systems BBC 2 January 2008

[31] BUPA exclusions bupa.co.uk, accessed 23 February 2009

[32] Bob Wachter, MD (January 16, 2012). "The Awkward World of Private Insurance in the UK". The Health Care Blog.

[33] Commissioning, NHS. "NHS Commissioning".

[34] Choices, NHS. "The structure of the NHS in England - NHS Choices". *www.nhs.uk*. Retrieved 2016-02-23.

[35] Lincoln, Taylor (April 8, 2014). "Severing the Tie That Binds: Why a Publicly Funded, Universal Health Care System Would Be a Boon to U.S. Businesses" (PDF). *Public Citizen*. Retrieved 1 July 2014.

[36] Institute of Medicine, Committee on the Consequences of Uninsurance; Board on Health Care Services (2003). *Hidden Costs, Value Lost: Uninsurance in America*. Washington, DC: The National Academies Press.

[37] Ungar, Rick (April 6, 2012). "A Dose Of Socialism Could Save Our States - State Sponsored, Single Payer Healthcare Would Bring In Business & Jobs". *Forbes*. Retrieved 20 May 2014.

[38] Hogg, W.; Baskerville, N.; Lemelin, J. (2005). "Cost savings associated with improving appropriate and reducing inappropriate preventive care: Cost-consequences analysis" (PDF). *BMC Health Services Research*. **5**: 20. doi:10.1186/1472-6963-5-20. PMC 1079830Ⓒ. PMID 15755330.

[39] Kao-Ping Chua; Flávio Casoy (June 16, 2007). "Single Payer 101". American Medical Student Association. Retrieved 20 May 2014.

[40] Hogg, W.; Baskerville, N; Lemelin, J (2005). "Cost savings associated with improving appropriate and reducing inappropriate preventive care: cost-consequences analysis". *BMC Health Services Research*. **5** (1): 20. doi:10.1186/1472-6963-5-20. PMC 1079830. PMID 15755330.

[41] PolitiFact: Barack Obama says preventive care 'saves money'. February 10, 2012.

[42] Krugman, Paul (June 13, 2005). "One Nation, Uninsured". *The New York Times*. Retrieved December 4, 2011.

[43] Physicians for a National Health Program (2008) "Single Payer System Cost?" *PNHP.org*

[44] Friedman, Gerald. "Funding a National Single-Payer System "Medicare for All" Would save Billions, and Could Be Redistributive.". Dollars & Sense.

[45] "State-Based Single-Payer Health Care — A Solution for the United States?" *New England Journal of Medicine* 364;13:1188-90, March 31, 2011

[46] *Vox*: Forget Obamacare: Vermont wants to bring single payer to America. April 9, 2014.

[47] Governor abandons single-payer health care plan, Associated Press, December 17, 2014

[48] HealthCare.gov: What is Medicare?.

[49] Appleby, Julie (2006-10-16). "Universal care appeals to USA". *USA Today*. Retrieved 2007-05-22.

[50] Health Affairs, July 2002. Woolhandler, Steffi

[51] "Letters: For Children's Sake, This 'Schip' Needs to Be Relaunched", Wall Street Journal, July 11, 2007, Uwe Reinhardt and others.

[52] Asch SM, McGlynn EA, Hogan MM, et al. (December 2004). "Comparison of quality of care for patients in the Veterans Health Administration and patients in a national sample". *Ann. Intern. Med.* **141** (12): 938–45. doi:10.7326/0003-4819-141-12-200412210-00010. PMID 15611491.

[53] "House Reps Introduce Medicare-for-All Bill" *Becker's Hospital Review*, Feb. 14, 2013

[54] "Single Payer Gets A Vote (Updated)". *Daily News*. New York. July 31, 2009.

[55] "H.R. 676: United States National Health Care Act or the Expanded and Improved Medicare for All Act (Govtrack.us)". Retrieved December 1, 2009.

[56] "Canadian Health Insurance: Lessons for the United States," General Accounting Office, June 1991.

[57] Universal Health Insurance Coverage Using Medicare's Payment Rates, Congressional Budget Office, December 1991.

[58] "Single-Payer and All-Payer Health Insurance Systems Using Medicare's Payment Rates" Congressional Budget Office, April 1993.

[59] "Estimates of Health Care Proposals from the 102nd Congress" Congressional Budget Office, July 1993.

[60] S.491, American Health Security Act of 1993, Congressional Budget Office, December 1993.

[61] Kahn, James (2014). "Billing and insurance-related administrative costs in US healthcare". *BMC Health Services Research*. **14**: 556. doi:10.1186/s12913-014-0556-7.

[62] Vermont moves toward single-payer | Arlene Karidis.

[63] "The California Single-Payer Debate, The Defeat of Proposition 186 – Kaiser Family Foundation". Kff.org. Retrieved November 20, 2011.

[64] "Healthcare for All Bill Passes — Governor Threatens Veto".

[65] *Marin Independent Journal*: "Leno reintroduces single-payer health plan." March 15, 2009.

[66] Latest News on SB 801 | Senator Mark Leno.

[67] Munro, Dan. "Colorado Puts Single-Payer Healthcare On 2016 Ballot".

[68] http://results.enr.clarityelections.com/CO/63746/183105/Web01/en/summary.html

[69] RealClearPolitics: Single-Payer Is Not Dead. January 14, 2014.

[70] "Illinois General Assembly Bill Status: HB 311".

[71] *New York Times*: State Referendums Seeking to Overhaul Health Care System. June 11, 2000.

[72] "Boston Globe: Ballot Questions (2010)". *Boston Globe*. Retrieved November 20, 2011.

[73] WBUR: Non-Binding Measure On Single-Payer System Passes In All 14 Districts. November 4, 2010.

[74] Committee on Health, Housing and Family Security Minutes, January 16, 2009.]

[75] Video of Senate committee session in which the bill was passed out of committee.

[76] Minutes of the House Health Care and Human Services Policy & Oversight Committee, February 25, 2009.

[77] Video of Senate committee session in which the bill was passed on a voice vote.

[78] Audio of House Health Care & Human Services Policy and Oversight Committee proceedings.

[79] Senate – Bill Number 0008.

[80] House – Bill number 0051.

[81] Senate – File number 18.

[82] House – File number 76.

[83] *Missoulan*: Schweitzer wants statewide universal health care program. September 28, 2011.

[84] Reuters: Brian Schweitzer, Montana Governor, Sees Big Savings With New State Health Clinic. September 30, 2012.

[85] Missoulan: Schweitzer's final budget proposal boosts education, health care. November 15, 2012.

[86] "New York State Assembly - Bill Search and Legislative Information".

[87] "Oregon Secretary of State: That Trail's Gone Cold!" (PDF).

[88] *Statesman Journal*: Demonstrators urge universal single-payer health care system. February 5, 2013.

[89] *Central Penn Business Journal*: State senator introduces Pa. health care plan. October 13, 2011.

[90] Co-sponsorship Memo Family and Business Health Care Security Act. Office of Representative Tony Payton, June 20, 2012.

[91] Lancaster Online: Universal interest in health care. January 13, 2008.

[92] "Vt. Senate approves single-payer plan – WCAX.COM Local Vermont News, Weather and Sports". Wcax.com. April 26, 2011. Retrieved November 20, 2011.

[93] Politico: Vermont could be first in line for single payer. September 17, 2012.

[94] American Medical News: Vermont approves universal health program. May 16, 2011.

[95] Owen Dyer (10 January 2014). "US Health Reforms: America's first single payer system". *BMJ*. **348**: g102. doi:10.1136/bmj.g102.

[96] Associated Press: [Governor abandons single-payer health care plan https://news.yahoo.com/governor-abandons-single-payer-health-223834879.html]. December 17, 2014.

[97] "Michael Moore claims a majority favor a single-payer health care system". PolitiFact. Retrieved November 20, 2011.

[98] Harvard/Harris poll: Robert J. Blendon et al., "Views on health care: Public opinion in three nations," *Health Affairs*, Spring 1989;8(1)149-157.

[99] *Los Angeles Times* poll: "Health Care in the United States," Poll no. 212, Storrs, Conn.: Administered by the Roper Center for Public Opinion Research, March 1990

[100] Wall Street Journal-NBC poll: Michael McQueen, "Voters, sick of the current health-care systems, want federal government to prescribe remedy," Wall Street Journal, June 28, 1991

[101] *Health Affairs*, Volume 20, No. 2. "Americans' Views on Health Policy: A Fifty-Year Historical Perspective." March/April 2001. http://content.healthaffairs.org/content/20/2/33.full.pdf+html

[102] AP/Yahoo poll: Administered by Knowledge Networks, December 2007: http://surveys.ap.org/data/KnowledgeNetworks/AP-Yahoo_2007-08_panel02.pdf

[103] TIME MAGAZINE/ABT SRBI – July 27–28, 2009 Survey: http://www.srbi.com/Research-Impacts/Polls/Time-Abt-SRBI-Poll-Most-Americans-Eager-for-Health.aspx

[104] Rasmussen Reports: Rasmussen Reports. January 1, 2010. Retrieved November 20, 2011.

[105] Rasmussen Reports: Rasmussen Reports. Retrieved December 30, 2012.

[106] "Proposal of the Physicians' Working Group for Single-Payer National Health Insurance". Physicians for a National Health Program.

[107] Chua, Kao-Ping (2006), *Single Payer 101* (PDF), Reston, Virginia: American Medical Student Association, retrieved 11 April 2012

[108] Single-payer, or Medicare for all, is the way to go from the California Nurses Association / National Nurses Organizing Committee.

[109] Carroll AE, Ackerman RT (April 2008). "Support for National Health Insurance among U.S. Physicians: 5 years later". *Ann. Intern. Med.* **148** (7): 566–7. doi:10.7326/0003-4819-148-7-200804010-00026. PMID 18378959.

[110] "List of Pros and Cons of Single Payer Health Care". *OccupyTheory*. 2015-01-02. Retrieved 2016-11-17.

[111] S.J. Katz, S. Zuckerman, and W.P. Welch. "Comparing Physician Fee Schedules in Canada and the United States," *Health Care Financing Review* 14 (1992):141–149; S.E.D. Shortt, *The Doctor Dilemma: Public Policy and the Changing Role of Physicians Under Ontario Medicare* (Montreal, Quebec: McGill-Queen's University Press, 1999); W.P. Welch, S.J. Katz, and S. Zuckerman, "Physician Fee Levels: Medicare Versus Canada," *Health Care Financing Review* 14, no. 3 (1993):41–54

1.3 Universal health care

See also: Universal health coverage by country

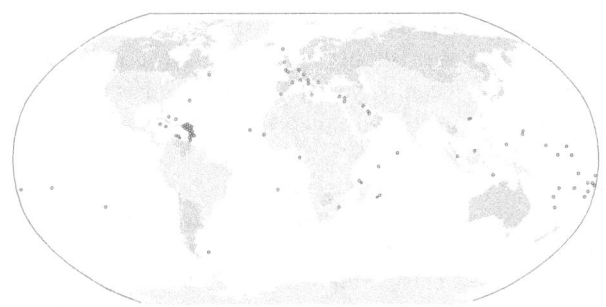

As of 2009, 58 countries have legislation mandating universal health care and have actually reached >90% health insurance coverage and >90% skilled birth attendance.[1]

Universal health care, sometimes referred to as **universal health coverage**, **universal coverage**, or **universal care**, usually refers to a health care system which provides health care and financial protection to all citizens of a particular country. It is organized around providing a specified package of benefits to all members of a society with the end goal of providing financial risk protection, improved access to health services, and improved health outcomes.[2] Universal health care is not one-size-fits-all and does not imply coverage for all people for everything. Universal health care can be determined by three critical dimensions: who is covered, what services are covered, and how much of the cost is covered.[2] It is described by the World Health Organization as a situation where citizens can access health services without incurring financial hardship.[3]

The health policy framework is of central importance. Thus, in the development of universal health systems, it is appropriate to recognize "healthy public policy" (Health in All Policies) as the overarching policy framework, with public health, primary health care, and community services as the cross-cutting framework for all health and health-related services operating across the spectrum from primary prevention to long term care and end-stage conditions. Although that perspective is both logical and well grounded in the social ecological model, the reality is different in most settings, and there is room for improvement everywhere.[4]

1.3.1   History

The first move towards a national health insurance system was launched in Germany in 1883, with the Sickness Insurance Law. Industrial employers were mandated to provide injury and illness insurance for their low-wage workers, and the system was funded and administered by employees and employers through "sick funds", which were drawn from deductions in workers' wages and from employers' contributions. Other countries soon began to follow suit. In the United Kingdom, the National Insurance Act

1911 provided coverage for primary care (but not specialist or hospital care) for wage earners, covering about one third of the population. The Russian Empire established a similar system in 1912, and other industrialized countries began following suit. By the 1930s, similar systems existed in virtually all of Western and Central Europe. Japan introduced an employee health insurance law in 1927, expanding further upon it in 1935 and 1940. Following the Russian Revolution of 1917, the Soviet Union established a fully public and centralized health care system in 1920.[5][6] However, it was not a truly universal system at that point, as rural residents were not covered.

In New Zealand, a universal health care system was created in a series of steps, from 1939 to 1941.[7][8] In Australia, the state of Queensland introduced a free public hospital system in the 1940s.

Following World War II, universal health care systems began to be set up around the world.   On July 5, 1948, the United Kingdom launched its universal National Health Service.   Universal health care was next introduced in the Nordic countries of Sweden (1955),[9] Iceland (1956),[10] Norway (1956),[11] Denmark (1961),[12] and Finland (1964).[13] Universal health insurance was then introduced in Japan (1961), and in Canada through stages, starting with the province of Saskatchewan in 1962, followed by the rest of Canada from 1968 to 1972.[7][14] The Soviet Union extended universal health care to its rural residents in 1969.[7][15] Italy introduced its *Servizio Sanitario Nazionale* (National Health Service) in 1978.   Universal health insurance was implemented in Australia beginning with the *Medibank* system in 1975, which led to universal coverage under the Medicare system, established in 1984.

From the 1970s to the 2000s, Southern and Western European countries began introducing universal coverage, most of them building upon previous health insurance programs to cover the whole population. For example, France built upon its 1928 national health insurance system, with subsequent legislation covering a larger and larger percentage of the population, until the remaining 1% of the population that was uninsured received coverage in 2000.[16][17] In addition, universal health coverage was introduced in some Asian countries, including South Korea (1989), Taiwan (1995), Israel (1995), and Thailand (2001).

Following the collapse of the Soviet Union, Russia retained and reformed its universal health care system,[18] as did other former Soviet nations and Eastern bloc countries.

Beyond the 1990s, many countries in Latin America, the Caribbean, Africa, and the Asia-Pacific region, including developing countries, took steps to bring their populations under universal health coverage, including China which has the largest universal health care system in the world.[19] A 2012 study examined progress being made by these countries, focusing on nine in particular: Ghana, Rwanda, Nigeria, Mali, Kenya, India, Indonesia, the Philippines, and Vietnam.[20][21]

1.3.2 Funding models

See also: Health care economics

Universal health care in most countries has been achieved by a mixed model of funding. General taxation revenue is the primary source of funding, but in many countries it is supplemented by specific levies (which may be charged to the individual and/or an employer) or with the option of private payments (by direct or optional insurance) for services beyond those covered by the public system.

Almost all European systems are financed through a mix of public and private contributions.[22] Most universal health care systems are funded primarily by tax revenue (like in Portugal[22] Spain, Denmark, and Sweden). Some nations, such as Germany and France[23] and Japan[24] employ a multipayer system in which health care is funded by private and public contributions. However, much of the non-government funding is by contributions by employers and employees to regulated non-profit sickness funds. Contributions are compulsory and defined according to law.

A distinction is also made between municipal and national healthcare funding. For example, one model is that the bulk of the healthcare is funded by the municipality, speciality healthcare is provided and possibly funded by a larger entity, such as a municipal co-operation board or the state, and the medications are paid by a state agency.

Universal health care systems are modestly redistributive. The progressivity of health care financing has limited implications for overall income inequality.[25]

Compulsory insurance

Main article: National health insurance

This is usually enforced via legislation requiring residents to purchase insurance, but sometimes the government provides the insurance. Sometimes, there may be a choice of multiple public and private funds providing a standard service (as in Germany) or sometimes just a single public fund (as in Canada). Healthcare in Switzerland and the US Patient Protection and Affordable Care Act are based on compulsory insurance.[26][27]

In some European countries in which private insurance and universal health care coexist, such as Germany, Belgium, and the Netherlands, the problem of adverse selection is overcome by using a risk compensation pool to equalize, as far as possible, the risks between funds. Thus, a fund with a predominantly healthy, younger population has to pay into a compensation pool and a fund with an older and predominantly less healthy population would receive funds from the pool. In this way, sickness funds compete on price, and there is no advantage to eliminate people with higher risks because they are compensated for by means of risk-adjusted capitation payments. Funds are not allowed to pick and choose their policyholders or deny coverage, but they compete mainly on price and service. In some countries, the basic coverage level is set by the government and cannot be modified.[28]

The Republic of Ireland at one time had a "community rating" system by VHI, effectively a single-payer or common risk pool. The government later opened VHI to competition but without a compensation pool. That resulted in foreign insurance companies entering the Irish market and offering cheap health insurance to relatively healthy segments of the market, which then made higher profits at VHI's expense. The government later reintroduced community rating by a pooling arrangement and at least one main major insurance company, BUPA, then withdrew from the Irish market.

Among the potential solutions posited by economists are single-payer systems as well as other methods of ensuring that health insurance is universal, such as by requiring all citizens to purchase insurance or limiting the ability of insurance companies to deny insurance to individuals or vary price between individuals.[29][30]

Single payer

Main article: Single-payer health care

Single-payer health care is a system in which the government, rather than private insurers, pays for all health care costs.[31] Single-payer systems may contract for healthcare services from private organizations (as is the case in Canada) or own and employ healthcare resources and personnel (as was the case in England before of the Health and Social Care Act). "Single-payer" thus describes only the funding mechanism and refers to health care financed by a single public body from a single fund and does not specify the type of delivery or for whom doctors work. Although the fund holder is usually the state, some forms of single-payer use a mixed public-private system.

Tax-based financing

In tax-based financing, individuals contribute to the provision of health services through various taxes. These are typically pooled across the whole population, unless local governments raise and retain tax revenues. Some countries (notably the United Kingdom, Canada, Ireland, Australia, New Zealand, Italy, Spain, Portugal and the Nordic countries) choose to fund health care directly from taxation alone. Other countries with insurance-based systems effectively meet the cost of insuring those unable to insure themselves via social security arrangements funded from taxation, either by directly paying their medical bills or by paying for insurance premiums for those affected.

Social health insurance

In social health insurance, contributions from workers, the self-employed, enterprises and government are pooled into a single or multiple funds on a compulsory basis. The funds typically contract with a mix of public and private providers for the provision of a specified benefit package. Preventive and public health care may be provided by these funds or responsibility kept solely by the Ministry of Health. Within social health insurance, a number of functions may be executed by parastatal or non-governmental sickness funds or in a few cases by private health insurance companies.

Private insurance

In private health insurance, premiums are paid directly from employers, associations, individuals and families to insurance companies, which pool risks across their membership base. Private insurance includes policies sold by commercial for profit firms, non-profit companies, and community health insurers. Generally, private insurance is voluntary in contrast to social insurance programs, which tend to be compulsory.[32]

In some countries with universal coverage, private insurance often excludes many health conditions that are expensive and the state health care system can provide. For example, in the United Kingdom, one of the largest private health care providers is BUPA, which has a long list of general exclusions even in its highest coverage policy,[33] most of which are routinely provided by the National Health Service. In the United States, dialysis treatment for end stage renal failure is generally paid for by government, not by the insurance industry. Those with privatized Medicare (Medicare Advantage) are the exception and must get their dialysis paid through their insurance company, but those with end stage renal failure generally cannot buy Medicare Advantage plans.[34]

The Planning Commission of India has also suggested that the country should embrace insurance to achieve universal health coverage.[35] General tax revenue is currently used to meet the essential health requirements of all people.

Community-based health insurance

A particular form of private health insurance that has often emerged if financial risk protection mechanisms have only a limited impact is community-based health insurance. Individual members of a specific community pay to a collective health fund, which they can draw from when they need of medical care. Contributions are not risk-related, and there is generally a high level of community involvement in the running of these plans.

1.3.3   Implementation and comparisons

Main article: Universal health coverage by country
See also: Health care system and Health systems by country
 Universal health care systems vary according to the degree

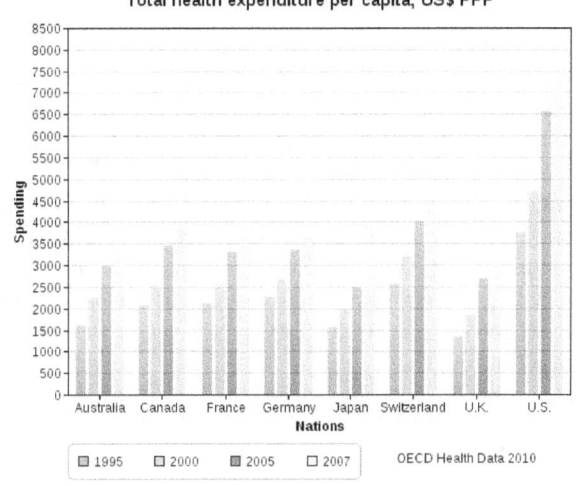

Health spending per capita, in US$ purchasing power parity-adjusted, among various OECD countries

of government involvement in providing care and/or health insurance. In some countries, such as the UK, Spain, Italy, Australia and the Nordic countries, the government has a high degree of involvement in the commissioning or delivery of health care services and access is based on residence rights, not on the purchase of insurance. Others have a much more pluralistic delivery system, based on obligatory health with contributory insurance rates related to salaries or income and usually funded by employers and beneficiaries jointly.

Sometimes, the health funds are derived from a mixture of insurance premiums, salary related mandatory contributions by employees and/or employers to regulated sickness funds, and by government taxes. These insurance based systems tend to reimburse private or public medical providers, often at heavily regulated rates, through mutual or publicly owned medical insurers. A few countries, such as the

Netherlands and Switzerland, operate via privately owned but heavily regulated private insurers, which are not allowed to make a profit from the mandatory element of insurance but can profit by selling supplemental insurance.

Universal health care is a broad concept that has been implemented in several ways. The common denominator for all such programs is some form of government action aimed at extending access to health care as widely as possible and setting minimum standards. Most implement universal health care through legislation, regulation and taxation. Legislation and regulation direct what care must be provided, to whom, and on what basis. Usually, some costs are borne by the patient at the time of consumption, but the bulk of costs come from a combination of compulsory insurance and tax revenues. Some programs are paid for entirely out of tax revenues. In others, tax revenues are used either to fund insurance for the very poor or for those needing long-term chronic care.

The United Kingdom National Audit Office in 2003 published an international comparison of ten different health care systems in ten developed countries, nine universal systems against one non-universal system (the United States), and their relative costs and key health outcomes.[36] A wider international comparison of 16 countries, each with universal health care, was published by the World Health Organization in 2004.[37] In some cases, government involvement also includes directly managing the health care system, but many countries use mixed public-private systems to deliver universal health care.

1.3.4   See also

- Health care reform debate in the United States

- Health insurance cooperative

- Health system

- List of countries by health insurance coverage

- National health insurance

- Primary health care

- Public health

- Publicly funded health care

- Right to health

- Single-payer health care

- Socialized medicine

- Two-tier health care

1.3.5   References

[1] Stuckler, David; Feigl, Andrea B.; Basu, Sanjay; McKee, Martin (November 2010). "The political economy of universal health coverage. Background paper for the First Global Symposium on Health Systems Research, 16–19 November 2010, Montreaux, Switzerland" (PDF). *Pacific Health Summit.* Seattle: National Bureau of Asian Research. p. 16. Figure 2. Global Prevalence of Universal Health Care in 2009; 58 countries: Andorra, Antigua, Argentina, Armenia, Australia, Austria, Azerbaijan, Bahrain, Belarus, Belgium, Bosnia and Herzegovina, Botswana, Brunei Darussalam, Bulgaria, Canada, Chile, Costa Rica, Croatia, Cuba, Cyprus, Czech Republic, Denmark, Estonia, Finland, France, Germany, Greece, Hungary, Iceland, Ireland, Israel, Italy, Japan, Kuwait, Luxembourg, Moldova, Mongolia, Netherlands, New Zealand, Norway, Oman, Panama, Portugal, Romania, Singapore, Slovakia, Slovenia, South Korea, Spain, Sweden, Switzerland, Taiwan, Thailand, Tunisia, UAE, Ukraine, United Kingdom, Venezuela.

[2] World Health Organization (November 22, 2010). "The world health report: health systems financing: the path to universal coverage". Geneva: World Health Organization. ISBN 978-92-4-156402-1. Retrieved April 11, 2012.

[3] "Universal health coverage (UHC)". Retrieved November 30, 2016.

[4] White F. Primary health care and public health: foundations of universal health systems. Med Princ Pract 2015;24:103-116. doi:10.1159/000370197

[5] http://content.healthaffairs.org/content/10/3/71.full.pdf

[6] *OECD Reviews of Health Systems OECD Reviews of Health Systems: Russian Federation 2012*, p. 38

[7] Abel-Smith, Brian (1987). "Social welfare; Social security; Benefits in kind; National health schemes". *The new Encyclopaedia Britannica* (15th ed.). Chicago: Encyclopaedia Britannica. ISBN 0-85229-443-3. Retrieved September 30, 2013.

[8] Richards, Raymond (1993). "Two Social Security Acts". *Closing the door to destitution: the shaping of the Social Security Acts of the United States and New Zealand.* University Park: Pennsylvania State University Press. p. 14. ISBN 978-0-271-02665-7. Retrieved March 11, 2013.
Mein Smith, Philippa (2012). "Making New Zealand 1930–1949". *A concise history of New Zealand* (2nd ed.). Cambridge: Cambridge University Press. pp. 164–165. ISBN 978-1-107-40217-1. Retrieved March 11, 2013.

[9] Serner, Uncas (1980). "Swedish health legislation: milestones in reorganisation since 1945". In Heidenheimer, Arnold J.; Elvander, Nils; Hultén, Charly. *The shaping of the Swedish health system.* New York: St. Martin's Press. p. 103. ISBN 0-312-71627-3. Universal and comprehensive

health insurance was debated at intervals all through the Second World War, and in 1946 such a bill was voted in Parliament. For financial and other reasons, its promulgation was delayed until 1955, at which time coverage was extended to include drugs and sickness compensation, as well.

[10] Kuhnle, Stein; Hort, Sven E.O. (September 1, 2004). "The developmental welfare state in Scandinavia: lessons to the developing world". Geneva: United Nations Research Institute for Social Development. p. 7. Retrieved March 11, 2013.

[11] Evang, Karl (1970). *Health services in Norway. English version by Dorothy Burton Skårdal* (3rd ed.). Oslo: Norwegian Joint Committee on International Social Policy. p. 23. OCLC 141033. Since 2 July 1956 the entire population of Norway has been included under the obligatory health national insurance program.

[12] Gannik, Dorte; Holst, Erik; Wagner, Mardsen (1976). "Primary health care". *The national health system in Denmark.* Bethesda: National Institutes of Health. pp. 43–44. Retrieved March 11, 2013.

[13] Alestalo, Matti; Uusitalo, Hannu (1987). "Finland". In Flora, Peter. *Growth to limits: the Western European welfare states since World War II, Vol. 4 Appendix (synopses, bibliographies, tables).* Berlin: Walter de Gruyter. pp. 137–140. ISBN 3-11-011133-0. Retrieved March 11, 2013.

[14] Taylor, Malcolm G. (1990). "Saskatchewan medical care insurance". *Insuring national health care: the Canadian experience.* Chapel Hill: University of North Carolina Press. pp. 96–130. ISBN 0-8078-1934-4.
Maioni, Antonia (1998). "The 1960s: the political battle". *Parting at the crossroads: the emergence of health insurance in the United States and Canada.* Princeton: Princeton University Press. pp. 121–122. ISBN 0-691-05796-6. Retrieved September 30, 2013.

[15] Kaser, Michael (1976). "The USSR". *Health care in the Soviet Union and Eastern Europe.* Boulder, Colo.: Westview Press. pp. 38–39, 43. ISBN 0-89158-604-0.
Roemer, Milton Irwin (1993). "Social security for medical care". *National health systems of the world: Volume II: The issues.* Oxford: Oxford University Press. p. 94. ISBN 0-19-507845-4. Retrieved September 30, 2013.
Denisova, Liubov N. (2010). "Protection of childhood and motherhood in the countryside". In Mukhina, Irina. *Rural women in the Soviet Union and post-Soviet Russia.* New York: Routledge. p. 167. ISBN 0-203-84684-2. Retrieved September 30, 2013.

[16] "Austerity and the Unraveling of European Universal Health Care - Dissent Magazine". Retrieved November 30, 2016.

[17] Bärnighausen, Till; Sauerborn, Rainer (May 2002). "One hundred and eighteen years of the German health insurance system: are there any lessons for middle- and low-income countries?". *Social Science & Medicine.* **54** (10): 1559–1587. doi:10.1016/S0277-9536(01)00137-X. PMID 12061488.

Busse, Reinhard; Riesberg, Annette (2004). "Germany" (PDF). *Health Care Systems in Transition.* Copenhagen: WHO Regional Office for Europe, European Observatory on Health Systems. **6** (9). ISSN 1020-9077. Retrieved October 8, 2013.
Carrin, Guy; James, Chris (January 2005). "Social health insurance: key factors affecting the transition towards universal coverage" (PDF). *International Social Security Review.* **58** (1): 45–64. doi:10.1111/j.1468-246X.2005.00209.x. Retrieved October 8, 2013.
Hassenteufel, Patrick; Palier, Bruno (December 2007). "Towards neo-Bismarckian health care states? Comparing health insurance reforms in Bismarckian welfare systems" (PDF). *Social Policy & Administration.* **41** (6): 574–596. doi:10.1111/j.1467-9515.2007.00573.x. Retrieved October 8, 2013.
Green, David; Irvine, Benedict; Clarke, Emily; Bidgood, Elliot (January 23, 2013). "Healthcare systems: Germany" (PDF). London: Civitas. Retrieved October 8, 2013.

[18] "WHO - Rocky road from the Semashko to a new health model". Retrieved November 30, 2016.

[19] "Universal health insurance coverage for 1.3 billion people: What accounts for China's success?". *Health Policy.* **119**: 1145–1152. doi:10.1016/j.healthpol.2015.07.008.

[20] Eagle, William. "Developing Countries Strive to Provide Universal Health Care". Retrieved November 30, 2016.

[21] "Universal Healthcare on the rise in Latin America". Retrieved November 30, 2016.

[22] Bentes, Margarida; Dias, Carlos Matias; Sakellarides, Sakellarides; Bankauskaite, Vaida (2004). "Health care systems in transition: Portugal" (PDF). Copenhagen: WHO Regional Office for Europe on behalf of the European Observatory on Health Systems and Policies. Retrieved August 30, 2006.

[23] Physicians for a National Health Program (2004). "International health systems". Chicago: Physicians for a National Health Program. Retrieved November 7, 2006.

[24] Chua, Kao-Ping (February 10, 2006). "Single payer 101" (PDF). Sterling, Virginia: American Medical Student Association. Archived from the original (PDF) on October 24, 2006. Retrieved November 7, 2006.

[25] Glied, Sherry A. (March 2008). "Health care financing, efficiency, and equity. Working Paper 13881" (PDF). Cambridge, Massachusetts: National Bureau of Economic Research. Retrieved March 25, 2008.

[26] Tomasky, Michael (March 21, 2010). "Healthcare vote: Barack Obama passes US health reform by narrow margin". *Michael Tomasky's blog.* London: The Guardian. Retrieved March 23, 2010.

[27] Roy, Avik. "Switzerland - a case study in consumer driven health care". *Forbes.*

[28] Varkevisser, Marco; van der Geest, Stéphanie (2002). "Competition among social health insurers: a case study for the Netherlands, Belgium and Germany" (PDF). *Research in Healthcare Financial Management.* **7** (1): 65–84. Retrieved November 28, 2007.

[29] Rothschild, Michael; Stiglitz, Joseph (November 1976). "Equilibrium in competitive insurance markets: an essay on the economics of imperfect information" (PDF). *Quarterly Journal of Economics.* **90** (4): 629–649. doi:10.2307/1885326. JSTOR 1885326. Retrieved March 20, 2007.

[30] Belli, Paolo (March 2001). "How adverse election affects the health insurance market. Policy Research Working Paper 2574" (PDF). Washington, D.C.: World Bank. Retrieved March 20, 2007.

[31] single-payer, Merriam Webster Dictionary

[32] World Health Organization (2008). "Health financing mechanisms: private health insurance". Geneva: World Health Organization. Archived from the original on October 9, 2010. Retrieved April 11, 2012.

[33] Bupa (2010). "Individuals: Health and life cover: Health care select 1: Key features of this health insurance plan: What's covered? What's not covered?". London: Bupa. Archived from the original on April 9, 2010. Retrieved April 11, 2010.

[34] Centers for Medicare & Medicaid Services (2010). "Medicare coverage of kidney dialysis & kidney transplant services" (PDF). Baltimore: Centers for Medicare & Medicaid Services. Retrieved April 11, 2010.

[35] Varshney, Vibha; Gupta, Alok; Pallavi, Aparna (September 30, 2012). "Universal health scare". *Down To Earth.* New Delhi: Society for Environmental Communications. Retrieved September 25, 2012.

[36] National Audit Office (February 1, 2003). "International health comparisons: a compendium of published information on healthcare systems, the provision of health care and health achievement in 10 countries". London: National Audit Office. Retrieved November 7, 2007.

[37] Grosse-Tebbe, Susanne; Figueras, Josep (2004). "Snapshots of health systems: the state of affairs in 16 countries in summer 2004" (PDF). Copenhagen: World Health Organization on behalf of the European Observatory on Health Systems and Policies. Archived from the original (PDF) on September 26, 2007. Retrieved November 7, 2007.

1.3.6   External links

- Achieving Universal Health Care (July 2011). *MEDICC Review: International Journal of Cuban Health and Medicine* **13** (3). Theme issue: authors from 19 countries on dimensions of the challenges of providing universal access to health care.

- Catalyzing Change: The System Reform Costs of Universal Health Coverage (November 15, 2010). New York: The Rockefeller Foundation. Report on the feasibility of establishing the systems and institutions needed to pursue UHC.

- Physicians for a National Health Program Chicago: PNHP. A group of physicians and health professionals who support single-payer reform.

- UHC Forward Washington, D.C.: Results for Development Institute. Portal on universal health coverage.

1.4   Health policy

This article is about policies, plans and strategies across the healthcare sector. For health insurance policies, see Health insurance. For the academic journal, see Health Policy (journal).

Health policy can be defined as the "decisions, plans, and

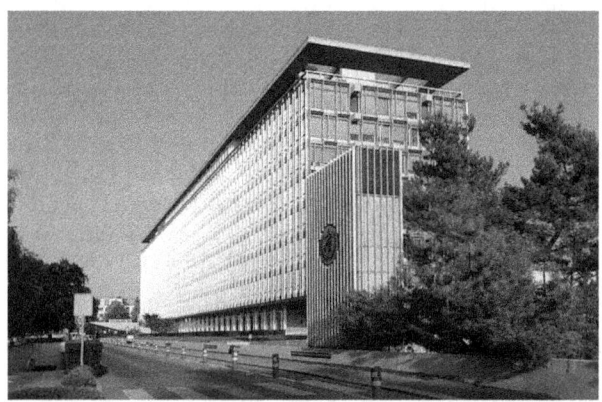

The headquarters of the World Health Organization in Geneva, Switzerland.

actions that are undertaken to achieve specific healthcare goals within a society. [1] According to the World Health Organization, an explicit health policy can achieve several things: it defines a vision for the future; it outlines priorities and the expected roles of different groups; and it builds consensus and informs people.[1]

There are many categories of health policies, including personal healthcare policy, pharmaceutical policy, and policies related to public health such as vaccination policy, tobacco control policy or breastfeeding promotion policy. They may cover topics of financing and delivery of healthcare, access to care, quality of care, and health equity.[2]

1.4.1 Background

Health-related policy and its implementation is complex. Conceptual models can help show the flow from health-related policy development to health-related policy and program implementation and to health systems and health outcomes. Policy should be understood as more than a national law or health policy that supports a program or intervention. Operational policies are the rules, regulations, guidelines, and administrative norms that governments use to translate national laws and policies into programs and services.[3] The policy process encompasses decisions made at a national or decentralized level (including funding decisions) that affect whether and how services are delivered. Thus, attention must be paid to policies at multiple levels of the health system and over time to ensure sustainable scale-up. A supportive policy environment will facilitate the scale-up of health interventions.[4]

There are many topics in the politics and evidence that can influence the decision of a government, private sector business or other group to adopt a specific policy. Evidence-based policy relies on the use of science and rigorous studies such as randomized controlled trials to identify programs and practices capable of improving policy relevant outcomes. Most political debates surround personal health care policies, especially those that seek to reform healthcare delivery, and can typically be categorized as either philosophical or economic. Philosophical debates center around questions about individual rights, ethics and government authority, while economic topics include how to maximize the efficiency of health care delivery and minimize costs.

The modern concept of healthcare involves access to medical professionals from various fields as well as medical technology, such as medications and surgical equipment. It also involves access to the latest information and evidence from research, including medical research and health services research.

In many countries it is left to the individual to gain access to healthcare goods and services by paying for them directly as out-of-pocket expenses, and to private sector players in the medical and pharmaceutical industries to develop research. Planning and production of health human resources is distributed among labour market participants.

Other countries have an explicit policy to ensure and support access for all of its citizens, to fund health research, and to plan for adequate numbers, distribution and quality of health workers to meet healthcare goals. Many governments around the world have established universal health care, which takes the burden of healthcare expenses off of private businesses or individuals through pooling of financial risk. There are a variety of arguments for and against universal healthcare and related health policies. Healthcare is an important part of health systems and therefore it often accounts for one of the largest areas of spending for both governments and individuals all over the world.

1.4.2 Personal healthcare policy options

Philosophy: right to health

See also: Philosophy of healthcare

Many countries and jurisdictions integrate a human rights philosophy in directing their healthcare policies. The World Health Organization reports that every country in the world is party to at least one human rights treaty that addresses health-related rights, including the right to health as well as other rights that relate to conditions necessary for good health.[5] The United Nations' Universal Declaration of Human Rights (UDHR) asserts that medical care is a right of all people:[6]

- *UDHR Article 25:* "Everyone has the right to a standard of living adequate for the health and well-being of himself and of his family, including food, clothing, housing and medical care and necessary social services, and the right to security in the event of unemployment, illness, disability, widowhood, old age or other lack of livelihood in circumstances beyond his control."

In some jurisdictions and among different faith-based organizations, health policies are influenced by the perceived obligation shaped by religious beliefs to care for those in less favorable circumstances, including the sick. Other jurisdictions and non-governmental organizations draw on the principles of humanism in defining their health policies, asserting the same perceived obligation and enshrined right to health.[7][8] In recent years, the worldwide human rights organization Amnesty International has focused on health as a human right, addressing inadequate access to HIV drugs and women's sexual and reproductive rights including wide disparities in maternal mortality within and across countries. Such increasing attention to health as a basic human right has been welcomed by the leading medical journal *The Lancet*.[9]

There remains considerable controversy regarding policies on who would be paying the costs of medical care for all people and under what circumstances. For example, government spending on healthcare is sometimes used as a global indicator of a government's commitment to the health of its people.[10] On the other hand, one school of thought emerging from the United States rejects the notion of health care financing through taxpayer funding as incompatible with the (considered no less important) right of the physician's professional judgment, and the related concerns that government involvement in overseeing the health of its citizens could erode the right to privacy between doctors and patients. The argument furthers that universal health insurance denies the right of individual patients to dispose of their own income as per their own will.[11][12]

Another issue in the rights debate is governments' use of legislation to control competition among private medical insurance providers against national social insurance systems, such as the case in Canada's national health insurance program. Laissez-faire supporters argue that this erodes the cost-effectiveness of the health system, as even those who can afford to pay for private healthcare services drain resources from the public system.[13] The issue here is whether investor-owned medical insurance companies or health maintenance organizations are in a better position to act in the best interests of their customers compared to government regulation and oversight. Another claim in the United States perceives government over-regulation of the healthcare and insurance industries as the effective end of charitable home visits from doctors among the poor and elderly.[14]

Economics: healthcare financing

Many types of health policies exist focusing on the financing of healthcare services to spread the economic risks of ill health. These include publicly funded health care (through taxation or insurance, also known as single-payer systems), mandatory or voluntary private health insurance, and complete capitalization of personal health care services through private companies, among others.[15][16] The debate is ongoing on which type of health financing policy results in better or worse quality of healthcare services provided, and how to ensure allocated funds are used effectively, efficiently and equitably.

There are many arguments on both sides of the issue of public versus private health financing policies:

Claims that publicly funded healthcare improves the quality and efficiency of personal health care delivery:

- Government spending on health is essential for the accessibility and sustainability of healthcare services and programmes.[10]

- For those people who would otherwise go without care due to lack of financial means, any quality care is an improvement.

- Since people perceive universal healthcare as *free* (if there is no insurance premium or co-payment), they

are more likely to seek preventive care which may reduce the disease burden and overall healthcare costs in the long run.

- Single-payer systems reduce wastefulness by removing the middle man, i.e. private insurance companies, thus reducing the amount of bureaucracy.[17] In particular, reducing the amount of paperwork that medical professionals have to deal with for insurance claims processing allows them to concentrate more on treating patients.

Claims that privately funded healthcare leads to greater quality and efficiencies in personal health care:

- Perceptions that publicly funded healthcare is *free* can lead to overuse of medical services, and hence raise overall costs compared to private health financing.[18][19]

- Privately funded medicine leads to greater quality and efficiencies through increased access to and reduced waiting times for specialized health care services and technologies.[11][20][21]

- Limiting the allocation of public funds for personal healthcare does not curtail the ability of uninsured citizens to pay for their healthcare as out-of-pocket expenses. Public funds can be better rationalized to provide emergency care services regardless of insured status or ability to pay, such as with the Emergency Medical Treatment and Active Labor Act in the United States.

- Privately funded and operated healthcare reduces the requirement for governments to increase taxes to cover healthcare costs, which may be compounded by the inefficiencies among government agencies due to their greater bureaucracy.[20][22]

1.4.3 Other health policy options

Health policy options extend beyond the financing and delivery of personal health care, to domains such as medical research and health workforce planning, both domestically and internationally.

Medical research policy

Medical research can be both the basis for defining evidence-based health policy, and the subject of health policy itself, particularly in terms of its sources of funding. Those in favor of government policies for publicly funded medical research posit that removing profit as a motive will increase the rate of medical innovation.[23] Those opposed argue that it will do the opposite, because removing the incentive of profit removes incentives to innovate and inhibits new technologies from being developed and utilized.[21][24]

The existence of sound medical research does not necessarily lead to evidence-based policymaking. For example, in South Africa, whose population sets the record for HIV infections, previous government policy limiting funding and access for AIDS treatments met with strong controversy given its basis on a refusal to accept scientific evidence on the means of transmission.[25] A change of government eventually led to a change in policy, with new policies implemented for widespread access to HIV services.[26] Another issue relates to intellectual property, as illustrated by the case of Brazil, where debates have arisen over government policy authorizing the domestic manufacture of antiretroviral drugs used in the treatment of HIV/AIDS in violation of drug patents.

Health workforce policy

Main article: Health workforce

Some countries and jurisdictions have an explicit policy or strategy to plan for adequate numbers, distribution and quality of health workers to meet healthcare goals, such as to address physician and nursing shortages. Elsewhere, workforce planning is distributed among labour market participants as a laissez-faire approach to health policy. Evidence-based policies for workforce development are typically based on findings from health services research.

Health in foreign policy

Many governments and agencies include a health dimension in their foreign policy in order to achieve global health goals. Promoting health in lower income countries has been seen as instrumental to achieve other goals on the global agenda, including:[27]

- Promoting global security – linked to fears of global pandemics, the intentional spread of pathogens, and a potential increase in humanitarian conflicts, natural disasters, and emergencies;

- Promoting economic development – including addressing the economic effect of poor health on development, of pandemic outbreaks on the global market place, and also the gain from the growing global market in health goods and services;

- Promoting social justice – reinforcing health as a social value and human right, including supporting the

United Nations' Millennium Development Goals.

Global health policy

Global health policy encompasses the global governance structures that create the policies underlying public health throughout the world. In addressing global health, global health policy "implies consideration of the health needs of the people of the whole planet above the concerns of particular nations."[28] Distinguished from both international health policy (agreements among sovereign states) and comparative health policy (analysis of health policy across states), global health policy institutions consist of the actors and norms that frame the global health response.[29]

1.4.4   See also

- Disease mongering

- Evidence-based policy

- Health care reform

- Health crisis

- Health economics

- Health insurance

- Health promotion

- Health law

- Inverse benefit law

- Inverse care law

- *Journal of Public Health Policy*

- Medical law

- National health insurance

- Patient safety

- Pharmaceutical policy

- Policy typologies

- Public health

- Public health law

- Quaternary prevention

- Two-tier health care

- Universal health care

- Unnecessary health care

- Vaccination policy

- *World Health Report* series on global health policy issues

1.4.5 References

[1] World Health Organization. *Health Policy*, accessed 22 March 2011.

[2] Harvard School of Public Health, Department of Health Policy and Management *About Health Care Policy*, accessed 25 March 2011.

[3] Cross, H, N Jewell and Karen Hardee. 2001. *Reforming Operational Policies: A Pathway to Improving Reproductive Health Programs* POLICY Occasional Paper. No. 7. Washington DC: The Futures Group International, POLICY Project

[4] K. Hardee, L. Ashford, E. Rottach, R. Jolivet, and R. Kiesel. 2012. *The Policy Dimensions of Scaling Up Health Initiatives.* Washington, DC: Futures Group, Health Policy Project

[5] World Health Organization. *Health and Human Rights.* Geneva. Accessed 27 May 2011.

[6] United Nations. *The Universal Declaration of Human Rights.* Adopted on December 10, 1948 by the General Assembly of the United Nations.

[7] National Health Care for the Homeless Council."Human Rights, Homelessness and Health Care."

[8] Center for Economic and Social Rights. "The Right to Health in the United States of America: What Does it Mean?" October 29, 2004.

[9] The Lancet (2011). "Half a century of Amnesty International". *The Lancet.* **377** (9780): 1808. doi:10.1016/S0140-6736(11)60768-X. PMID 21621708.

[10] Lu, C.; Schneider, M. T.; Gubbins, P.; Leach-Kemon, K.; Jamison, D.; Murray, C. J. (2010). "Public financing of health in developing countries: A cross-national systematic analysis". *The Lancet.* **375** (9723): 1375–1387. doi:10.1016/S0140-6736(10)60233-4. PMID 20381856.

[11] Sade, R. M. (1971). "Medical Care as a Right: A Refutation". *New England Journal of Medicine.* **285** (23): 1288–1292. doi:10.1056/NEJM197112022852304. PMID 5113728. (Reprinted as "The Political Fallacy that Medical Care is a Right.")

[12] The Cato Institute. *Universal Health Care Won't Work – Witness Medicare.*

[13] Tanner MD. *Revolt Against Canadian Health Care System Continues.* "Cato-at-liberty" – The Cato Institute, August 2006.

[14] David E. Kelley, "A Life of One's Own: Individual Rights and the Welfare State." Cato Institute, October 1998, ISBN 1-882577-70-1

[15] Kereiakes, D. J.; Willerson, J. T. (2004). "US Health Care: Entitlement or Privilege?". *Circulation.* **109** (12): 1460–1462. doi:10.1161/01.CIR.0000124795.36864.78. PMID 15051650.

[16] World Health Organization. *Health financing policy.* Geneva. Accessed 27 May 2011.

[17] William F May. "The Ethical Foundations of Health Care Reform." *The Christian Century*, June 1–8, 1994, pp. 572–76.

[18] Heritage Foundation News Release, "British, Canadian Experience Shows Folly of Socialized Medicine, Analyst Says." Sept. 29, 2000

[19] Heritage Foundation News Release,"The Cure: How Capitalism Can Save American Health Care." December 18, 2006.

[20] Goodman, John. "Five Myths of Socialized Medicine." Cato Institute: *Cato's Letter.* Winter, 2005.

[21] Friedmen, David. *The Machinery of Freedom.* Arlington House Publishers: New York, 1978. pp. 65–9.

[22] The Cato Institute. *Cato Handbook on Policy, 6th Edition –* Chapter 7: "Health Care." Washington, 2005.

[23] For example, the recent discovery that dichloroacetate (DCA) can cause regression in several cancers, including lung, breast and brain tumors.Alberta scientists test chemotherapy alternative Last Updated: Wednesday, January 17, 2007 The DCA compound is not patented or owned by any pharmaceutical company, and, therefore, would likely be an inexpensive drug to administer, Michelakis added. The bad news, is that while DCA is not patented, Michelakis is concerned that it may be difficult to find funding from private investors to test DCA in clinical trials.University of Alberta – Small molecule offers big hope against cancer. January 16, 2007

[24] Miller RL; DK Benjamin; DC North (2003). *The Economics of Public Issues* (13th ed.). Boston: Addison-Wesley. ISBN 0321118731.

[25] "Controversy dogs Aids forum." *BBC News*, 10 July 2000.

[26] "HIV and AIDS in South Africa." *Avert.* Accessed 23 June 2011.

[27] Kickbusch, I. (2011). "Global health diplomacy: How foreign policy can influence health". *BMJ.* **342**: d3154. doi:10.1136/bmj.d3154. PMID 21665931.

[28] Brown, T. M.; Cueto, M.; Fee, E. (2006). "The World Health Organization and the Transition from "International" to "Global" Public Health". *American Journal of Public Health.* **96** (1): 62–72. doi:10.2105/AJPH.2004.050831. PMC 1470434. PMID 16322464.

[29] Szlezák, N. A.; Bloom, B. R.; Jamison, D. T.; Keusch, G. T.; Michaud, C. M.; Moon, S.; Clark, W. C. (2010). Walt, Gill, ed. "The Global Health System: Actors, Norms, and Expectations in Transition". *PLoS Medicine*. **7** (1): e1000183. doi:10.1371/journal.pmed.1000183. PMC 2796301. PMID 20052277.

1.4.6 Further reading

- Morrisey, Michael A. (2008), "Health Care", in David R. Henderson (ed.), *Concise Encyclopedia of Economics* (2nd ed.), Indianapolis: Library of Economics and Liberty, ISBN 978-0865976658, OCLC 237794267

1.4.7 External links

- Alliance for Health Policy and Systems Research

- *Health Policy and Planning* journal

- Centre for History in Public Health, London School of Hygiene and Tropical Medicine

- https://www.mcmasterhealthforum. org/docs/default-source/Misc/ gha---student-publication-(2010-08-12-final-low-res) .pdf?sfvrsn=2

1.5 Health economics

For the journal, see Health Economics.

Health economics is a branch of economics concerned with issues related to efficiency, effectiveness, value and behavior in the production and consumption of health and healthcare. In broad terms, health economists study the functioning of healthcare systems and health-affecting behaviors such as smoking.

A seminal 1963 article by Kenneth Arrow, often credited with giving rise to health economics as a discipline, drew conceptual distinctions between health and other goods.[1] Factors that distinguish health economics from other areas include extensive government intervention, intractable uncertainty in several dimensions, asymmetric information, barriers to entry, externalities and the presence of a third-party agent.[2] In healthcare, the third-party agent is the physician, who makes purchasing decisions (e.g., whether to order a lab test, prescribe a medication, perform a surgery, etc.) while being insulated from the price of the product or service.

Health economists evaluate multiple types of financial information: costs, charges and expenditures.

Uncertainty is intrinsic to health, both in patient outcomes and financial concerns. The knowledge gap that exists between a physician and a patient creates a situation of distinct advantage for the physician, which is called *asymmetric information*.

Externalities arise frequently when considering health and health care, notably in the context of infectious disease. For example, making an effort to avoid catching the common cold affects people other than the decision maker.[3][4][5][6]

1.5.1 Scope

The scope of health economics is neatly encapsulated by Alan Williams' "plumbing diagram"[7] dividing the discipline into eight distinct topics:

- What influences health? (other than healthcare)

- What is health and what is its value?

- The demand for healthcare

- The supply of healthcare

- Micro-economic evaluation at treatment level

- Market equilibrium

- Evaluation at whole system level

- Planning, budgeting and monitoring mechanisms.

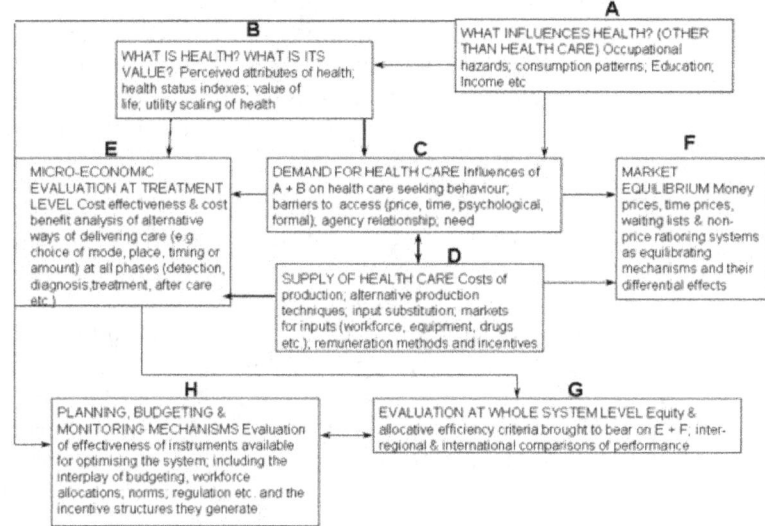

1.5.2 Healthcare demand

The demand for healthcare is a derived demand from the demand for health. Healthcare is demanded as a means for consumers to achieve a larger stock of "health capital." The demand for health is unlike most other goods because individuals allocate resources in order to both consume and produce health.

The above description gives three roles of persons in health economics. The World Health Report (p. 52) states that people take four roles in the healthcare:

1. Contributors

2. Citizens

3. Provider

4. Consumers

Michael Grossman's 1972 model of health production[8] has been extremely influential in this field of study and has several unique elements that make it notable. Grossman's model views each individual as both a producer and a consumer of health. Health is treated as a stock which degrades over time in the absence of "investments" in health, so that health is viewed as a sort of capital. The model acknowledges that health is both a consumption good that yields direct satisfaction and utility, and an investment good, which yields satisfaction to consumers indirectly through fewer sick days. Investment in health is costly as consumers must trade off time and resources devoted to health, such as exercising at a local gym, against other goals. These factors are used to determine the optimal level of health that an individual will demand. The model makes predictions over the effects of changes in prices of healthcare and other goods, labour market outcomes such as employment and wages, and technological changes. These predictions and other predictions from models extending Grossman's 1972 paper form the basis of much of the econometric research conducted by health economists.

In Grossman's model, the optimal level of investment in health occurs where the marginal cost of health capital is equal to the marginal benefit. With the passing of time, health depreciates at some rate δ. The interest rate faced by the consumer is denoted by r. The marginal cost of health capital can be found by adding these variables: $MC_{HK} = r + \delta$. The marginal benefit of health capital is the rate of return from this capital in both market and non-market sectors. In this model, the optimal health stock can be impacted by factors like age, wages and education. As an example, δ increases with age, so it becomes more and more costly to attain the same level of health capital or health

stock as one ages. Age also decreases the marginal benefit of health stock. The optimal health stock will therefore decrease as one ages.

Beyond issues of the fundamental, "real" demand for medical care derived from the desire to have good health (and thus influenced by the production function for health) is the important distinction between the "marginal benefit" of medical care (which is always associated with this "real demand" curve based on derived demand), and a separate "effective demand" curve, which summarizes the amount of medical care demanded at particular market prices. Because most medical care is not purchased from providers directly, but is rather obtained at subsidized prices due to insurance, the out-of-pocket prices faced by consumers are typically much lower than the market price. The consumer sets MB=MC out of pocket, and so the "effective demand" will have a separate relationship between price and quantity than will the "marginal benefit curve" or real demand relationship. This distinction is often described under the rubric of "ex-post moral hazard" (which is again distinct from ex-ante moral hazard, which is found in any type of market with insurance).

1.5.3 Health technology assessment

Economic evaluation, and in particular cost-effectiveness analysis, has become a fundamental part of technology appraisal processes for agencies in a number of countries. The Institute for Quality and Economy in Health Services (Institut für Qualität und Wirtschaftlichkeit im Gesundheitswesen — IQWiG) in Germany and the National Institute for Health and Care Excellence (NICE) in the United Kingdom, for example, both consider the cost-effectiveness of new pharmaceuticals entering the market.

Some agencies, including NICE, recommend the use of cost–utility analysis (CUA). This approach measures outcomes in a composite metric of both length and quality of life, the Quality-adjusted life year (QALY).

1.5.4 Healthcare markets

The five health markets typically analyzed are:

- Healthcare financing market

- Physician and nurses services market

- Institutional services market

- Input factors markets

- Professional education market

Although assumptions of textbook models of economic markets apply reasonably well to healthcare markets, there are important deviations. Many states have created risk pools in which relatively healthy enrollees subsidise the care of the rest. Insurers must cope with adverse selection which occurs when they are unable to fully predict the medical expenses of enrollees; adverse selection can destroy the risk pool. Features of insurance market risk pools, such as group purchases, preferential selection ("cherry-picking"), and preexisting condition exclusions are meant to cope with adverse selection.

Insured patients are naturally less concerned about healthcare costs than they would if they paid the full price of care. The resulting moral hazard drives up costs, as shown by the famous RAND Health Insurance Experiment. Insurers use several techniques to limit the costs of moral hazard, including imposing copayments on patients and limiting physician incentives to provide costly care. Insurers often compete by their choice of service offerings, cost sharing requirements, and limitations on physicians.

Consumers in healthcare markets often suffer from a lack of adequate information about what services they need to buy and which providers offer the best value proposition. Health economists have documented a problem with supplier induced demand, whereby providers base treatment recommendations on economic, rather than medical criteria. Researchers have also documented substantial "practice variations", whereby the treatment also on service availability to rein in inducement and practice variations.

Some economists argue that requiring doctors to have a medical license constrains inputs, inhibits innovation, and increases cost to consumers while largely only benefiting the doctors themselves.[9]

1.5.5   Other issues

Medical economics

Often used synonymously with health economics, *medical economics*, according to Culyer,[10] is the branch of economics concerned with the application of economic theory to phenomena and problems associated typically with the second and third health market outlined above. Typically, however, it pertains to cost–benefit analysis of pharmaceutical products and cost-effectiveness of various medical treatments. Medical economics often uses mathematical models to synthesise data from biostatistics and epidemiology for support of medical decision-making, both for individuals and for wider health policy.

Behavioral economics

Peter Orszag has suggested that behavioral economics is an important factor for improving the healthcare system, but that relatively little progress has been made when compared to retirement policy.[11]

Mental health economics

Mental health economics incorporates a vast array of subject matters, ranging from pharmacoeconomics to labor economics and welfare economics. Mental health can be directly related to economics by the potential of affected individuals to contribute as human capital. In 2009 Currie and Stabile published "Mental Health in Childhood and Human Capital" in which they assessed how common childhood mental health problems may alter the human capital accumulation of affected children.[12] Externalities may include the influence that affected individuals have on surrounding human capital, such as at the workplace or in the home.[13] In turn, the economy also affects the individual, particularly in light of globalization. For example, studies in India, where there is an increasingly high occurrence of western outsourcing, have demonstrated a growing hybrid identity in young professionals who face very different sociocultural expectations at the workplace and in at home.[14]

Mental health economics presents a unique set of challenges to researchers. Individuals with cognitive disabilities may not be able to communicate preferences. These factors represent challenges in terms of placing value on the mental health status of an individual, especially in relation to the individual's potential as human capital. Further, employment statistics are often used in mental health economic studies as a means of evaluating individual productivity; however, these statistics do not capture "presenteeism", when an individual is at work with a lowered productivity level, quantify the loss of non-paid working time, or capture externalities such as having an affected family member. Also, considering the variation in global wage rates or in societal values, statistics used may be contextually, geographically confined, and study results may not be internationally applicable.[13]

Though studies have demonstrated mental healthcare to reduce overall healthcare costs, demonstrate efficacy, and reduce employee absenteeism while improving employee functioning, the availability of comprehensive mental health services is in decline. Petrasek and Rapin (2002) cite the three main reasons for this decline as (1) stigma and privacy concerns, (2) the difficulty of quantifying medical savings and (3) physician incentive to medicate without specialist referral.[15] Evers et al. (2009) have suggested that improvements could be made by promoting more active dissemination of mental health economic analysis, building partnerships through policy-makers and researchers, and employing greater use of knowledge brokers.[13]

1.5.6 See also

1.5.7 References

[1] Arrow 1963

[2] Phelps, Charles E. (2003), *Health Economics* (3rd ed.), Boston: Addison Wesley, ISBN 0-321-06898-X Description and 2nd ed. preview.

[3] Fuchs, Victor R. (1987). "health economics" *The New Palgrave: A Dictionary of Economics*, v. 2, pp. 614–19.

[4] Fuchs, Victor R. (1996). "Economics, Values, and Health Care Reform," *American Economic Review*, 86(1), pp. 1–24 (press **+**).

[5] Fuchs, Victor R. ([1974] 1998). *Who Shall Live? Health, Economics, and Social Choice*, Expanded edition. Chapter-preview links, pp. vii–xi.

[6] Wolfe, Barbara (2008). "health economics." *The New Palgrave Dictionary of Economics', 2nd Edition. Abstract & TOC.*

[7] Williams, A. (1987), "Health economics: the cheerful face of a dismal science", in Williams, A., *Health and Economics*, London: Macmillan

[8] Grossman, Michael (1972), "On the Concept of Health Capital and the Demand for Health", *Journal of Political Economy*, **80** (2): 223–255, doi:10.1086/259880

[9] Svorny, Shirley (2004), "Licensing Doctors: Do Economists Agree?", *Econ Journal Watch*, **1** (2): 279–305

[10] A.J. Culyer (1989) "A Glossary of the more common terms encountered in health economics" in MS Hersh-Cochran and KP Cochran (Eds.) *Compendium of English Language Course Syllabi and Textbooks in Health Economics*, Copenhagen, WHO, 215–34

[11] Peter Orszag, "Behavioral Economics: Lessons from Retirement Research for Health Care and Beyond," Presentation to the Retirement Research Consortium, August 7, 2008

[12] Currie, Janet and Mark Stabile. "Mental Health in Childhood and Human Capital". *The Problems of Disadvantaged Youth: An Economic Perspective* ed. J. Gruber. Chicago: University of Chicago Press, 2009.

[13] Evers, S.; Salvador–Carulla, L.; Halsteinli, V.; McDaid, D.; MHEEN Group (April 2007), "Implementing mental health economic evaluation evidence: Building a Bridge between theory and practice", *Journal of Mental Health*, **16** (2): 223–241, doi:10.1080/09638230701279881

[14] Bhavsar, V.; Bhugra, D. (December 2008), "Globalization: Mental health and social economic factors", *Global Social Policy*, **8** (3): 378–396, doi:10.1177/1468018108095634

[15] Petrasek M, Rapin L; Rapin (2002), "The mental health paradox", *Benefits Q*, **18** (2): 73–7, PMID 12004583

1.5.8 Further reading

- Alastair M. Gray, Philip M. Clarke, Jane Wolstenholme, Sarah Wordsworth (2010) *Applied Methods of Cost-effectiveness Analysis in Healthcare*, Oxford University Press. Preview ISBN 0-19-922728-4

- Arrow, K. (December 1963), "Uncertainty and the welfare economics of medical care" (PDF), *American Economic Review*, **53** (5): 941–973

- Drummond, Michael F. (2005) *Methods for the Economic Evaluation of Health Care Programmes*, Oxford University Press. Preview. ISBN 0-19-852945-7

- Fuchs, Victor R. (1998) *Who Shall Live? Health, Economics, and Social Choice*, Wspc.

- Mahar, Maggie, *Money-Driven Medicine: The Real Reason Health Care Costs So Much*, Harper/Collins, 2006. ISBN 978-0-06-076533-0

- Morrisey, Michael A. (2008), "Health Care", in David R. Henderson (ed.), *Concise Encyclopedia of Economics* (2nd ed.), Indianapolis: Library of Economics and Liberty, ISBN 978-0865976658, OCLC 237794267

- Siegel, Joanna E.; Russell, Louise B.; Weinstein, Milton C.; Gold, Marthe R. (1996), *Cost-effectiveness in health and medicine*, New York [u.a.]: Oxford Univ. Press, ISBN 978-0-19-510824-8

- Starr, Paul, *The Social Transformation of American Medicine*, Basic Books, 1982. ISBN 0-465-07934-2

- Wennberg J, Gittelsohn; Gittelsohn, A. (December 1973), "Small area variations in health care delivery", *Science*, **182** (4117): 1102–8, Bibcode:1973Sci...182.1102W, doi:10.1126/science.182.4117.1102, PMID 4750608

- Whittington, Ruth (2008). *Introduction to Health Economics: A Beginners Guide* Preview. ISBN 978-0-9545494-5-9.

- Wise, David A. (2009), *Developments in the Economics of Aging*, University of Chicago Press, ISBN 978-0-226-90335-4

- A.J. Culyer and J.P. Newhouse, ed. (2000). *Handbook of Health Economics*, Elsevier. 1A. *Description. Elsevier.*

- _____ (2000). *Handbook of Health Economics*, 1B. *Description. Elsevier.*

1.5.9 Journals

- *Health Economics.*[1] Aims & scope and links back-issue titles and abstracts.

- *Journal of Health Economics* Aims & scope and links to back-issue titles and abstracts.

- *Review of Economics of the Household*

1.5.10 External links

Associations

- International Health Economics Association

- Health Economics education (HEe) – UK-based site for teachers of Health Economics

- International Society for Pharmacoeconomics and Outcomes Research

Links/Terminology/Discussion

- Health Economics Online Glossary of Terms – maintained by the University of Groningen, The Netherlands

- HealthEconomics.Com

1.6 Public health

Public health refers to "the science and art of preventing disease, prolonging life and promoting human health through organized efforts and informed choices of society, organizations, public and private, communities and individuals."[1] It is concerned with threats to health based on population health analysis.[2] The population in question can be as small as a handful of people, or as large as all the inhabitants of several continents (for instance, in the case of a pandemic). The dimensions of health can encompass "a state of complete physical, mental and social well-being and not merely the absence of disease or infirmity," as defined by the United Nations' World Health Organization.[3] Public health incorporates the interdisciplinary approaches of epidemiology, biostatistics

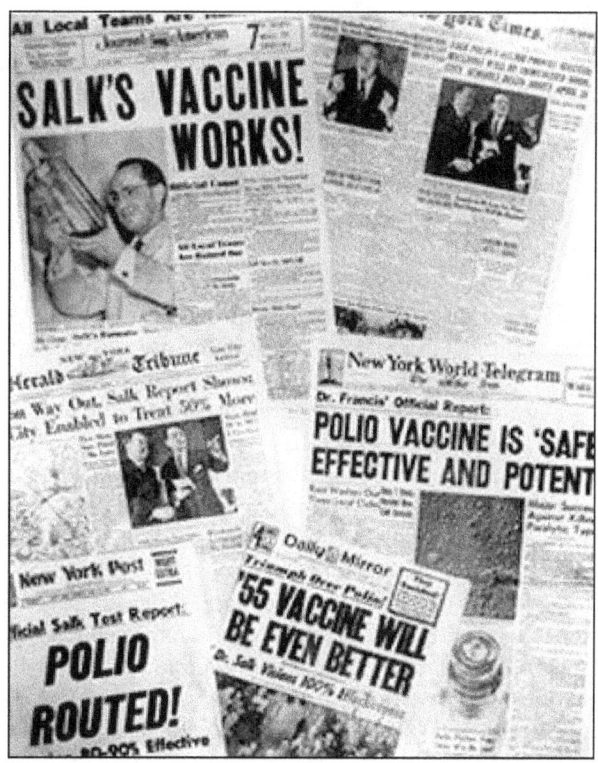

Newspaper headlines from around the world about polio vaccine tests (13 April 1955)

and health services. Environmental health, community health, behavioral health, health economics, public policy, insurance medicine, mental health and occupational safety and health are other important subfields.

The focus of public health intervention is to improve health and quality of life through prevention and treatment of disease and other physical and mental health conditions. This is done through surveillance of cases and health indicators, and through promotion of healthy behaviors. Examples of common public health measures include promotion of hand washing, breastfeeding, delivery of vaccinations, suicide prevention and distribution of condoms to control the spread of sexually transmitted diseases.

Modern public health practice requires multidisciplinary teams of public health workers and professionals including the following: physicians specializing in public health, community medicine, or infectious disease; psychologists; epidemiologists; biostatisticians; medical assistants or Assistant Medical Officers; public health nurses; midwives; medical microbiologists; environmental health officers or public health inspectors; pharmacists; dentists; dietitians and nutritionists; veterinarians; public health engineers; public health lawyers; sociologists; community development workers; communications experts; bioethicists; and others.[4]

There is a great disparity in access to health care and public health initiatives between developed nations and developing nations. In the developing world, public health infrastructures are still forming.

1.6.1 Background

The focus of a public health intervention is to prevent and manage diseases, injuries and other health conditions through surveillance of cases and the promotion of healthy behaviors, communities and environments. Many diseases are preventable through simple, nonmedical methods. For example, research has shown that the simple act of hand washing with soap can prevent many contagious diseases.[5] In other cases, treating a disease or controlling a pathogen can be vital to preventing its spread to others, either during an outbreak of infectious disease or through contamination of food or water supplies. Public health communications programs, vaccination programs and distribution of condoms are examples of common public health measures. Measures such as these have contributed greatly to the health of populations and increases in life expectancy.

Public health plays an important role in disease prevention efforts in both the developing world and in developed countries, through local health systems and non-governmental organizations. The World Health Organization (WHO) is the international agency that coordinates and acts on global public health issues. Most countries have their own government public health agencies, sometimes known as ministries of health, to respond to domestic health issues. For example, in the United States, the front line of public health initiatives are state and local health departments. The United States Public Health Service (PHS), led by the Surgeon General of the United States, and the Centers for Disease Control and Prevention, headquartered in Atlanta, are involved with several international health activities, in addition to their national duties. In Canada, the Public Health Agency of Canada is the national agency responsible for public health, emergency preparedness and response, and infectious and chronic disease control and prevention. The Public health system in India is managed by the Ministry of Health & Family Welfare of the government of India with state-owned health care facilities.

1.6.2 Current practice

Public health programs

Most governments recognize the importance of public health programs in reducing the incidence of disease, disability, and the effects of aging and other physical and mental health conditions, although public health generally re-

ceives significantly less government funding compared with medicine.[6] Public health programs providing vaccinations have made strides in promoting health, including the eradication of smallpox, a disease that plagued humanity for thousands of years.

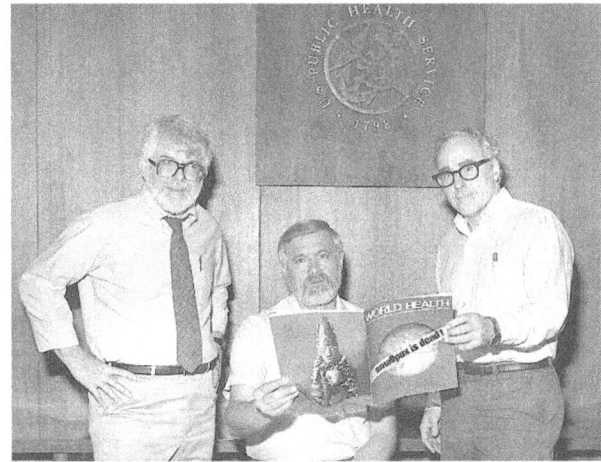

Three former directors of the Global Smallpox Eradication Programme read the news that smallpox had been globally eradicated, 1980

The World Health Organization (WHO) identifies core functions of public health programs including:[7]

- providing leadership on matters critical to health and engaging in partnerships where joint action is needed;

- shaping a research agenda and stimulating the generation, translation and dissemination of valuable knowledge;

- setting norms and standards and promoting and monitoring their implementation;

- articulating ethical and evidence-based policy options;

- monitoring the health situation and assessing health trends.

In particular, public health surveillance programs can:[8]

- serve as an early warning system for impending public health emergencies;

- document the impact of an intervention, or track progress towards specified goals; and

- monitor and clarify the epidemiology of health problems, allow priorities to be set, and inform health policy and strategies.

- diagnose, investigate, and monitor health problems and health hazards of the community

Public health surveillance has led to the identification and prioritization of many public health issues facing the world today, including HIV/AIDS, diabetes, waterborne diseases, zoonotic diseases, and antibiotic resistance leading to the reemergence of infectious diseases such as tuberculosis. Antibiotic resistance, also known as drug resistance, was the theme of World Health Day 2011. Although the prioritization of pressing public health issues is important, Laurie Garrett argues that there are following consequences.[9] When foreign aid is funnelled into disease-specific programs, the importance of public health in general is disregarded. This public health problem of stovepiping is thought to create a lack of funds to combat other existing diseases in a given country.

For example, the WHO reports that at least 220 million people worldwide suffer from diabetes. Its incidence is increasing rapidly, and it is projected that the number of diabetes deaths will double by the year 2030.[10] In a June 2010 editorial in the medical journal *The Lancet*, the authors opined that "The fact that type 2 diabetes, a largely preventable disorder, has reached epidemic proportion is a public health humiliation."[11] The risk of type 2 diabetes is closely linked with the growing problem of obesity. The WHO's latest estimates highlighted that globally approximately 1.5 billion adults were overweight in 2008, and nearly 43 million children under the age of five were overweight in 2010.[12] The United States is the leading country with 30.6% of its population being obese. Mexico follows behind with 24.2% and the United Kingdom with 23%. Once considered a problem in high-income countries, it is now on the rise in low-income countries, especially in urban settings. Many public health programs are increasingly dedicating attention and resources to the issue of obesity, with objectives to address the underlying causes including healthy diet and physical exercise.

Some programs and policies associated with public health promotion and prevention can be controversial. One such example is programs focusing on the prevention of HIV transmission through safe sex campaigns and needle-exchange programmes. Another is the control of tobacco smoking. Changing smoking behavior requires long-term strategies, unlike the fight against communicable diseases, which usually takes a shorter period for effects to be observed. Many nations have implemented major initiatives to cut smoking, such as increased taxation and bans on smoking in some or all public places. Proponents argue by presenting evidence that smoking is one of the major killers, and that therefore governments have a duty to reduce the death rate, both through limiting passive (secondhand) smoking and by providing fewer opportunities for people to smoke. Opponents say that this undermines individual freedom and personal responsibility, and worry that the state may be emboldened to remove more and more

choice in the name of better population health overall.

Simultaneously, while communicable diseases have historically ranged uppermost as a global health priority, noncommunicable diseases and the underlying behavior-related risk factors have been at the bottom. This is changing however, as illustrated by the United Nations hosting its first General Assembly Special Summit on the issue of noncommunicable diseases in September 2011.[13]

Many health problems are due to maladaptive personal behaviors. From an evolutionary psychology perspective, over consumption of novel substances that are harmful is due to the activation of an evolved reward system for substances such as drugs, tobacco, alcohol, refined salt, fat, and carbohydrates. New technologies such as modern transportation also cause reduced physical activity. Research has found that behavior is more effectively changed by taking evolutionary motivations into consideration instead of only presenting information about health effects. Thus, the increased use of soap and hand-washing to prevent diarrhea is much more effectively promoted if its lack of use is associated with the emotion of disgust. Disgust is an evolved system for avoiding contact with substances that spread infectious diseases. Examples might include films that show how fecal matter contaminates food. The marketing industry has long known the importance of associating products with high status and attractiveness to others. Conversely, it has been argued that emphasizing the harmful and undesirable effects of tobacco smoking on other persons and imposing smoking bans in public places have been particularly effective in reducing tobacco smoking.[14]

Applications in health care

As well as seeking to improve population health through the implementation of specific population-level interventions, public health contributes to medical care by identifying and assessing population needs for health care services, including:[15][16][17][18]

- Assessing current services and evaluating whether they are meeting the objectives of the health care system

- Ascertaining requirements as expressed by health professionals, the public and other stakeholders

- Identifying the most appropriate interventions

- Considering the effect on resources for proposed interventions and assessing their cost-effectiveness

- Supporting decision making in health care and planning health services including any necessary changes.

- Informing, educating, and empowering people about health issues

Implementing effective improvement strategies

To improve public health, one important strategy is to promote modern medicine and scientific neutrality to drive the public health policy and campaign, which is recommended by Armanda Solorzana, through a case study of the Rockefeller Foundation's hookworm campaign in Mexico in the 1920s. Soloranza argues that public health policy can't concern only politics or economics. Political concerns can lead government officials to hide the real numbers of people affected by disease in their regions, such as upcoming elections. Therefore, scientific neutrality in making public health policy is critical; it can ensure treatment needs are met regardless of political and economic conditions.[19]

The history of public health care clearly shows the global effort to improve health care for all. However, in modern-day medicine, real, measurable change has not been clearly seen, and critics argue that this lack of improvement is due to ineffective methods that are being implemented. As argued by Paul E. Farmer, structural interventions could possibly have a large impact, and yet there are numerous problems as to why this strategy has yet to be incorporated into the health system. One of the main reasons that he suggests could be the fact that physicians are not properly trained to carry out structural interventions, meaning that the ground level health care professionals cannot implement these improvements. While structural interventions can not be the only area for improvement, the lack of coordination between socioeconomic factors and health care for the poor could be counterproductive, and end up causing greater inequity between the health care services received by the rich and by the poor. Unless health care is no longer treated as a commodity, global public health can ultimately not be achieved. This being the case, without changing the way in which health care is delivered to those who have less access to it, the universal goal of public health care cannot be achieved.[20]

Public Health 2.0

Public Health 2.0 is a movement within public health that aims to make the field more accessible to the general public and more user-driven. The term is used in three senses. In the first sense, "Public Health 2.0" is similar to "Health 2.0" and describes the ways in which traditional public health practitioners and institutions are reaching out (or could reach out) to the public through social media and health blogs.[21][22]

In the second sense, "Public Health 2.0" describes public health research that uses data gathered from social networking sites, search engine queries, cell phones, or other technologies.[23] A recent example is the proposal of statistical framework that utilizes online user-generated content (from social media or search engine queries) to estimate the impact of an influenza vaccination campaign in the UK.[24]

In the third sense, "Public Health 2.0" is used to describe public health activities that are completely user-driven.[25] An example is the collection and sharing of information about environmental radiation levels after the March 2011 tsunami in Japan.[26] In all cases, Public Health 2.0 draws on ideas from Web 2.0, such as crowdsourcing, information sharing, and user-centred design.[27] While many individual healthcare providers have started making their own personal contributions to "Public Health 2.0" through personal blogs, social profiles, and websites, other larger organizations, such as the American Heart Association (AHA) and United Medical Education (UME), have a larger team of employees centered around online driven health education, research, and training. These private organizations recognize the need for free and easy to access health materials often building libraries of educational articles.

1.6.3 Developing countries

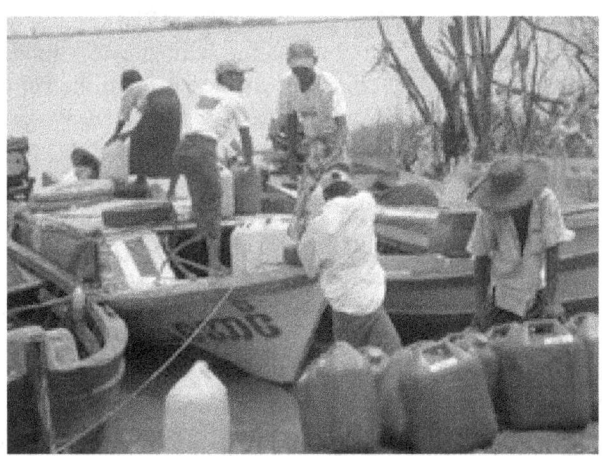

Emergency Response Team in Burma after Cyclone Nargis in 2008

There is a great disparity in access to health care and public health initiatives between developed nations and developing nations. In the developing world, public health infrastructures are still forming. There may not be enough trained health workers or monetary resources to provide even a basic level of medical care and disease prevention.[28] As a result, a large majority of disease and mortality in the developing world results from and contributes to extreme poverty. For example, many African governments spend less than US$10 per person per year on health care, while, in the United States, the federal government spent approximately US$4,500 per capita in 2000. However, expenditures on health care should not be confused with spending on public health. Public health measures may not generally be considered "health care" in the strictest sense. For example, mandating the use of seat belts in cars can save countless lives and contribute to the health of a population, but typically money spent enforcing this rule would not count as money spent on health care.

Large parts of the developing world remained plagued by largely preventable or treatable infectious diseases and poor maternal and child health, exacerbated by malnutrition and poverty. The WHO reports that a lack of exclusive breastfeeding during the first six months of life contributes to over a million avoidable child deaths each year.[29] Intermittent preventive therapy aimed at treating and preventing malaria episodes among pregnant women and young children is one public health measure in endemic countries.

Each day brings new front-page headlines about public health: emerging infectious diseases such as SARS, rapidly making its way from China (see Public health in China) to Canada, the United States and other geographically distant countries; reducing inequities in health care access through publicly funded health insurance programs; the HIV/AIDS pandemic and its spread from certain high-risk groups to the general population in many countries, such as in South Africa; the increase of childhood obesity and the concomitant increase in type II diabetes among children; the social, economic and health effects of adolescent pregnancy; and the public health challenges related to natural disasters such as the 2004 Indian Ocean tsunami, 2005's Hurricane Katrina in the United States and the 2010 Haiti earthquake.

Since the 1980s, the growing field of population health has broadened the focus of public health from individual behaviors and risk factors to population-level issues such as inequality, poverty, and education. Modern public health is often concerned with addressing determinants of health across a population. There is a recognition that our health is affected by many factors including where we live, genetics, our income, our educational status and our social relationships; these are known as "social determinants of health." A social gradient in health runs through society. The poorest generally suffer the worst health, but even the middle classes will generally have worse health outcomes than those of a higher social stratum.[30] The new public health advocates for population-based policies that improve health in an equitable manner.

Sustainable Development Goals

Further information: Sustainable Development Goals

To address current and future challenges in addressing health issues in the world, the United Nations have developed the Sustainable Development Goals 2015 building off of the Millennium Development Goals of 2000 to be completed by 2030.[31] These goals in their entirety encompass

the entire spectrum of development across nations, however Goals 1-6 directly address health disparities, primarily in developing countries.[32] These six goals address key issues in global public health: Poverty, Hunger and food security, Health, Education, Gender equality and women's empowerment, and water and sanitation.[32] Public health officials can use these goals to set their own agenda and plan for smaller scale initiatives for their organizations. These goals hope to lessen the burden of disease and inequality faced by developing countries and lead to a healthier future.

The links between the various sustainable development goals and public health are numerous and well established:

- Living below the poverty line is attributed to poorer health outcomes and can be even worse for persons living in developing countries where extreme poverty is more common.[33] A child born into poverty is twice as likely to die before the age of five compared to a child from a wealthier family.[34]

- The detrimental effects of hunger and malnutrition that can arise from systemic challenges with food security are enormous. The World Health Organization estimates that 12.9 percent of the population in developing countries is undernourished.[35]

- Health challenges in the developing world are enormous, with "only half of the women in developing nations receiving the recommended amount of healthcare they need.[34]

- Educational equity has yet to be reached in the world. Public health efforts are impeded by this, as a lack of education can lead to poorer health outcomes. This is shown by children of mothers who have no education having a lower survival rate compared to children born to mothers with primary or greater levels of education.[34] Cultural differences in the role of women vary by country, many gender inequalities are found in developing nations. Combating these inequalities has shown to also lead to better public health outcome.

- In studies done by the World Bank on populations in developing countries, it was found that when women had more control over household resources, the children benefit through better access to food, healthcare, and education.[36]

- Basic sanitation resources and access to clean sources of water are a basic human right. However, 1.8 billion people globally use a source of drinking water that is fecally contaminated, and 2.4 billion people lack access to basic sanitation facilities like toilets or pit latrines.[37] A lack of these resources is what causes approximately 1000 children a day to die from diarrhoel diseases that could have been prevented from better water and sanitation infrastructure.[37]

1.6.4 Education and training

Education and training of public health professionals is available throughout the world in Schools of Public Health, Medical Schools, Veterinary Schools, Schools of Nursing, and Schools of Public Affairs. The training typically requires a university degree with a focus on core disciplines of biostatistics, epidemiology, health services administration, health policy, health education, behavioral science and environmental health.[38][39] In the global context, the field of public health education has evolved enormously in recent decades, supported by institutions such as the World Health Organization and the World Bank, among others. Operational structures are formulated by strategic principles, with educational and career pathways guided by competency frameworks, all requiring modulation according to local, national and global realities. It is critically important for the health of populations that nations assess their public health human resource needs and develop their ability to deliver this capacity, and not depend on other countries to supply it.[40]

Schools of public health - a U.S. Perspective

In the United States, the Welch-Rose Report of 1915[41] has been viewed as the basis for the critical movement in the history of the institutional schism between public health and medicine because it led to the establishment of schools of public health supported by the Rockefeller Foundation.[42] The report was authored by William Welch, founding dean of the Johns Hopkins Bloomberg School of Public Health, and Wickliffe Rose of the Rockefeller Foundation. The report focused more on research than practical education.[42][43] Some have blamed the Rockefeller Foundation's 1916 decision to support the establishment of schools of public health for creating the schism between public health and medicine and legitimizing the rift between medicine's laboratory investigation of the mechanisms of disease and public health's nonclinical concern with environmental and social influences on health and wellness.[42][44]

Even though schools of public health had already been established in Canada, Europe and North Africa, the United States had still maintained the traditional system of housing faculties of public health within their medical institutions. A $25,000 donation from businessman Samuel Zemurray instituted the School of Public Health and Tropical Medicine at Tulane University in 1912 conferring its first doctor of public health degree in 1914.[45][46] The Johns Hopkins School of Hygiene and Public Health became an independent, degree-granting institution for research and training in public health, and the largest public health training facility in the United States,[47][48][49][50] when it was founded in 1916. By 1922, schools of public health were established at Columbia, Harvard and Yale on the Hopkins model. By 1999 there were twenty nine schools of public health in the US, enrolling around fifteen thousand students.[38][42]

Over the years, the types of students and training provided have also changed. In the beginning, students who enrolled in public health schools typically had already obtained a medical degree; public health school training was largely a second degree for medical professionals. However, in 1978, 69% of American students enrolled in public health schools had only a bachelor's degree.[38]

Degrees in public health

Main article: Professional degrees of public health

Schools of public health offer a variety of degrees which generally fall into two categories: professional or academic.[51] The two major postgraduate degrees are the Master of Public Health (M.P.H.) or the Master of Science in Public Health (MSPH). Doctoral studies in this field include Doctor of Public Health (DrPH) and Doctor of Philosophy (Ph.D.) in a subspeciality of greater Public Health disciplines. DrPH is regarded as a professional degree and Ph.D. as more of an academic degree.

Professional degrees are oriented towards practice in public health settings. The Master of Public Health, Doctor of Public Health, Doctor of Health Science (DHSc) and the Master of Health Care Administration are examples of degrees which are geared towards people who want careers as practitioners of public health in health departments, managed care and community-based organizations, hospitals and consulting firms among others. Master of Public Health degrees broadly fall into two categories, those that put more emphasis on an understanding of epidemiology and statistics as the scientific basis of public health practice and those that include a more eclectic range of methodologies. A Master of Science of Public Health is similar to an MPH but is considered an academic degree (as opposed to a professional degree) and places more emphasis on scientific methods and research. The same distinction can be made between the DrPH and the DHSc. The DrPH is considered a professional degree and the DHSc is an academic degree.

Academic degrees are more oriented towards those with interests in the scientific basis of public health and preventive medicine who wish to pursue careers in research, university teaching in graduate programs, policy analysis and development, and other high-level public health positions. Examples of academic degrees are the Master of Science, Doctor of Philosophy, Doctor of Science (ScD), and Doctor of Health Science (DHSc). The doctoral programs are distinct from the MPH and other professional programs by the addition of advanced coursework and the nature and scope of a dissertation research project.

In the United States, the Association of Schools of Public Health[52] represents Council on Education for Public Health (CEPH) accredited schools of public health.[53] Delta Omega is the honor society for graduate studies in public health. The society was founded in 1924 at the Johns Hopkins School of Hygiene and Public Health. Currently, there are approximately 68 chapters throughout the United States and Puerto Rico.[54]

1.6.5   History

Early history

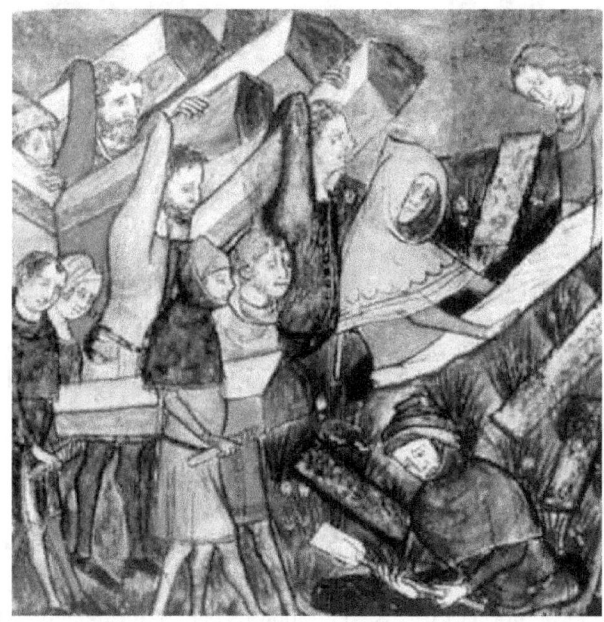

The primitive nature of medieval medicine rendered Europe helpless to the onslaught of the Black Death in the 14th century. Fragment of a miniature from "The Chronicles of Gilles Li Muisis" (1272-1352). Bibliothèque royale de Belgique, MS 13076-77, f. 24v.

Public health has early roots in antiquity. From the beginnings of human civilization, it was recognized that polluted water and lack of proper waste disposal spread communicable diseases (theory of miasma). Early religions attempted to regulate behavior that specifically related to health, from types of food eaten, to regulating certain indulgent behaviors, such as drinking alcohol or sexual relations. Leaders

were responsible for the health of their subjects to ensure social stability, prosperity, and maintain order.

By Roman times, it was well understood that proper diversion of human waste was a necessary tenet of public health in urban areas. The ancient Chinese medical doctors developed the practice of variolation following a smallpox epidemic around 1000 BC. An individual without the disease could gain some measure of immunity against it by inhaling the dried crusts that formed around lesions of infected individuals. Also, children were protected by inoculating a scratch on their forearms with the pus from a lesion.

In 1485 the Republic of Venice established a Permanent Court of supervisors of health with special attention to the prevention of the spread of epidemics in the territory from abroad. The three supervisors were initially appointed by the Venetian Senate. In 1537 it was assumed by the Grand Council, and in 1556 added two judges, with the task of control, on behalf of the Republic, the efforts of the supervisors.[55]

However, according to Michel Foucault, the plague model of governmentality was later controverted by the cholera model. A Cholera pandemic devastated Europe between 1829 and 1851, and was first fought by the use of what Foucault called "social medicine", which focused on flux, circulation of air, location of cemeteries, etc. All those concerns, born of the miasma theory of disease, were mixed with urbanistic concerns for the management of populations, which Foucault designated as the concept of "biopower". The German conceptualized this in the *Polizeiwissenschaft* ("Police science").

Modern public health

The 18th century saw rapid growth in voluntary hospitals in England.[56] The latter part of the century brought the establishment of the basic pattern of improvements in public health over the next two centuries: a social evil was identified, private philanthropists brought attention to it, and changing public opinion led to government action.[57]

The practice of vaccination became prevalent in the 1800s, following the pioneering work of Edward Jenner in treating smallpox. James Lind's discovery of the causes of scurvy amongst sailors and its mitigation via the introduction of fruit on lengthy voyages was published in 1754 and led to the adoption of this idea by the Royal Navy.[58] Efforts were also made to promulgate health matters to the broader public; in 1752 the British physician Sir John Pringle published *Observations on the Diseases of the Army in Camp and Garrison*, in which he advocated for the importance of adequate ventilation in the military barracks and the provision of latrines for the soldiers.[59]

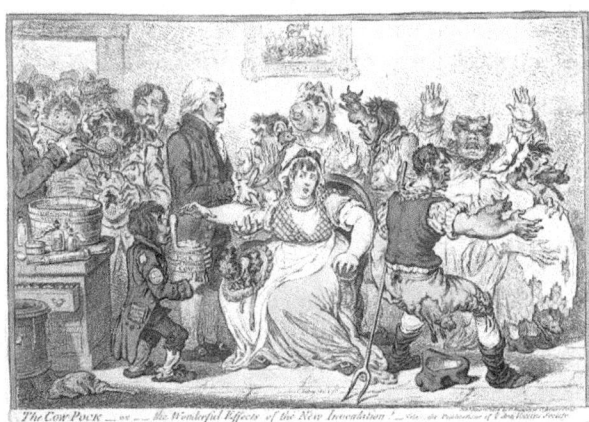

1802 caricature of Edward Jenner vaccinating patients who feared it would make them sprout cowlike appendages.

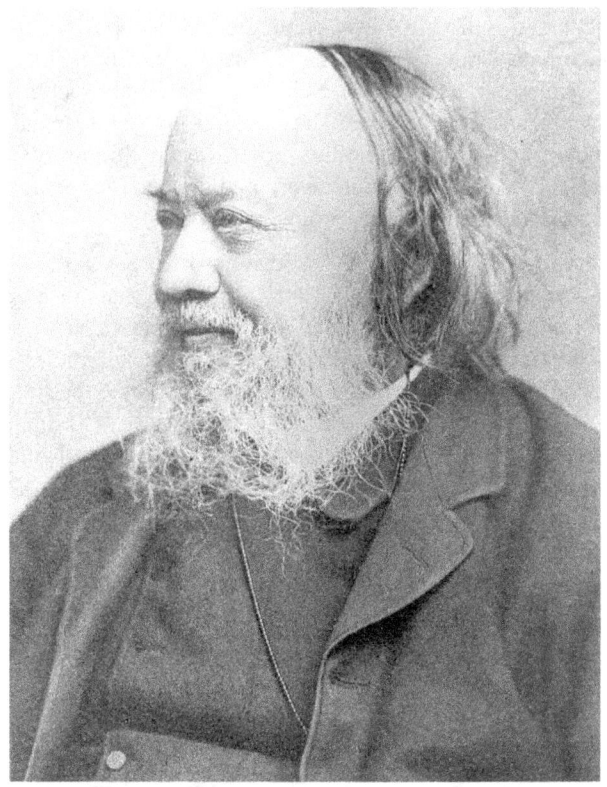

Sir Edwin Chadwick was a pivotal influence on the early public health campaign.

With the onset of the Industrial Revolution, living standards amongst the working population began to worsen, with cramped and unsanitary urban conditions. In the first four decades of the 19th century alone, London's population doubled and even greater growth rates were recorded in the new industrial towns, such as Leeds and Manchester. This rapid urbanisation exacerbated the spread of disease in the large conurbations that built up around the workhouses and factories. These settlements were cramped and primitive with no organized sanitation. Disease was inevitable and its incubation in these areas was encouraged by the poor lifestyle of the inhabitants. Unavailable housing led to the rapid growth of slums and the per capita death rate began to rise alarmingly, almost doubling in Birmingham and Liverpool. Thomas Malthus warned of the dangers of overpopulation in 1798. His ideas, as well as those of Jeremy Bentham, became very influential in government circles in the early years of the 19th century.[57]

Public health legislation The first attempts at sanitary reform and the establishment of public health institutions were made in the 1840s. Thomas Southwood Smith, physician at the London Fever Hospital, began to write papers on the importance of public health, and was one of the first physicians brought in to give evidence before the Poor Law Commission in the 1830s, along with Neil Arnott and James Phillips Kay.[60] Smith advised the government on the importance of quarantine and sanitary improvement for limiting the spread of infectious diseases such as cholera and yellow fever.[61][62]

The Poor Law Commission reported in 1838 that "the expenditures necessary to the adoption and maintenance of measures of prevention would ultimately amount to less than the cost of the disease now constantly engendered". It recommended the implementation of large scale govern-

ment engineering projects to alleviate the conditions that allowed for the propagation of disease.[57] The Health of Towns Association was formed in Exeter on 11 December 1844, and vigorously campaigned for the development of public health in the United Kingdom.[63] Its formation followed the 1843 establishment of the Health of Towns Commission, chaired by Sir Edwin Chadwick, which produced a series of reports on poor and insanitary conditions in British cities.[63]

These national and local movements led to the Public Health Act, finally passed in 1848. It aimed to improve the sanitary condition of towns and populous places in England and Wales by placing the supply of water, sewerage, drainage, cleansing and paving under a single local body with the General Board of Health as a central authority. The Act was passed by the Liberal government of Lord John Russell, in response to the urging of Edwin Chadwick. Chadwick's seminal report on *The Sanitary Condition of the Labouring Population* was published in 1842[64] and was followed up with a supplementary report a year later.[65]

Vaccination for various diseases was made compulsory in the United Kingdom in 1851, and by 1871 legislation required a comprehensive system of registration run by appointed vaccination officers.[66]

Further interventions were made by a series of subsequent Public Health Acts, notably the 1875 Act. Reforms included latrinization, the building of sewers, the regular collection of garbage followed by incineration or disposal in a landfill, the provision of clean water and the draining of standing water to prevent the breeding of mosquitoes.

The Infectious Disease (Notification) Act 1889 mandated the reporting of infectious diseases to the local sanitary authority, which could then pursue measures such as the removal of the patient to hospital and the disinfection of homes and properties.[67]

In the U.S., the first public health organization based on a state health department and local boards of health was founded in New York City in 1866.[68]

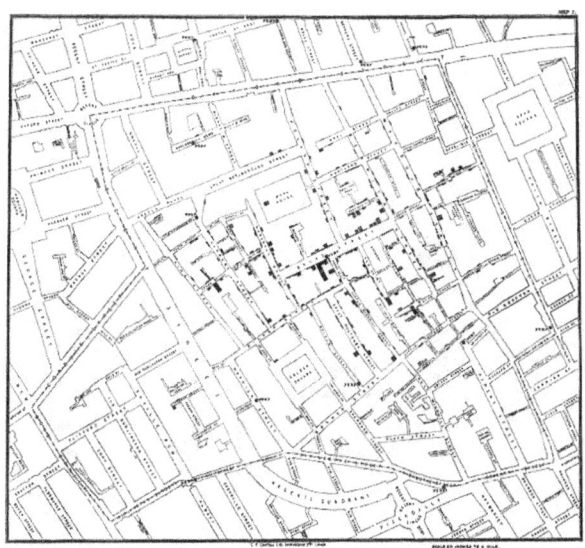

John Snow's dot map, showing the clusters of cholera cases in the London epidemic of 1854.

Epidemiology The science of epidemiology was founded by John Snow's identification of a polluted public water well as the source of an 1854 cholera outbreak in London. Dr. Snow believed in the germ theory of disease as opposed to the prevailing miasma theory. He first publicized his theory in an essay, *On the Mode of Communication of Cholera*, in 1849, followed by a more detailed treatise in 1855 incorporating the results of his investigation of the role of the water supply in the Soho epidemic of 1854.[69]

By talking to local residents (with the help of Reverend Henry Whitehead), he identified the source of the outbreak as the public water pump on Broad Street (now Broadwick Street). Although Snow's chemical and microscope examination of a water sample from the Broad Street pump did not conclusively prove its danger, his studies of the pattern of the disease were convincing enough to persuade the local

council to disable the well pump by removing its handle.[70]

Snow later used a dot map to illustrate the cluster of cholera cases around the pump. He also used statistics to illustrate the connection between the quality of the water source and cholera cases. He showed that the Southwark and Vauxhall Waterworks Company was taking water from sewage-polluted sections of the Thames and delivering the water to homes, leading to an increased incidence of cholera. Snow's study was a major event in the history of public health and geography. It is regarded as the founding event of the science of epidemiology.[71]

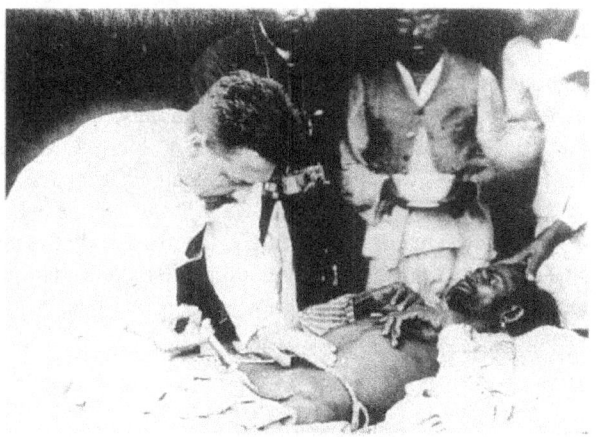

Paul-Louis Simond injecting a plague vaccine in Karachi, 1898.

Disease control With the pioneering work in bacteriology of French chemist Louis Pasteur and German scientist Robert Koch, methods for isolating the bacteria responsible for a given disease and vaccines for remedy were developed at the turn of the 20th century. British physician Ronald Ross identified the mosquito as the carrier of malaria and laid the foundations for combating the disease.[72] Joseph Lister revolutionized surgery by the introduction of antiseptic surgery to eliminate infection. French epidemiologist Paul-Louis Simond proved that plague was carried by fleas on the back of rats,[73] and the Americans Walter Reed and James Carroll demonstrated that mosquitoes carry the virus responsible for yellow fever.[74]

With onset of the epidemiological transition and as the prevalence of infectious diseases decreased through the 20th century, public health began to put more focus on chronic diseases such as cancer and heart disease. Previous efforts in many developed countries had already led to dramatic reductions in the infant mortality rate using preventative methods. In Britain, the infant mortality rate fell from over 15% in 1870 to 7% by 1930.[75]

Country examples

France   France 1871-1914 followed well behind Bismarckian Germany, as well as Great Britain, in developing the welfare state including public health. Tuberculosis was the most dreaded disease of the day, especially striking young people in their 20s. Germany set up vigorous measures of public hygiene and public sanatoria, but France let private physicians handle the problem, which left it with a much higher death rate.[76] The French medical profession jealously guarded its prerogatives, and public health activists were not as well organized or as influential as in Germany, Britain or the United States.[77][78] For example, there was a long battle over a public health law which began in the 1880s as a campaign to reorganize the nation's health services, to require the registration of infectious diseases, to mandate quarantines, and to improve the deficient health and housing legislation of 1850. However the reformers met opposition from bureaucrats, politicians, and physicians. Because it was so threatening to so many interests, the proposal was debated and postponed for 20 years before becoming law in 1902. Success finally came when the government realized that contagious diseases had a national security impact in weakening military recruits, and keeping the population population growth rate well below Germany's.[79]

States John Adams, the Congress authorized the creation of hospitals for mariners. As the U.S. expanded, the scope of the governmental health agency expanded.

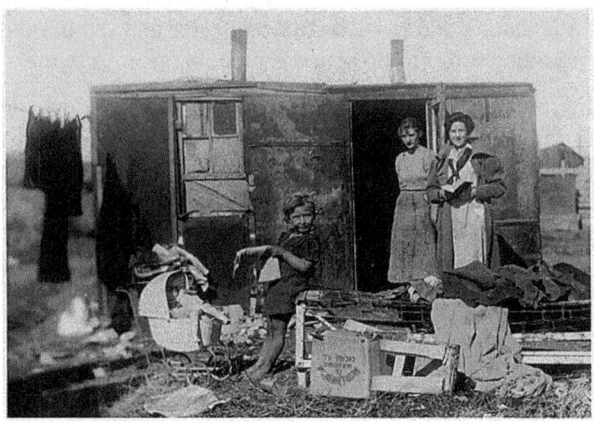

Public health nursing made available through child welfare services in U.S. (c. 1930s)

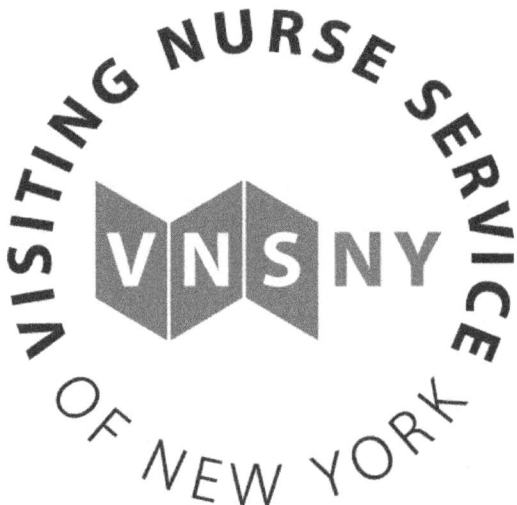

Logo of the Visiting Nurse Service of New York, founded by nursing pioneer Lillian Wald in 1893

In the United States, public health worker Sara Josephine Baker, M.D. established many programs to help the poor in New York City keep their infants healthy, leading teams of nurses into the crowded neighborhoods of Hell's Kitchen and teaching mothers how to dress, feed, and bathe their babies.

Another key pioneer of public health in the U.S. was Lillian Wald, who founded the Henry Street Settlement house in New York. The Visiting Nurse Service of New York was a significant organization for bringing health care to the urban poor.

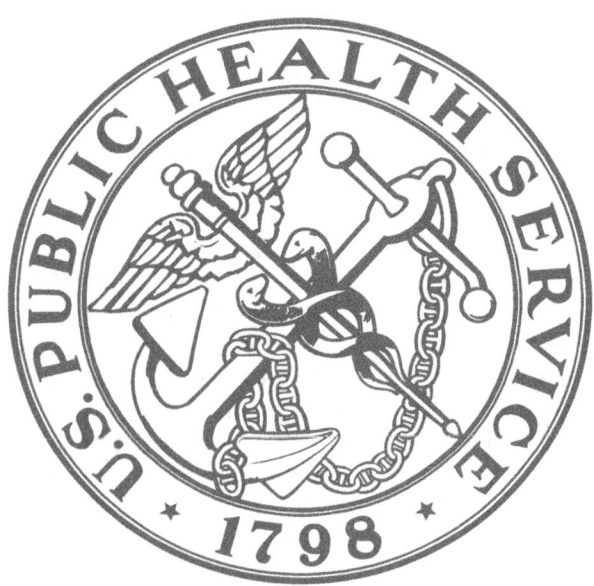

Seal of the United States Public Health Service

United States   Most of the Public health activity in the United States took place at the municipal level before the mid-20th century. There was some activity at the national and state level as well.[80]

In the administration of the second president of the United

Dramatic increases in average life span in the late 19th century and 20th century, is widely credited to public health achievements, such as vaccination programs and control of many infectious diseases including polio, diphtheria, yellow fever and smallpox; effective health and safety policies such as road traffic safety and occupational safety; improved family planning; tobacco control measures; and programs designed to decrease non-communicable diseases by acting on known risk factors such as a person's background, lifestyle and environment.

Another major public health improvement was the decline in the "urban penalty" brought about by improvements in sanitation. These improvements included chlorination of drinking water, filtration and sewage treatment which led to the decline in deaths caused by infectious waterborne diseases such as cholera and intestinal diseases.[81] The federal Office of Indian Affairs (OIA) operated a large-scale field nursing program. Field nurses targeted native women for health education, emphasizing personal hygiene and infant care and nutrition.[82]

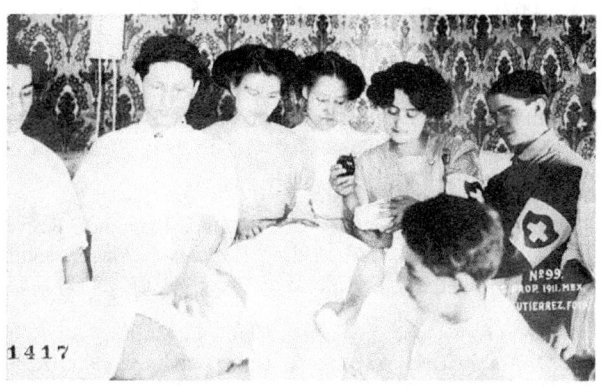

Elena Arizmendi Mejia and volunteers of the Mexican Neutral White Cross, 1911

Latin America   Public health issues were important for the Spanish empire during the colonial era. Epidemic disease was the main factor in the decline of indigenous populations in the era immediately following the sixteenth-century conquest era and was a problem during the colonial era. The Spanish crown took steps in eighteenth-century Mexico to bring in regulations to make populations healthier.[83] In the late nineteenth century, Mexico was in the process of modernization, and public health issues were again tackled from a scientific point of view.[84][85][86][87] Even during the Mexican Revolution (1910–20), public health was an important concern, with a text on hygiene published in 1916.[88] During the Mexican Revolution, feminist and trained nurse Elena Arizmendi Mejia founded the Neutral White Cross, treating wounded soldiers no matter for what faction they fought. In the post-revolutionary

period after 1920, improved public health was a revolutionary goal of the Mexican government.[89][90]

Public health was important elsewhere in Latin America in consolidating state power and integrating marginalized populations into the nation-state. In Colombia, public health was a means for creating and implementing ideas of citizenship.[91] In Bolivia, the push came after their 1952 revolution.[92]

1.6.6   See also

- 10 Essential Public Health Services
- American Board of Preventive Medicine
- American Osteopathic Board of Preventive Medicine
- Behavioral medicine
- Breastfeeding promotion
- Diseases of affluence / Diseases of poverty
- Environmental epidemiology
- Epidemiology
- Evidence-based medicine
- Molecular epidemiology
- Molecular pathological epidemiology
- GIS and public health
- Global health
- Global Mental Health
- Health care delivery
- Health care providers
- Health Officers
- Health profession
- List of preventable causes of death
- National public health institutes
- Nutrition psychology
- One Health
- Personalized medicine
- Precision medicine
- Preventive medicine
- Public health journals

- Public health law

- Timeline of global health

- Universal health care

- Veterinary equivalency

- *World Health Report*

International public health strategies and programs

- Global Strategy for Women's and Children's Health

- International Code of Marketing of Breast-milk Substitutes

- Millennium Development Goals

- The Global Fund to Fight AIDS, Tuberculosis and Malaria

- WHO Framework Convention on Tobacco Control

- Social determinants of health in poverty

1.6.7 References

[1] Winslow, Charles-Edward Amory (1920). "The Untilled Field of Public Health". *Modern Medicine*. **2**: 183–191.

[2] "What is Public Health". *Centers for Disease Control Foundation*. Atlanta, GA: Centers for Disease Control. Retrieved 27 January 2017.

[3] Frequently asked questions from the "Preamble to the Constitution of the World Health Organization" as adopted by the International Health Conference, 1946

[4] Joint Task Group on Public Health Human Resources; Advisory Committee on Health Delivery & Human Resources; Advisory Committee on Population Health & Health Security (2005). *Building the public health workforce for the 21st century*. Ottawa: Public Health Agency of Canada. OCLC 144167975.

[5] Global Public-Private Partnership for Handwashing with Soap. *Handwashing research*, accessed 19 April 2011.

[6] World Health Organization. "Public health principles and neurological disorders. In: *Neurological Disorders: Public Health Challenges*. Geneva; 2006 - http://www.who.int/mental_health/neurology/neurodiso/en/index.html

[7] World Health Organization. *The role of WHO in public health*, accessed 19 April 2011.

[8] World Health Organization. *Public health surveillance*, accessed 19 April 2011.

[9] Garrett Laurie (2007). "The Challenge of Global Health". *Foreign Affairs*. **86** (1): 14–38.

[10] World Health Organization. *Diabetes Fact Sheet N°312*, January 2011. Accessed 19 April 2011.

[11] The Lancet (2010). "Type 2 diabetes—time to change our approach". *The Lancet*. **375** (9733): 2193. doi:10.1016/S0140-6736(10)61011-2. PMID 20609952.

[12] World Health Organization. *Obesity and overweight Fact sheet N°311*, Updated March 2011. Accessed 19 April 2011.

[13] United Nations. *Press Conference on General Assembly Decision to Convene Summit in September 2011 on Non-Communicable Diseases*. New York, 13 May 2010.

[14] Valerie Curtis and Robert Aunger. "Motivational mismatch: evolved motives as the source of—and solution to—global public health problems". In Roberts, S. C. (2011). Roberts, S. Craig, ed. "Applied Evolutionary Psychology". Oxford University Press. doi:10.1093/acprof:oso/9780199586073.001.0001. ISBN 9780199586073.

[15] Gillam Stephen; Yates, Jan; Badrinath, Padmanabhan (2007). *Essential Public Health : theory and practice*. Cambridge University Press. OCLC 144228591.

[16] Pencheon, David; Guest, Charles; Melzer, David; Gray, JA Muir (2006). Pencheon, David, ed. *Oxford Handbook of Public Health Practice*. Oxford University Press. OCLC 663666786.

[17] Smith, Sarah; Sinclair, Don; Raine, Rosalind; Reeves, Barnarby (2005). *Health Care Evaluation*. Understanding Public Health. Open University Press. OCLC 228171855.

[18] Sanderson, Colin J.; Gruen, Reinhold (2006). *Analytical Models for Decision Making*. Understanding Public Health. Open University Press. OCLC 182531015.

[19] Birn, A. E.; Solórzano, A. (1999). "Public health policy paradoxes: Science and politics in the Rockefeller Foundation's hookworm campaign in Mexico in the 1920s". *Social Science & Medicine*. **49** (9): 1197–1213. doi:10.1016/S0277-9536(99)00160-4. PMID 10501641.

[20] Farmer, P. E.; Nizeye, B.; Stulac, S.; Keshavjee, S. (2006). "Structural Violence and Clinical Medicine". *PLoS Medicine*. **3** (10): e449. doi:10.1371/journal.pmed.0030449. PMC 1621099. PMID 17076568.

[21] Wilson, Kumanan; Keelan, Jennifer (May 2009). "Coping with public health 2.0". *Canadian Medical Association Journal*. **180** (10): 1080. doi:10.1503/cmaj.090696. PMC 2679846. PMID 19433834.

[22] Vance, K.; Howe, W.; Dellavalle, R.P. (April 2009). "Social internet sites as a source of public health information". *Dermatologic Clinics*. **27** (2): 133–136. doi:10.1016/j.det.2008.11.010. PMID 19254656.

[23] "Public Health 2.0: Spreading like a virus" (PDF). 24 April 2007. Retrieved 2011-06-13.

[24] Lampos, Vasileios; Yom-Tov, Elad; Pebody, Richard; Cox, Ingemar J. (2 July 2015). "Assessing the impact of a health intervention via user-generated Internet content". *Data Mining and Knowledge Discovery*. **29**: 1434–1457. doi:10.1007/s10618-015-0427-9.

[25] DLSPH Conference Planning Committee. "Public Health 2.0 FAQs". Public Health 2.0 Conference. Retrieved 2011-06-13.

[26] D. Parvaz (26 April 2011). "Crowdsourcing Japan's radiation levels". Al Jazeera. Retrieved 2011-06-13.

[27] Hardey, Michael (July 2008). "Public health and Web 2.0". *Perspectives in Public Health*. **128** (4): 181–189. doi:10.1177/1466424008092228.

[28] Lincoln C Chen; David Evans; Tim Evans; Ritu Sadana; Barbara Stilwell; Phylida Travis; Wim Van Lerberghe; Pascal Zurn (2006). *World Health Report 2006: working together for health*. Geneva: WHO. OCLC 71199185.

[29] "10 facts on breastfeeding". World Health Organization. Retrieved 20 April 2011.

[30] Richard G. Wilkinson; Michael G. Marmot, eds. (2003). *The Solid Facts: Social Determinants of Health*. WHO. OCLC 54966941.

[31] "2015 - United Nations sustainable development agenda". *United Nations Sustainable Development*. Retrieved 2015-11-25.

[32] "Sustainable development goals - United Nations". *United Nations Sustainable Development*. Retrieved 2015-11-25.

[33] "NCCP | Child Poverty". *www.nccp.org*. Retrieved 2015-11-25.

[34] "Health - United Nations Sustainable Development". *United Nations Sustainable Development*. Retrieved 2015-11-25.

[35] "Hunger and food security - United Nations Sustainable Development". *United Nations Sustainable Development*. Retrieved 2015-11-25.

[36] "World Development Report". *openknowledge.worldbank.org*. Retrieved 2015-11-25.

[37] "Water and Sanitation - United Nations Sustainable Development". *United Nations Sustainable Development*. Retrieved 2015-11-25.

[38] U.S. Department of Health & Human Services. (1999). *Achievements in Public Health, 1900–1999* - http://www.cdc.gov/mmwr/PDF/wk/mm4850.pdf

[39] Public Health Agency of Canada. Canadian Public Health Workforce Core Competencies, accessed 19 April 2011.

[40] White F. The imperative of public health education: a global perspective. Med Princ Pract 2013;22:515-529 doi:10.1159/000354198</

[41] Welch, William H.; Rose, Wickliffe (1915). "Institute of Hygiene: Being a report by Dr. William H. Welch and Wickliffe Rose to the General Education Board, Rockefeller Foundation": 660–668 reprinted in Fee, Elizabeth (1992). *The Welch-Rose Report: Blueprint for Public Health Education in America* (PDF). Washington, DC: Delta Omega Honorary Public Health Society.

[42] Patel, Kant; Rushefsky, Mark E.; McFarlane, Deborah R. (2005). *The Politics of Public Health in the United States*. M.E. Sharpe. p. 91. ISBN 0-7656-1135-X.

[43] Brandt AM, Gardner M (2000). "Antagonism and accommodation: interpreting the relationship between public health and medicine in the United States during the 20th century". *American Journal of Public Health*. **90** (5): 707–15. doi:10.2105/AJPH.90.5.707. PMC 1446218. PMID 10800418.

[44] White, Kerr L. (1991). *Healing the schism: Epidemiology, medicine, and the public's health*. New York: Springer-Verlag. ISBN 0-387-97574-8.

[45] Darnell, Regna (2008). *Histories of anthropology annual*. University of Nebraska Press. p. 36. ISBN 0-8032-6664-2.

[46] Dyer, John Percy (1966). *Tulane: the biography of a university, 1834-1965*. Harper & Row. p. 136.

[47] The World Book Encyclopedia, 1994, p. 135.

[48] Education of the Physician: International Dimensions. *Education Commission for Foreign Medical Graduates.*, Association of American Medical Colleges. Meeting. (1984 : Chicago, Ill), p. v.

[49] Milton Terris, "The Profession of Public Health", *Conference on Education, Training, and the Future of Public Health*. March 22–24, 1987. Board on Health Care Services. Washington, DC: National Academy Press, p. 53.

[50] JSTOR.org

[51] "Schools of Public Health and Public Health Programs" (PDF). Council on Education for Public Health. 11 March 2011. Retrieved 30 March 2011.

[52] Association of Schools of Public Health

[53] Council on Education for Public Health

[54] Delta Omega website (primary source)

[55] [[:it:Magistrato alla Sanità]] [Magistrato alla Sanità]

[56] Carruthers, G. Barry. *History of Britain's Hospitals* (2005)

[57] "public health". Encyclopedia Britannica.

[58] Vale, Brian. "The Conquest of Scurvy in the Royal Navy 1793–1800: A Challenge to Current Orthodoxy". *The Mariners' Mirror*, volume 94, number 2, May 2008, pp. 160–175.

[59] Selwyn, S (1966), "Sir John Pringle: hospital reformer, moral philosopher and pioneer of antiseptics", *Medical History* (published July 1966), **10** (3), pp. 266–74, doi:10.1017/s0025727300011133, PMC 1033606, PMID 5330009

[60] Amanda J. Thomas (2010). *The Lambeth cholera outbreak of 1848-1849: the setting, causes, course and aftermath of an epidemic in London*. McFarland. pp. 55–6. ISBN 978-0-7864-3989-8. Retrieved 5 April 2012.

[61] Margaret Stacey (1 June 2004). *The Sociology of Health and Healing*. Taylor and Francis. p. 69. ISBN 978-0-203-38004-8. Retrieved 5 April 2012.

[62] Samuel Edward Finer (1952). *The Life and Times of Sir Edwin Chadwick*. Methuen. pp. 424–5. ISBN 978-0-416-17350-5.

[63] Ashton, John; Ubido, Janet (1991). "The Healthy City and the Ecological Idea" (PDF). *Journal of the Society for the Social History of Medicine*. **4** (1): 173–181. doi:10.1093/shm/4.1.173. Retrieved 8 July 2013.

[64] Chadwick, Edwin (1842). "Chadwick's Report on Sanitary Conditions". *excerpt from* Report...from the Poor Law Commissioners on an Inquiry into the Sanitary Conditions of the Labouring Population of Great Britain *(pp.369-372) (online source)*. added by Laura Del Col: to The Victorian Web. Retrieved 2009-11-08.

[65] Chadwick, Edwin (1843). *Report on the Sanitary Condition of the Labouring Population of Great Britain. A Supplementary Report on the results of a Special Inquiry into The Practice of Interment in Towns*. London: Printed by R. Clowes & Sons, for Her Majesty's Stationery Office. Retrieved 2009-11-08. Full text at Internet Archive (archive.org)

[66] "Decline of Infant Mortality in England and Wales, 1871-1948 : a Medical Conundrum". Retrieved 2012-12-17.

[67] Mooney, Graham (2015). *Intrusive Interventions: Public Health, Domestic Space, and Infectious Disease Surveillance in England, 1840-1914*. Rochester, NY: University of Rochester Press. ISBN 9781580465274.

[68] United States Public Health Service, *Municipal Health Department Practice for the Year 1923* (Public Health Bulletin # 164, July 1926), pp. 348, 357, 364

[69] *Concepts and practice of humanitarian medicine* (2008) Par S. William Gunn, M. Masellis ISBN 0-387-72263-7

[70] Vinten-Johansen, Peter, *et al.* (2003). *Cholera, Chloroform, and the Science of Medicine: A Life of John Snow*. Oxford University Press. ISBN 0-19-513544-X

[71] Johnson, Steven (2006). *The Ghost Map: The Story of London's Most Terrifying Epidemic – and How it Changed Science, Cities and the Modern World*. Riverhead Books. ISBN 1-59448-925-4

[72] ":: Laboc Hospital - A Noble Prize Winner's Workplace". easternpanorama.in. Retrieved 2013-07-11.

[73] Edward Marriott (1966) in "Plague. A Story of Science, Rivalry and the Scourge That Won't Go Away" ISBN 978-1-4223-5652-4

[74] Pierce J.R., J, Writer. 2005. *Yellow Jack: How Yellow Fever Ravaged America and Walter Reed Discovered its Deadly Secrets*. John Wiley and Sons. ISBN 0-471-47261-1

[75] "The declines in infant mortality and fertility: Evidence from British cities in demographic transition" (PDF). Retrieved 2012-12-17.

[76] Allan Mitchell, *The Divided Path: The German Influence on Social Reform in France After 1870* (1991) pp 252-75 excerpt

[77] Martha L. Hildreth, *Doctors, Bureaucrats & Public Health in France, 1888-1902* (1987)

[78] Alisa Klaus, *Every Child a Lion: The Origins of Maternal & Infant Health Policy in the United States & France, 1890-1920* (1993).

[79] Ann-Louise Shapiro, "Private Rights, Public Interest, and Professional Jurisdiction: The French Public Health Law of 1902." *Bulletin of the History of Medicine* 54.1 (1980): 4+

[80] John Duffy, *The sanitarians: a history of American public health* (1992).

[81] Cuter, David; Grant Miller (February 2005). "The Role of Public Health Improvements in Health Advances: The Twentieth Century United States". *Demography*. **42** (1): 1–22. doi:10.1353/dem.2005.0002. OCLC 703811616. PMID 15782893.

[82] Hancock Christin L (2001). "Healthy Vocatoons: Field Nursing and the Religious Overtones of Public Health". *Journal of Women's History*. **23** (3): 113–137.

[83] Donald Cooper, *Epidemic Disease in Mexico City, 1761-1813: An Administrative, Social, and Medical History*. Austin: University of Texas Press 1965.

[84] Claudia Agostoni, *Monuments of Progess: Modernization and Public Health in Mexico City, 1876-1910*. Calgary: University of Calgary Press; Boulder: University of Colorado Press; Mexico City: Instituto de Investigaciones Históricos 2003.

[85] Claudia Agostoni, "Discurso médico, cultura higiénica y la mjuer en la ciudad de México al cambio de siglo (XIX-XX)", *Mexican Studies / Estudios Mexicanos* vol. 18, no. 1. Winter 2002, pp. 1-22.

[86] Ana María Carrillo, "Economía, Política, y Saludo Pública en el México Porfiriana, 1876-1910", *Historia, Ciencias, Saúde - Maginguinhos* 9, suplemento 2002, pp. 67-87.

[87] Patience A. Schell. "Nationalizing children through schools and hypgiene: Porfirian and Revolutionary Mexico City". *The Americas* 60:4, April 2004, pp. 559-587.

[88] Alberto J. Pani, *La higiene en México.* Mexico: Imprenta de J. Ballescá 1916.

[89] Katherine Elaine Bliss, "The Science of Redemption: Syphilis, Sexual Promiscuity, and Reformism in Revolutionary Mexico City" *Hispanic American Historical Review* 79:1 1999, pp. 1-40.

[90] Ernesto Aréchiga Córdoba, "Educación, propaganda o 'Dictadura sanitaria'. Estrategias discursivas de higiene y salubridad pública en el México posrevolucionario, 1917-1934". Dynamis 25, 2005, pp. 117-143.

[91] Hanni Jalil, "Curing a Sick Nation: Public Health and Citizenship in Colombia, 1930-1940." PhD dissertation, University of California, Santa Barbara 2015.

[92] Nicole Pacino, "Prescription for a Nation: Public Health in Post-Revolutionary Bolivia, 1952-1964." PhD dissertation, University of California, Santa Barbara 2013.

1.6.8   Further reading

- Berridge, Virginia. *Public Health: A Very Short Introduction* (Oxford University Press, 2016).

- Berridge, Virginia, et al. *Public Health in History* (2011).

- Breslow, Lester, ed. (2002). *Encyclopedia of Public Health.* New York: Macmillan Reference USA. ISBN 978-0-02-865354-9.

- Garrett, Laurie (2000). *Betrayal of Trust: the Collapse of Global Public Health.* New York: Hyperion. ISBN 0-7868-6522-9.

- Heymann, David L., ed. (2008). *Control of Communicable Diseases Manual.* Washington, D.C.: American Public Health Association. ISBN 978-0-87553-189-2.

- Heggenhougen, Kris; Stella R Quah, eds. (2008). *International Encyclopedia of Public Health.* Amsterdam Boston: Elsevier/Academic Press. ISBN 978-0-12-227225-7.

- Jalil, Hanni. "Curing a Sick Nation: Public Health and Citizenship in Colombia, 1930-1940." PhD dissertation, University of California, Santa Barbara, 2015.

- La Berge, Ann F. *Mission and Method: The Early Nineteenth-Century French Public Health Movement.* New York: Cambridge University Press 1992.

- Novick, Lloyd F; Cynthia B Morrow; Glen P Mays (2008). *Public Health Administration: Principles for Population-Based Management* (2nd ed.). Sudbury, MA: Jones and Bartlett Pub. ISBN 978-0-7637-3842-6.

- Pacino, Nicole. "Prescription for a Nation: Public Health in Post-Revolutionary Bolivia, 1952-1964." PhD dissertation, University of California, Santa Barbara 2013.

- Schneider, Dona; David E Lilienfeld (2008). *Public Health: the Development of a Discipline.* New Brunswick, NJ: Rutgers University Press. ISBN 978-0-8135-4231-7.

- Rosen, George. *A History of Public Health.* New York: MD Publications 1958.

- Stokols, D.; Hall, K.L.; Vogel, A.L. (2013). "Transdisciplinary public health: Core characteristics, definitions, and strategies for success". In Haire-Joshu, D.; McBride, T.D. *Transdisciplinary public health: Research, methods, and practice* (PDF). San Francisco: Jossey-Bass. pp. 3–30.

- Tausch, Arno (2012). *Globalization, the Human Condition, and Sustainable Development in the Twenty-first Century: Cross-national Perspectives and European Implications. With Almas Heshmati and a Foreword by Ulrich Brand* (1st ed.). Anthem Press, London. ISBN 9780857284105.

- Turnock, Bernard (2009). *Public Health: What It Is and How It Works* (4th ed.). Sudbury, MA: Jones and Bartlett Publishers. ISBN 978-0-7637-5444-0.

- *Oxford Textbook of Public Health* (5th ed.). Oxford and New York: Oxford University Press. 2009. ISBN 978-0-19-921870-7.

- White, Franklin; Stallones, Lorann; Last, John M. (2013). *Global Public Health: Ecological Foundations.* Oxford University Press. ISBN 978-0-19-975190-7.

1.6.9   External links

- Health-EU, the official public health portal of the European Union

- The Healthy Village, Public Health Awareness and Advocacy

- Public Health - Educational Articles by United Medical Education; a public resource for health related educational articles and emergency training in ACLS, PALS, and BLS certification online.

- What Is Public Health? by the Association of Schools and Programs of Public Health

Chapter 2

Publicly Funded Healthcare Topics (in Alphabetical Order)

2.1 All-payer rate setting

All-payer rate setting is a price setting mechanism in which all third parties pay the same price for services at a given hospital.[1] The system does not imply that charges are the same for every hospital. It can be used to increase the market power of payers (such as private and/or public insurance companies) to mitigate inflation in health care costs. All-payer characteristics are found in the health systems of France, Germany, Japan, and the Netherlands.[2] Maryland also uses such a model.[1]

2.1.1 Maryland

Main article: Maryland hospital payment system

Since the late 1970s, Maryland has operated an all-payer system for hospital services. An independent commission establishes the rate structure for each hospital. That eliminated hospital cost shifting across payers and spread more equitably the costs of uncompensated care and medical education and limited cost growth, but per capita Medicare hospital costs are among the country's highest.[3] It appears that the system eliminated price competition between hospitals and led them to divert high-cost patients to alternative settings, where prices remained unregulated.[4]

Medicare's participation in the system is authorized by the Social Security Act and is tied to a growth limit in payment per admission. The Medicare waiver created incentives to increase the volume of services. Medicare pays higher rates for hospital services in Maryland than it does under the national prospective payment systems.[3]

On January 10, 2014, the Centers for Medicare and Medicaid Services (CMS) and the State announced a new model that will focus on overall per capita expenditures for hospital services as well as on improvements in the quality of care

and population health outcomes. For 5 years beginning in 2014, Maryland will limit the growth of per capita hospital costs to the lesser of 3.58% or 0.5% less than the actual national growth rate for 2015 through 2018. The change is forecast to save Medicare at least \$330 million. 3.58% is Maryland's historical 10-year growth rate of per capita gross state product.[3]

2.1.2 See also

- Capitation (healthcare)

- Fee-for-service

- Single-payer health care

2.1.3 References

[1] "Maryland receives OK for healthcare overhaul that caps hospital spending". Modern Healthcare. 2012-02-06. Retrieved 2014-01-10.

[2] Joseph White (May 12, 2009). "Cost Control and Health Care Reform — The Case for All-Payer Regulation" (PDF). Retrieved June 29, 2011.

[3] Rajkumar, R.; Patel, A.; Murphy, K.; Colmers, J. M.; Blum, J. D.; Conway, P. H.; Sharfstein, J. M. (2014). "Maryland's All-Payer Approach to Delivery-System Reform". *New England Journal of Medicine*. **370**: 140110110008004. doi:10.1056/NEJMp1314868. PMID 24410022.

[4] Pope, Christopher. "Legislating Low Prices: Cutting Costs or Care?". Heritage Foundation. Retrieved 8 September 2014.

2.2 Brian Day

Brian Day MRCP (UK), FRCS (Eng), FRCS (C), (born January 29, 1947) is an orthopedic surgeon and health researcher in Canada, a past president of the Canadian Medical Association, and a prominent sometimes controversial advocate[1] for patient access to a hybrid of Canada's health system.

As the founder and medical director of a private clinic Cambie Surgery Centre and Specialist Referral Centre[2] in Vancouver, British Columbia, Dr. Day is a spokesperson for a high-profile, multi-year and ongoing lawsuit against the provincial government, *Cambie Surgeries Corporation v. British Columbia (Medical Services Commission)*.[3] that is sometimes cited publicly as 'The Day Case'.[4]

2.2.1 Early life and education

Day was raised in Toxteth, a working-class area of post-war Liverpool, England. He was the eldest of four children in a family with strong Labour views. Both his mother and father were socialists.[1] Day credited his personal shift from the political left to the political center-right by his disenchantment with the British labour movement's jurisdictional inertia and contributions to inefficiency in health care.[5]

Day attended the Liverpool Institute, the same high school attended by Paul McCartney and George Harrison.[1] His family's neighbourhood could be tough. Day has a permanent scar on a finger from a knife fight when he was 10 years old.[1][6] His father, a pharmacist, was killed in 1981 by hooligans looking for drugs during riots in the neighbourhood.[1] The possible contribution of misdiagnosis by British doctors for the death of Day's mother in 1986 is cited as his dissatisfaction with the British health system.[7][8]

Day entered medical school at age 18 at the University of Manchester, where he graduated in 1970. After an initial interest in general surgery, which he pursued as a postgraduate in Manchester and at the Hammersmith Hospital in London, he focused on orthopaedics.[1] He obtained his medical degrees, MB ChB from the University of Manchester, and post-graduate qualifications in both internal medicine and general surgery. In July 1973, Day moved to Vancouver, British Columbia, Canada.[1] In 1978, Day completed his training and a M.Sc. degree at the University of British Columbia (UBC).

2.2.2 Medical career

In 1979, Day received the Canadian Orthopaedic Association's Edouard Samson Award, for outstanding orthopaedic research in Canada. Following a fellowship in traumatology, in Basel, Switzerland, Oxford, and Los Angeles, he began practice at the Vancouver General Hospital. After starting in trauma, he developed an interest and expertise in orthopaedic sports medicine and arthroscopy.

As an orthopedic surgeon, he earned an international reputation for performing arthroscopic surgery on hips, knees, shoulders and elbows. Day is regarded as being instrumental in the introduction of arthroscopic joint surgery in Canada.[5]

From 1970 to 2014, Day wrote more than 150 scientific articles or book chapters, in areas of orthopaedics and arthroscopic surgery / sports medicine, and on the topic of health policy.

Medical association leadership (Canada and North America)

Day is a founding member and was 2004 president of the Arthroscopy Association of North America, being the second Canadian elected to that position.

In August 2006, Day was elected president of the Canadian Medical Association (CMA) for the 2007/08 term, despite a challenge at the convention floor by another British Columbian physician (whom Day had beaten in the nomination process) regarding Day's views about for-profit health care.[1] He was the first orthopaedic surgeon in the 148-year history of the CMA to be elected president.[9] Day states that his advocacy as president of CMA was for a hybrid public-private system, not a full replacement by private hospitals.[10] The CMA policy drafted in 2007 was "When access to timely care cannot be provided in the publicly funded system, Canadians should be able to use private health insurance to reimburse the cost of care obtained in the private sector."[3]

Two losses at Doctors of BC

In 2015, Day was temporarily announced as the president-elect for Doctors of BC, the provincial medical association in British Columbia, because of a win by a single vote difference. The election was then rescinded because of an error found in properly categorizing one ballot. Dr. Day then lost the subsequent run-off election in June 2015 to DR. Alan Ruddiman by 603 votes after the publicity about the single-vote win escalated participation to the highest turnout by physician members of the association.[11] In May 2016, Day was defeated 1,896 to 1,674 votes by Dr. Trina

Larsen Soles in the election for the 2017–18 Doctors of BC presidency.[12] Day is a member of the editorial board for the BC Medical Journal.[2]

2.2.3 Advocacy for access to private care

In 2003, *Maclean's Magazine* named Day one its top 50 Canadians "to watch", describing him as "an iconoclast, whose time is now."[13] He is referred to as Dr. Profit by opponents who believe his legal challenges will threaten Canada's publicly funded medicare system, and Dr. Prophet by supporters for his advocacy of a role for patient choice and the right to obtain private insurance in the face of long government wait lists for care.[5]

Dr. Day has argued many Canadians are being hypocritical towards private healthcare, because 70 per cent of Canadians buy healthcare insurance. Many with such insurance themselves claim to oppose private healthcare, while embracing it for themselves. The other 30 per cent of Canadians who cannot afford the extra healthcare insurance receive poorer access to care.[14]

Day cites the Canada Health Act of 1984 being responsible for rationing of care that has resulted in over a million Canadians suffering on wait lists, and to more than 5 million without a doctor. In the 2005 Chaoulli v Quebec (AG) decision, the Supreme Court of Canada struck down prohibitions on private insurance in that province because it was an infringement of the Quebec Charter of Human Rights and Freedoms; the decision did not extend to the rest of Canada, but constitutional experts opined that it would certainly have major impact on similar cases brought to court elsewhere. Day also supports the end of block funding for hospitals and a change to "Patient Focused Funding" where revenue follows the patient. He advocates a patient-centered system with a greater role for competition in Canadian healthcare as a means to reduce waiting times and save government money by treating people before their condition worsens.[1] He is a frequent spokesman for the topic with news media and submits position papers with government. For instance, his submission to Roy Romanow's Commission on the Future of Health Care in Canada made 10 recommendations:

1. De-politicize the debate

2. Repeal the Canada Health Act

3. Eliminate global budgets and reward productivity

4. Incorporate business methods

5. Increase privatization and contracting out

6. Introduce competition, choice and accountability

7. Massively reduce bureaucracy

8. Reduce influence of public sector health unions

9. Accept economic reality, and introduce user fees

10. Rank "core services" and deinsure unnecessary services[15]

US 'Conservatives For Patient Rights' commercial controversy

In May 2009, Day drew criticism after he was shown in a series of television ads for a US lobby group called Conservatives for Patients' Rights that opposed President Obama's health care reforms. Day appeared on the television program BNN on May 11, 2009, to clarify that he issued a letter distancing himself from the ad. He also pointed out that Obamacare was based on private insurance and private delivery, the opposite of what many Canadians believe in.[16]

2.2.4 Cambie Surgery Centre and Constitutional Legal Challenge

In 1995, Day founded Cambie Surgery Centre, a for-profit Vancouver clinic. Day is the facility's medical director, and one of its 40-plus shareholders. The Cambie Surgery Centre has 50 full- and part-time nurses and 125 doctors performing operations and other procedures for up to 5,000 patients a year which may be the busiest private hospital in Canada.[17]

Day has said he decided to set up the Cambie Surgical Centre, which is non-union, after government funding decreased in the mid-90s cut his operating time at UBC from 17 hours a week to about six. The start-up was during the province's premiership of Michael Harcourt.[8] To demolish an old nursing home and build a surgery centre on the site, Day needed to raise about $5 million.[8] He succeeded in convincing notable Vancouverites such as the late Milan Ilich and Jack Poole, as well as Kip Woodward (chair of Providence Health Care and future chair of Vancouver Coastal Health), and 19 others including Jim Wyse and Hugh Magee,[8] to commit $100,000 each with the remainder financed by the Royal Bank of Canada.

Cambie Surgeries Corporation v. British Columbia (Medical Services Commission)

In 2009, the Cambie Surgery Centre and patients filed a lawsuit versus the province's Medical Services Commission. The lawsuit continues to be a court case in late 2016 with the Supreme Court of British Columbia with possibly 200 witnesses.[7] Six of the eight plaintiffs are patients, two of whom died before the conclusion of the court case.[3]

In 2012, the British Columbia Medical Services Commission confirmed what the clinics had openly admitted to doing since 1996—namely allowing patients, in violation of the Medicare Protection Act, to spend their own funds to jump the queue and access the clinic.[18][19]

The Commission asked the Cambie Surgery Centre not to permit patients access to earlier treatment.[20] The plaintiffs pointed out the constitutional challenge had been brought before the courts 3 years earlier. In the Supreme Court of British Columbia, the plaintiffs are challenging the prohibition against patients being prohibited from using their own funds to access care, instead of receiving it in order based on medical priority. Specifically, they are challenging the ban on private health insurance to cover medically necessary care, and the ban preventing doctors from working in both the public and private health systems at the same time. The proceedings are expected to continue in September 2016.[21][22]

Proponents of publicly funded healthcare in Canada argue that this legal challenge against medicare could set a dangerous precedent. Proponents of for-profit care argue the opposite and that patients will be protected from the dangers of waiting for care. In the Chaoulli decision (2005) the Supreme Court of Canada declared it was a fact that Canadians were suffering and dying on wait lists. If the case is decided at trial in B.C., as is expected, either side may seek an appeal of the outcome at the Supreme Court of Canada. A decision at this level would mean the outcome would be binding in all provinces and territories across the country. Some legal experts have described this case as one of the most significant legal challenges in Canadian history.[23]

2.2.5 Recognition

- 1993 to 2001: Associate Editor, *Journal of Arthroscopic Surgery*

- 2001: 80th Annual Osler Lecturer, Vancouver Medical Association

- 2004: President, Arthroscopy Association of North America (AANA)

- 2004: Honorary Member, Cuban Orthopaedic Association

- 2004: Member, Board of Trustees, *Journal of Arthroscopy*

- 2005/06: President, Canadian Independent Medical Clinics Association (CIMCA)

- 2012: jointly listed as #38 in the Power50 list for influencers in sport in Canada by The Globe and Mail[24]

- 2014: Doctors of BC Don Rix Leadership Award

2.2.6 References

[1] Mason, Gary (August 1, 2007). "Brian Day: Day in Your Life". *'BC Business Magazine'*. Vancouver. Retrieved August 1, 2014.

[2] "Editorial Board". BC Medical Journal. Retrieved 2016-09-02.

[3] Fayerman, Pamela (2016-09-01). "B.C. trial over private health care could reshape Canadian medicare". *The Vancouver Sun*.

[4] Peden, Alex. "Backgrounder: Court challenges to one-tier medicare". *EvidenceNetwork.ca*. University of Manitoba. Retrieved 2016-09-02.

[5] Ward, Doug (April 8, 2002). "A new Day for health care". *Vancouver Sun*. Retrieved 2 August 2014.

[6] Mickleburgh, Rod (2010-11-05). "Part 1: Is this private clinic surgeon a crusader or criminal?". *The Globe and Mail*. Retrieved 2016-09-02.

[7] Mason, Gary (2016-09-02). "Changing Canada's healthcare system is a life-long fight". *The Globe and Mail*.

[8] Fayerman, Pamela (2015-02-24). "Dr. Brian Day #3: his dad's murder, mom's misdiagnosis, Beatles connection and the prominent families who were his investors". *The Vancouver Sun*. Retrieved 2016-09-03.

[9] "First orthopedic surgeon voted CMA president-elect calls for health care reform". *healio.com*. Orthopedics Today 2006. Retrieved 2016-09-02.

[10] Day, Brian (June 18, 2015). "Rebuttal from Brian Day: my prescription for Canada's health care". *Opinion: National Observer*. Retrieved 5 July 2015.

[11] Canadian Press (June 19, 2015). "B.C. doctors elect new president; Dr. Brian Day loses by 600 votes". *Global BC*. Retrieved 5 July 2015.

[12] Britten, Liam (2016-05-16). "Brian Day, private medical care advocate, loses Doctors of B.C. election". *CBC News*.

[13] 50 Canadians to watch in 2003, *Maclean's Magazine*, January 20, 2003

[14] Brian Day's diagnosis: The president of the Canadian Medical Association explains how to fix our health-care system - Full Comment Archived October 29, 2007, at the Wayback Machine.

[15] Dr. Brian Day - Submission to the Commission on the Future of Health Care in Canada

[16] Ward, Doug (October 10, 2009). "Canadian critics slam Obamacare in U.S.". *Vancouver Sun*. Retrieved 2 August 2014.

[17] Fayerman, Pamela (2015-02-15). "Dr. Brian Day #1: Everything you need to know about him and his legal case against the government health care "monopoly"". *The Vancouver Sun staff blog*. Retrieved 2016-09-02.

[18] Ministry of Health Billing Integrity Program (June 2012). *Specialist Referral Clinic (Vancouver) Inc. and Cambie Surgeries Corporation: Audit Report* (PDF).

[19] Brend, Yvette. "Epic court battle over private health care rages in B.C. courts". *cbc news*.

[20] "Medical Services Commission releases audit". *gov.bc.ca*.

[21] "Injunction sought against private clinic operating in Vancouver". *The Globe and Mail*.

[22] "B.C. doctors urge provincial ministers to take a stand on public health care". *The Globe and Mail*.

[23] Macleod, Andrew (17 April 2014). "For-Profit Clinic Lawsuit May Transform Health Care". *TheTyee.ca*. Retrieved 22 April 2014.

[24] "The Globe's Power 50 list- 2012". *Globe and Mail*. Feb 6, 2012. Retrieved 2 August 2014.

2.2.7 Further reading

- Brian Day: CMA's next president supports private health care, By Michael McCarthy, *The Lancet*, Oct 14, 2006, Vol 368, p. 1321

2.2.8 External links

- BrianDay.ca - Official site

- 2010 BCSC 396 *Cambie Surgeries Corp. v. British Columbia (Medical Services Commission)*

2.3 Healthcare reform in the United States

Health care reform in the United States has a long history. Reforms have often been proposed but have rarely been accomplished. In 2010, landmark reform was passed through two federal statutes enacted in 2010: the Patient Protection and Affordable Care Act (PPACA), signed March 23, 2010,[1][2] and the Health Care and Education Reconciliation Act of 2010 (H.R. 4872), which amended the PPACA and became law on March 30, 2010.[3][4]

Future reforms of the American health care system continue to be proposed, with notable proposals including a single-payer system and a reduction in fee-for-service medical care.[5] The PPACA includes a new agency, the Center for Medicare and Medicaid Innovation, which is intended to research reform ideas through pilot projects.

2.3.1 History of national reform efforts

Main article: History of health care reform in the United States

Here is a summary of reform achievements at the national level in the United States. For failed efforts, state-based efforts, native tribes services and more details generally, see the main article History of health care reform in the United States.

- **1965** President Lyndon Johnson enacted legislation that introduced Medicare, covering both hospital (Part A) and supplemental medical (Part B) insurance for senior citizens. The legislation also introduced Medicaid, which permitted the Federal government to partially fund a program for the poor, with the program managed and co-financed by the individual states.[6][7]

- **1985** The Consolidated Omnibus Budget Reconciliation Act of 1985 (COBRA) amended the Employee Retirement Income Security Act of 1974 (ERISA) to give some employees the ability to continue health insurance coverage after leaving employment.[8]

- **1996** The Health Insurance Portability and Accountability Act (HIPAA) not only protects health insurance coverage for workers and their families when they change or lose their jobs, it also made health insurance companies cover pre-existing conditions. If such condition had been diagnosed before purchasing insurance, insurance companies are required to cover it after patient has one year of continuous coverage. If such condition was already covered on their current policy, new insurance policies due to changing jobs, etc... have to cover the condition immediately.[9]

- **1997** The Balanced Budget Act of 1997 introduced two new major Federal healthcare insurance programs, Part C of Medicare and the State Children's Health Insurance Program, or SCHIP. Part C formalized longstanding "Managed Medicare" (HMO, etc.) demonstration projects and SCHIP was established to provide health insurance to children in families at or below 200 percent of the federal poverty line. Many other "entitlement" changes and additions were made to Parts A and B of fee for service (FFS) Medicare and to Medicaid within an omnibus law that also made changes to the Food Stamp and other Federal programs. [10]

- **2000** The Medicare, Medicaid, and SCHIP Benefits Improvement and Protection Act (BIPA) effectively reversed some of the cuts to the three named programs in the Balanced Budget Act of 1997 because of Congressional concern that providers would stop providing services.

- **2003** The Medicare Prescription Drug, Improvement and Modernization Act (also known as the Medicare Modernization Act or MMA) introduced supplementary optional coverage within Medicare for self-administered prescription drugs and as the name suggests also changed the other three existing Parts of Medicare law.

- **2010** The Patient Protection and Affordable Care Act, called PPACA or ACA but also known as Obamacare, was enacted, providing for the phased introduction over multiple years of a comprehensive system of mandated health insurance reforms designed to eliminate "some of the worst practices of the insurance companies"—pre-existing condition screening and premium loadings, policy cancellations on technicalities when illness seems imminent, annual and lifetime coverage caps. It also sets a minimum ratio of direct health care spending to premium income, and creates price competition bolstered by the creation of three standard insurance coverage levels to enable like-for-like comparisons by consumers, and a web-based health insurance exchange where consumers can compare prices and purchase plans. The system preserves private insurance and private health care providers and provides subsidies in the form of income tax reductions to enable lower income Americans to buy insurance. PPACA also made many changes to the 1997, 2000 and 2003 laws that had previously changed Medicare and further expanded eligibility for Medicaid (that expansion was later ruled by the Supreme Court to be at the discretion of the states)

- **2015** The Medicare Access & CHIP Reauthorization Act (MACRA) made significant changes to the process by which many Medicare Part B services are reimbursed and also extended SCHIP

2.3.2 Motivation

Main article: Health care reform debate in the United States
International comparisons of healthcare have found that the United States spends more per-capita than other similarly

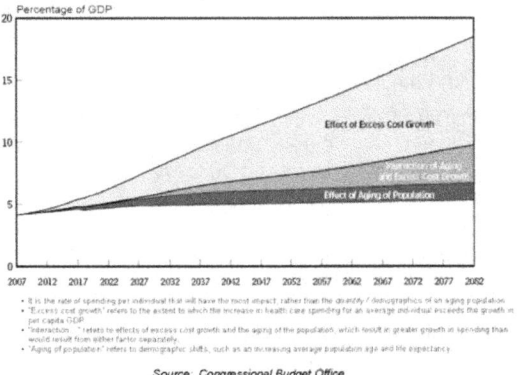

Projected Federal Spending on Medicare and Medicaid (% GDP)

Source: Congressional Budget Office

Medicare and Medicaid Spending as % GDP (data from the CBO)

developed nations but falls below similar countries in various health metrics, suggesting inefficiency and waste. In addition, the United States has significant underinsurance and significant impending unfunded liabilities from its aging demographic and its social insurance programs Medicare and Medicaid (Medicaid provides free long-term care to the elderly poor). The fiscal and human impact of these issues have motivated reform proposals.

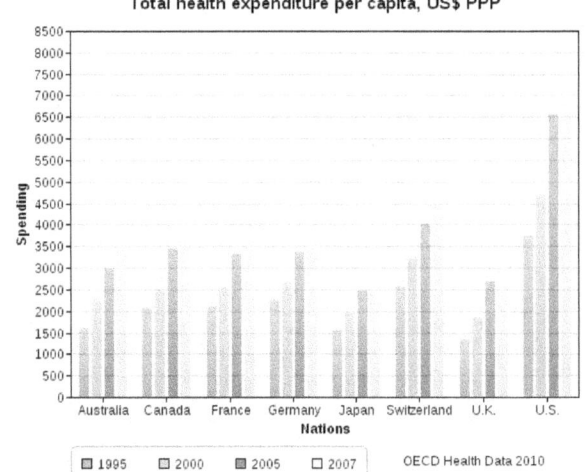

Total health expenditure per capita, US$ PPP

Health spending per capita, in US$ PPP-adjusted, compared amongst various first world nations.

According to 2009 World Bank statistics, the U.S. had the highest healthcare costs relative to the size of the economy (GDP) in the world, even though estimated 50.2 million citizens (approximately 15.6% of the September 2011 estimated population of 312 million) lacked insurance.[11] In March 2010, billionaire Warren Buffett commented that the high costs paid by U.S. companies for their employees' health care put them at a competitive disadvantage.[12]

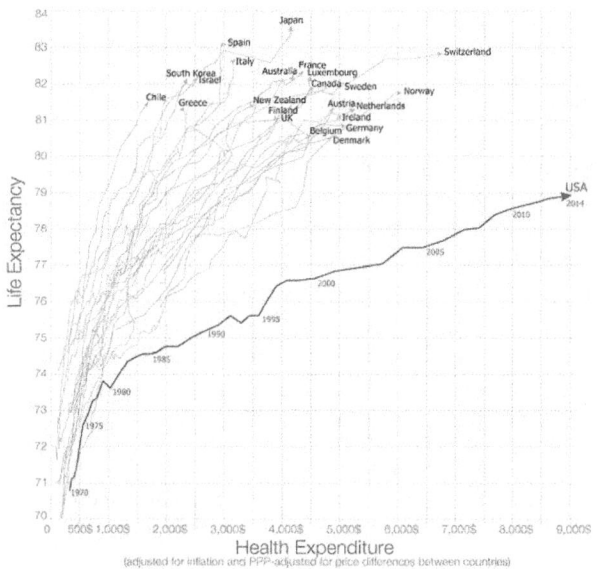

Life expectancy compared to healthcare spending from 1970 to 2008, in the US and the next 19 most wealthy countries by total GDP.[13]

Further, an estimated 77 million Baby Boomers are reaching retirement age, which combined with significant annual increases in healthcare costs per person will place enormous budgetary strain on U.S. state and federal governments, particularly through Medicare and Medicaid spending (Medicaid provides long-term care for the elderly poor).[14] Maintaining the long-term fiscal health of the U.S. federal government is significantly dependent on healthcare costs being controlled.[15]

Insurance cost and availability

Further information: Health insurance coverage in the United States

In addition, the number of employers who offer health insurance has declined and costs for employer-paid health insurance are rising: from 2001 to 2007, premiums for family coverage increased 78%, while wages rose 19% and prices rose 17%, according to the Kaiser Family Foundation.[16] Even for those who are employed, the private insurance in the US varies greatly in its coverage; one study by the Commonwealth Fund published in Health Affairs estimated that 16 million U.S. adults were underinsured in 2003. The underinsured were significantly more likely than those with adequate insurance to forgo health care, report financial stress because of medical bills, and experience coverage gaps for such items as prescription drugs. The study found that underinsurance disproportionately affects those with lower incomes — 73% of the underinsured in the study

population had annual incomes below 200% of the federal poverty level.[17] However, a study published by the Kaiser Family Foundation in 2008 found that the typical large employer preferred provider organization (PPO) plan in 2007 was more generous than either Medicare or the Federal Employees Health Benefits Program Standard Option.[18] One indicator of the consequences of Americans' inconsistent health care coverage is a study in *Health Affairs* that concluded that half of personal bankruptcys involved medical bills,[19] although other sources dispute this.[20]

There are health losses from insufficient health insurance. A 2009 Harvard study published in the American Journal of Public Health found more than 44,800 excess deaths annually in the United States due to Americans lacking health insurance.[21][22] More broadly, estimates of the total number of people in the United States, whether insured or uninsured, who die because of lack of medical care were estimated in a 1997 analysis to be nearly 100,000 per year.[23] A study of the effects of the Massachusetts universal health care law (which took effect in 2006) found a 3% drop in mortality among people 20–64 years old – 1 death per 830 people with insurance. Other studies, just as those examining the randomized distribution of Medicaid insurance to low-income people in Oregon in 2008, found no change in death rate.[24]

The cost of insurance has been a primary motivation in the reform of the US healthcare system, and many different explanations have been proposed in the reasons for high insurance costs and how to remedy them. One critique and motivation for healthcare reform has been the development of the medical–industrial complex. This relates to moral arguments for health care reform, framing healthcare as a social good, one that is fundamentally immoral to deny to people based on economic status. [25] The motivation behind healthcare reform in response to the medical-industrial complex also stems from issues of social inequity, promotion of medicine over preventative care. [26] The medical-industrial complex, defined as a network of health insurance companies, pharmaceutical companies, and the like, plays a role in the complexity of the US insurance market and a fine line between government and industry within it. [27] Likewise, critiques of insurance markets being conducted under a capitalistic, free-market model also include that medical solutions, as opposed to preventative healthcare measures, are promoted to maintain this medical-industrial complex. [27] Arguments for a market-based approach to health insurance include the Grossman model, which is based on an ideal competitive model, but others have critiqued this, arguing that fundamentally, this means that people in higher socioeconomic levels will receive a better quality of healthcare. [26]

Uninsured rate

Another concern is the rate of uninsured people in the US. In June 2014, Gallup–Healthways Well–Being conducted a survey and found that the uninsured rate is going down. 13.4 percent of U.S. adults are uninsured in 2014. This is a decrease from the percentage at 17.1 percent in January 2014 and translates to roughly 10 million to 11 million individuals who gained coverage. The survey also looked at the major demographic groups and found each is making progress towards getting health insurance. However, Hispanics, who have the highest uninsured rate of any racial or ethnic group, are lagging in their progress. Under the new health care reform, Latinos were expected to be major beneficiaries of the new health care law. Gallup found that the biggest drop in the uninsured rate (2.8 percentage points) was among households making less than $36,000 a year.[28][29][30]

Waste and fraud

In December 2011 the outgoing Administrator of the Centers for Medicare & Medicaid Services, Donald Berwick, asserted that 20% to 30% of health care spending is waste. He listed five causes for the waste: (1) overtreatment of patients, (2) the failure to coordinate care, (3) the administrative complexity of the health care system, (4) burdensome rules and (5) fraud.[31]

An estimated 3%–10% of all health care expenditures in the U.S. are fraudulent. In 2011, Medicare and Medicaid made $65 billion in improper payments (including both error and fraud). Government efforts to reduce fraud include $4.2 billion in fraudulent payments recovered by the Department of Justice and the FBI in 2012, longer jail sentences specified by the Affordable Care Act, and Senior Medicare Patrols—volunteers trained to identify and report fraud.[32]

In 2007, the Department of Justice and Health and Human Services formed the Medicare Fraud Strike Force to combat fraud through data analysis and increased community policing. As of May 2013, the Strike Force has charged more than 1,500 people for false billings of more than $5 billion. Medicare fraud often takes the form of kickbacks and money-laundering. Fraud schemes often take the form of billing for medically unnecessary services or services not rendered.[33]

Quality of care

There is significant debate regarding the quality of the U.S. healthcare system relative to those of other countries. Physicians for a National Health Program, a political advocacy group, has claimed that a free market solution to health care provides a lower quality of care, with higher mortality rates, than publicly funded systems.[34] The quality of

health maintenance organizations and managed care have also been criticized by this same group.[35]

According to a 2000 study of the World Health Organization, publicly funded systems of industrial nations spend less on health care, both as a percentage of their GDP and per capita, and enjoy superior population-based health care outcomes.[36] However, conservative commentator David Gratzer and the Cato Institute, a libertarian think tank, have both criticized the WHO's comparison method for being biased; the WHO study marked down countries for having private or fee-paying health treatment and rated countries by comparison to their expected health care performance, rather than objectively comparing quality of care.[37][38]

Some medical researchers say that patient satisfaction surveys are a poor way to evaluate medical care. Researchers at the RAND Corporation and the Department of Veterans Affairs asked 236 elderly patients in two different managed care plans to rate their care, then examined care in medical records, as reported in Annals of Internal Medicine. There was no correlation. "Patient ratings of health care are easy to obtain and report, but do not accurately measure the technical quality of medical care," said John T. Chang, UCLA, lead author.[39][40][41]

2.3.3 Public opinion

Public opinion polls have shown a majority of the public supports various levels of government involvement in health care in the United States,[42] with stated preferences depending on how the question is asked.[43] Polls from Harvard University in 1988,[44] the Los Angeles Times in 1990,[45] and the Wall Street Journal in 1991[46] all showed strong support for a health care system compared to the system in Canada. More recently, however, polling support has declined for that sort of health care system,[42][43] with a 2007 Yahoo/AP poll showing a majority of respondents considered themselves supporters of "single-payer health care,"[47] a majority in favor of a number of reforms according to a joint poll with the *Los Angeles Times* and *Bloomberg*,[48] and a plurality of respondents in a 2009 poll for Time Magazine showed support for "a national single-payer plan similar to Medicare for all."[49] Polls by Rasmussen Reports in 2011[50] and 2012[51] showed pluralities opposed to single-payer health care. Many other polls show support for various levels of government involvement in health care, including polls from *New York Times*/CBS News[52][53] and *Washington Post*/ABC News,[54] showing favorability for a form of national health insurance. The Kaiser Family Foundation[55] showed a majority in favor of a form of national health insurance, often compared to Medicare, and a Quinnipiac poll in three states in 2008 found majority support for the government ensuring "that

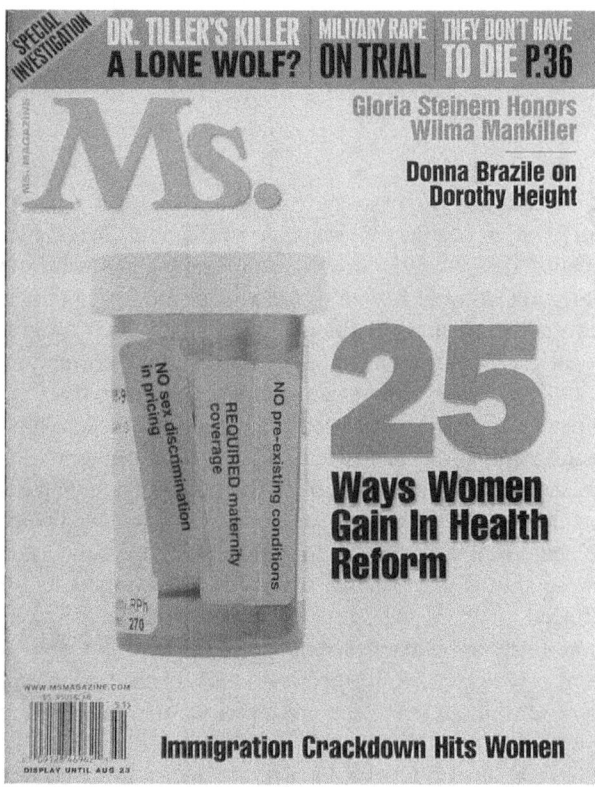

The spring 2010 healthcare reform issue of Ms. *magazine*

everyone in the United States has adequate health-care" among likely Democratic primary voters.[56]

A 2001 article in the public health journal *Health Affairs* studied fifty years of American public opinion of various health care plans and concluded that, while there appears to be general support of a "national health care plan," poll respondents "remain satisfied with their current medical arrangements, do not trust the federal government to do what is right, and do not favor a single-payer type of national health plan."[42] Politifact rated a statement by Michael Moore "false" when he stated that "[t]he majority actually want single-payer health care." According to Politifact, responses on these polls largely depend on the wording. For example, people respond more favorably when they are asked if they want a system "like Medicare".[43]

2.3.4 Patient Protection and Affordable Care Act

Main articles: Patient Protection and Affordable Care Act and Health Care and Education Reconciliation Act of 2010

After campaigning on the promise of health care reform, President Barack Obama gave a speech in March 2010 at a rally in Pennsylvania explaining the necessity of health insurance reform and calling on Congress to hold a final up or down vote on reform.[57] The result of his efforts was the Patient Protection and Affordable Care Act. Because Obama's party did not have a filibuster-proof majority in the Senate, the law was amended by the Health Care and Education Reconciliation Act of 2010 using the reconciliation process in which debate in the Senate is limited and the filibuster is therefore not permitted.

The legislation remains controversial,[58][59][60] with some states challenging it in federal court[61] and opposition from some voters.[62] In June 2012, in a 5–4 decision, the U.S. Supreme Court found major portions of the law to be constitutional.[63] However, the law continues to face legal challenges. The latest attempt at reversing the Affordable Care Act occurred during the Government Shutdown on October 1, 2013. Government officials that oppose the ACA tried to make approval of a bill to reopen the government contingent on the demise of the ACA. This attempt met with failure and the government reopened on November 16, 2013.[64]

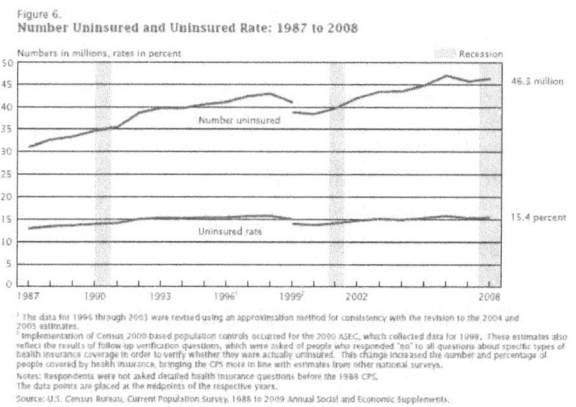

Uninsured Americans, with the numbers shown here from 1987 to 2008, are a major driver for reform efforts

As a result of the law, insurance companies can no longer charge members based on gender, burdening men with the health care costs of women. A study by the National Institutes of Health reported that the lifetime per capita expenditure at birth, using year 2000 dollars, showed a large difference between health care costs of females ($361,192) and males ($268,679). A large portion of this cost difference is in the shorter lifespan of men, but even after adjustment for age (assume men live as long as women), there still is a 20% difference in lifetime health care expenditures.[65]

The act's provisions become effective over time. The most significant changes, particularly affecting the availability and terms of insurance become effective January 1, 2014. These include an expansion of Medicaid (at the option of each state) to those without dependent children and subsidized healthcare exchanges. Changes which occur earlier include allowing dependents to remain on their plan until 26, limitations on rescission (dropping insureds when they get sick), removal of lifetime coverage limits, mandates that insurers fully cover certain preventative services, high-risk pools for uninsureds, tax credits for businesses to provide insurance to employees, an insurance company rate review program, and minimum medical loss ratios.[3]

The law creates the Patient-Centered Outcomes Research Institute to study comparative effectiveness research funded by a fee on insurers per covered life (starting at $1, increasing to $2 and thereafter adjusted according to an index[66]). It also allowed the FDA to approve generic biologic drugs and specifically allows for 12 years of exclusive use for newly developed biologic drugs.

In addition, the law explores some programs intended to increase incentives to provide quality and collaborative care, such as accountable care organizations. The Center for Medicare and Medicaid Innovation was created to fund pilot programs which may reduce costs;[67] the experiments cover nearly every idea healthcare experts advocate, except malpractice/tort reform.[68] The law also requires for reduced Medicare reimbursements for hospitals with excess readmissions and eventually ties physician Medicare reimbursements to quality of care metrics.

The law is also designed to complement the 2009 HITECH Act which encourages the "meaningful use" of electronic health records; for example, the law directs the government to make use of these records for analyzing healthcare provider quality.[69]

The Affordable Care Act also aims to promote access to preventative healthcare. Through providing access to screenings for diseases like breast cancer, promoting health in the workplace, and community preventative health, the Affordable Care Act contains sections that advance and promote preventative health initiatives. [70]

2.3.5 Alternatives and research directions

There are alternatives to the exchange-based market system which was enacted by the Patient Protection and Affordable Care Act which have been proposed in the past and continue to be proposed, such as a single-payer system and allowing health insurance to be regulated at the federal level.

In addition, the Patient Protection and Affordable Health Care Act of 2010 contained provisions which allows the Centers for Medicare and Medicaid Services (CMS) to undertake pilot projects which, if they are successful could be implemented in future.

Single-payer health care

Further information: Single-payer healthcare § United States

A number of proposals have been made for a universal single-payer healthcare system in the United States, most recently the United States National Health Care Act, (popularly known as H.R. 676 or "Medicare for All") but none have achieved more political support than 20% congressional co-sponsorship. Advocates argue that preventative health care expenditures can save several hundreds of billions of dollars per year because publicly funded universal health care would benefit employers and consumers, that employers would benefit from a bigger pool of potential customers and that employers would likely pay less, and would be spared administrative costs of health care benefits. It is also argued that inequities between employers would be reduced.[71][72][73] Also, for example, cancer patients are more likely to be diagnosed at Stage I where curative treatment is typically a few outpatient visits, instead of at Stage III or later in an emergency room where treatment can involve years of hospitalization and is often terminal.[74][75] Others have estimated a long-term savings amounting to 40% of all national health expenditures due to preventative health care,[76] although estimates from the Congressional Budget Office and *The New England Journal of Medicine* have found that preventative care is more expensive.[77]

Any national system would be paid for in part through taxes replacing insurance premiums, but advocates also believe savings would be realized through preventative care and the elimination of insurance company overhead and hospital billing costs.[78] An analysis of a single-payer bill by Physicians for a National Health Program estimated the immediate savings at $350 billion per year.[79] The Commonwealth Fund believes that, if the United States adopted a universal health care system, the mortality rate would improve and the country would save approximately $570 billion a year.[80]

Recent enactments of single-payer systems within individual states, such as in Vermont in 2011, may serve as living models supporting federal single-payer coverage.[81] The plan in Vermont, however, has failed.[82]

Public option

Main article: Public health insurance option

In January 2013, Representative Jan Schakowsky and 44 other U.S. House of Representatives Democrats introduced H.R. 261, the "Public Option Deficit Reduction Act" which would amend the 2010 Affordable Care Act to create a public option. The bill would set up a government-run health insurance plan with premiums 5% to 7% percent lower than private insurance. The Congressional Budget Office estimated it would reduce the United States public debt by $104 billion over 10 years.[83]

Balancing doctor supply and demand

The Medicare Graduate Medical Education program regulates the supply of medical doctors in the U.S.[84] By adjusting the reimbursement rates to establish more income equality among the medical professions, the effective cost of medical care can be lowered.

Bundled payments

A key project is one that could radically change the way the medical profession is paid for services under Medicare and Medicaid. The current system, which is also the prime system used by medical insurers is known as fee-for-service because the medical practitioner is paid only for the performance of medical procedures which, it is argued means that doctors have a financial incentive to do more tests (which generates more income) which may not be in the patients' best long-term interest. The current system encourages medical interventions such as surgeries and prescribed medicines (all of which carry some risk for the patient but increase revenues for the medical care industry) and does not reward other activities such as encouraging behavioral changes such as modifying dietary habits and quitting smoking, or follow-ups regarding prescribed regimes which could have better outcomes for the patient at a lower cost. The current fee-for-service system also rewards bad hospitals for bad service. Some have noted that the best hospitals have fewer re-admission rates than others, which benefits patients, but some of the worst hospitals have high re-admission rates which is bad for patients but is perversely rewarded under the fee-for-service system.

Projects at CMS are examining the possibility of rewarding health care providers through a process known as "bundled payments"[85] by which local doctors and hospitals in an area would be paid not on a fee for service basis but on a capitation system linked to outcomes. The areas with the best outcomes would get more. This system, it is argued, makes medical practitioners much more concerned to focus on activities that deliver real health benefits at a lower cost to the system by removing the perversities inherent in the fee-for-service system.

Though aimed as a model for health care funded by CMS, if the project is successful it is thought that the model could be followed by the commercial health insurance industry also.

2.3.6 See also

- Health care reform

- Health care reforms proposed during the Obama administration

- Health care system § International comparisons

- Health economics

- Health policy

- List of healthcare reform advocacy groups in the United States

- McCarran–Ferguson Act

- Medicare Sustainable Growth Rate

2.3.7 References

[1] Stolberg, Sheryl Gay; Pear, Robert (March 24, 2010). "Obama signs health care overhaul bill, with a flourish". *The New York Times*. p. A19. Retrieved March 23, 2010.

[2] Pear, Robert; Herszenhorn, David M. (March 22, 2010). "Obama hails vote on health care as answering 'the call of history'". *The New York Times*. p. A1. Retrieved March 22, 2010. With the 219-to-212 vote, the House gave final approval to legislation passed by the Senate on Christmas Eve.

[3] Smith, Donna; Alexander, David; Beech, Eric (March 19, 2010). "Factbox-U.S. healthcare bill would provide immediate benefits". Reuters. Retrieved March 24, 2010.

[4] "Timeline: when healthcare reform will affect you". CNN. March 26, 2010. Retrieved March 24, 2010.

[5] Rosenthal, Elisabeth (December 21, 2013). "News Analysis – Health Care's Road to Ruin". *The New York Times*. Retrieved December 22, 2013.

[6] "Brief history of the Medicare program". San Antonio, Tex.: New Tech Media. 2010. Retrieved August 31, 2010.

[7] Ball, Robert M. (October 24, 1961). "The role of social insurance in preventing economic dependency (address at the Second National Conference on the Churches and Social Welfare, Cleveland, Ohio)". Washington, D.C.: U.S. Social Security Administration. Retrieved August 31, 2010.

  - Robert M. Ball, the then Deputy Director of the Bureau of Old-Age and Survivors Insurance in the Social Security Administration, had defined the major obstacle to financing health insurance for the elderly several years earlier: the high cost of care for the aged and the generally low incomes of retired people. Because retired older people use much more medical care than younger, employed people, an insurance premium related to the risk for older people needed to be high, but if the high premium had to be paid after retirement, when incomes are low, it was an almost impossible burden for the average person. The only feasible approach, he said, was to finance health insurance in the same way as cash benefits for retirement, by contributions paid while at work, when the payments are least burdensome, with the protection furnished in retirement without further payment.

[8] "An employee's guide to health benefits under COBRA – The Consolidated Omnibus Budget Reconciliation Act of 1986" (PDF). Washington, D.C.: Employee Benefits Security Administration, U.S. Department of Labor. 2010. Retrieved November 8, 2009.

[9] http://www.gpo.gov/fdsys/pkg/PLAW-104publ191/html/PLAW-104publ191.htm

[10] "What is SCHIP?". Washington, D.C.: National Center for Public Policy Research. 2007. Retrieved September 1, 2010.

[11] WHO (May 2009). "World Health Statistics 2009". World Health Organization. Retrieved August 2, 2009.

[12] Funk, Josh (March 1, 2010). "Buffett says economy recovering but at slow rate". *San Francisco Chronicle*. SFGate.com. Retrieved April 3, 2010.

[13] Kenworthy, Lane (July 10, 2011). "America's inefficient health-care system: another look". *Consider the Evidence* (blog). Retrieved September 11, 2012.

[14] "coming_gen_storm_e.indd" (PDF). *The Economist*. Retrieved January 12, 2012.

[15] "Charlie Rose-Peter Orszag Interview Transcript". November 3, 2009. Retrieved January 12, 2012.

[16] "Health Insurance Premiums Rise 6.1% In 2007, Less Rapidly Than In Recent Years But Still Faster Than Wages And Inflation" (Press release). Kaiser Family Foundation. September 11, 2007. Retrieved September 13, 2007.

[17] Cathy Schoen; Michelle M. Doty; Sara R. Collins; Alyssa L. Holmgren (June 14, 2005). "Insured But Not Protected: How Many Adults Are Underinsured?". *Health Affairs Web Exclusive*. Suppl Web Exclusives: W5–289–W5–302. doi:10.1377/hlthaff.w5.289. PMID 15956055.

[18] Dale Yamamoto, Tricia Neuman and Michelle Kitchman Strollo, *How Does the Benefit Value of Medicare Compare to the Benefit Value of Typical Large Employer Plans?*, Kaiser Family Foundation, September 2008

[19] Himmelstein DU, Warren E, Thorne D, Woolhandler S (2005). "Illness and injury as contributors to bankruptcy". *Health Aff (Millwood)*. Suppl Web Exclusives: W5–63–W5–73. doi:10.1377/hlthaff.w5.63. PMID 15689369.

[20] Todd Zywicki, "An Economic Analysis of the Consumer Bankruptcy Crisis", 99 NWU L. Rev. 1463 (2005)

[21] "American Journal of Public Health | December 2009, Vol 99, No.12" (PDF).

[22] "State-by-state breakout of excess deaths from lack of insurance" (PDF).

[23] A 1997 study carried out by Professors David Himmelstein and Steffie Woolhandler (*New England Journal of Medicine* 336, no. 11 1997) "concluded that almost 100,000 people died in the United States each year because of lack of needed care—three times the number of people who died of AIDs." The Inhuman State of U.S. Health Care, *Monthly Review*, Vicente Navarro, September 2003. Retrieved September 10, 2009

[24] "Study calls wide Mass. coverage a lifesaver". Boston Globe. May 5, 2014.

[25] CRAIG, DAVID M., ed. (2014-01-01). *Health Care as a Social Good*. Religious Values and American Democracy. Georgetown University Press. pp. 85–120. ISBN 9781626160774.

[26] Chernomas, Robert; Hudson, Ian (2013-01-01). *To Live and Die in America: Class, Power, Health and Healthcare*. Pluto Books. ISBN 9780745332123.

[27] Ehrenreich, John, ed. (2016-01-01). *Third Wave Capitalism*. How Money, Power, and the Pursuit of Self-Interest Have Imperiled the American Dream. Cornell University Press. pp. 39–77. doi:10.7591/j.ctt1h4mjdm.6#page_scan_tab_contents. ISBN 9781501702310.

[28] ALONSO-ZALDIVAR, RICARDO (March 10, 2014). "SURVEY: UNINSURED RATE DROPS; HEALTH LAW CITED". *The Associated Press*. Retrieved March 10, 2014.

[29] Easley, Jason (March 10, 2014). "Republicans Darkest Fears Realized: ACA Causes Number of Uninsured to Drop Across All Ages". *Politicus USA*. Retrieved March 10, 2014.

[30] Howell, Tom (March 10, 2014). "Rate of uninsured Americans is dropping: Gallup". *Washington Times*. Retrieved March 10, 2014.

[31] Pear, Robert (December 3, 2011). "Health Official Takes Parting Shot at 'Waste'". *New York Times*. Retrieved December 20, 2011.

[32] Phipps, Jennie L. (February 21, 2013). "How big is Medicare fraud?". *Retirement Blog*. Bankrate. Retrieved November 28, 2013.

[33] "Medicare Fraud Strike Force Charges 89 Individuals for Approximately $223 Million in False Billing". U.S. Department of Justice. May 14, 2013. Retrieved November 28, 2013.

[34] For-Profit Hospitals Cost More and Have Higher Death Rates, *Physicians for a National Health Program*

[35] For-Profit HMOs Provide Worse Quality Care, *Physicians for a National Health Program*

[36] "Prelims i-ixx/E" (PDF). Retrieved January 12, 2012.

[37] David Gratzer, Why Is not Government Health Care The Answer?, *Free Market Cure*, July 16, 2007

[38] Glen Whitman, "WHO's Fooling Who? The World Health Organization's Problematic Ranking of Health Care Systems", Cato Institute, February 28, 2008

[39] Capital: In health care, consumer theory falls flat David Wessel, Wall Street Journal, September 7, 2006.

[40] "Rand study finds patients' ratings of their medical care do not reflect the technical quality of their care" (Press release). RAND Corporation. May 1, 2006. Retrieved August 27, 2007.

[41] Chang JT, Hays RD, Shekelle PG, et al. (May 2006). "Patients' global ratings of their health care are not associated with the technical quality of their care". *Ann. Intern. Med.* **144** (9): 665–72. doi:10.7326/0003-4819-144-9-200605020-00010. PMID 16670136.

[42] *Health Affairs*, Volume 20, No. 2. "Americans' Views on Health Policy: A Fifty-Year Historical Perspective." March/April 2001. http://content.healthaffairs.org/content/20/2/33.full.pdf+html

[43] "Michael Moore claims a majority favor a single-payer health care system". PolitiFact. Retrieved November 20, 2011.

[44] Blendon Robert J.; et al. (1989). "Views on health care: Public opinion in three nations". *Health Affairs*. **8** (1): 149–57. doi:10.1377/hlthaff.8.1.149.

[45] *Los Angeles Times* poll: "Health Care in the United States," Poll no. 212, Storrs, Conn.: Administered by the Roper Center for Public Opinion Research, March 1990

[46] Wall Street Journal-NBC poll: Michael McQueen, "Voters, sick of the current health –care systems, want federal government to prescribe remedy," Wall Street Journal, June 28, 1991

[47] AP/Yahoo poll: Administered by Knowledge Networks, December 2007: http://surveys.ap.org/data/KnowledgeNetworks/AP-Yahoo_2007-08_panel02.pdf

[48] *Los Angeles Times/Bloomberg*: President Bush, Health Care, The Economy. October 25, 2007.

[49] TIME MAGAZINE/ABT SRBI – July 27–28, 2009 Survey: http://www.srbi.com/TimePoll4794_Final_%20Report.pdf

[50] Rasmussen Reports: Rasmussen Reports. January 1, 2010. Retrieved November 20, 2011.

[51] Rasmussen Reports: Rasmussen Reports. Retrieved December 30, 2012.

[52] Sack, Kevin (June 20, 2009). "In Poll, Wide Support for Government-Run Health". *The New York Times*. Retrieved January 12, 2012.

[53] "CBS News/New York Times Poll, For Release: Sunday, February 1, 2009, 9:00 AM, American Public Opinion: Today Vs. 30 Years Ago, January 11–15, 2009" (PDF). *CBS News*. Retrieved February 19, 2015.

[54] "Here's an initial summary of headlines from our health care poll, followed by the full trended results" (PDF). Retrieved January 12, 2012.

[55] "Kaiser Health Tracking Poll: July 2009 – Topline" (PDF). Retrieved January 12, 2012.

[56] Quinnipiac University – Office of Public Affairs (April 2, 2008). "Question 9: "Do you think it's the government's responsibility to make sure that everyone in the United States has adequate health-care, or don't you think so?"". Quinnipiac.edu. Retrieved January 12, 2012.

[57] President's speech prior to passage of the legislation

[58] NewsHour Extra: Democrats Push Through Historic, Controversial Health Care Legislation | March 23, 2010 | PBS

[59] One Year Later, Health-Care Reform Still Controversial | Some lawmakers still pushing to nullify federal policy | Unda' the Rotunda | Boise Weekly

[60] http://www.npr.org/blogs/thetwo-way/2013/05/16/184611542/house-republicans-vote-again-to-defund-obamacare

[61] Florida's lawsuit over health care law swells to 26 states – Tampa Bay Times

[62] RealClearPolitics – Election Other – Obama and Democrats' Health Care Plan

[63] Liptak, Adam (June 28, 2012). "Supreme Court Lets Health Law Largely Stand, in Victory for Obama". *The New York Times*. Retrieved June 29, 2012.

[64] "Obama signs bill to end partial shutdown, avert debt default - CNN.com". *CNN*. October 17, 2013.

[65] Alemayehu B, Warner KE (2004). "The lifetime distribution of health care costs". *Health Serv Res.* **39**: 627–42. doi:10.1111/j.1475-6773.2004.00248.x. PMC 1361028. PMID 15149482.

[66] Primer on PPACA's New Fees and Taxes. Cigna.

[67] Kuraitis V. (2010). Pilots, Demonstrations & Innovation in the PPACA Healthcare Reform Legislation. e-CareManagement.com.

[68] Gawande A (December 2009). "Testing, Testing". *The New Yorker*. Retrieved March 22, 2010.

[69] PPACA Emphasizes Use of Health Information Technology. Foley & Lardner LLP.

[70] Koh, Howard K.; Sebelius, Kathleen G. (2010-09-30). "Promoting Prevention through the Affordable Care Act". *New England Journal of Medicine*. **363** (14): 1296–1299. doi:10.1056/NEJMp1008560. ISSN 0028-4793. PMID 20879876.

[71] Institute of Medicine, Committee on the Consequences of Uninsurance; Board on Health Care Services (2003). *Hidden Costs, Value Lost: Uninsurance in America*. Washington, DC: The National Academies Press.

[72] Lincoln, Taylor (April 8, 2014). "Severing the Tie That Binds: Why a Publicly Funded, Universal Health Care System Would Be a Boon to U.S. Businesses" (PDF). Public Citizen. Retrieved May 20, 2014.

[73] Ungar, Rick (April 6, 2012). "A Dose Of Socialism Could Save Our States – State Sponsored, Single Payer Healthcare Would Bring In Business & Jobs". *Forbes*. Retrieved May 20, 2014.

[74] Hogg, W.; Baskerville, N.; Lemelin, J. (2005). "Cost savings associated with improving appropriate and reducing inappropriate preventive care: Cost-consequences analysis" (PDF). *BMC Health Services Research*. **5**: 20. doi:10.1186/1472-6963-5-20. PMC 1079830. PMID 15755330.

[75] Kao-Ping Chua; Flávio Casoy (June 16, 2007). "Single Payer 101". American Medical Student Association. Retrieved May 20, 2014.

[76] Hogg, W.; Baskerville, N; Lemelin, J (2005). "Cost savings associated with improving appropriate and reducing inappropriate preventive care: cost-consequences analysis". *BMC Health Services Research*. **5** (1): 20. doi:10.1186/1472-6963-5-20. PMC 1079830. PMID 15755330.

[77] PolitiFact: Barack Obama says preventive care 'saves money'. February 10, 2012.

[78] Krugman, Paul (June 13, 2005). "One Nation, Uninsured". *The New York Times*. Retrieved December 4, 2011.

[79] Physicians for a National Health Program (2008) "Single Payer System Cost?" *PNHP.org*

[80] Friedman, Gerald. "Funding a National Single-Payer System "Medicare for All" Would save Billions, and Could Be Redistributive.". Dollars & Sense.

[81] "State-Based Single-Payer Health Care — A Solution for the United States?" *New England Journal of Medicine* 364;13:1188–90, March 31, 2011

[82] Politico (20 Dec 2014). Accessed 20 May 2015.

[83] "House Dems push again for creation of government-run health insurance option" *The Hill*, January 16, 2013

[84] "Graduate Medical Education Funding Is Not Helping Solve Primary Care, Rural Provider Shortages, Study Finds". Robert Wood Johnson Foundation. June 19, 2013.

[85] The Medicare Bundled Payment Pilot Program: Participation Considerations

2.3.8 Further reading

- Christensen, Clayton Hwang, Jason, Grossman, Jerome, *The Innovator's Prescription*, McGraw Hill, 2009. ISBN 978-0-07-159208-6

- Terry L. Leap, *Phantom Billing, Fake Prescriptions, and the High Cost of Medicine: Health Care Fraud and What to do about It* (Cornell University Press, 2011).

- Mahar, Maggie, *Money-Driven Medicine: The Real Reason Health Care Costs So Much*, HarperCollins, 2006. ISBN 978-0-06-076533-0

- Morrisey, Michael A. (2008). "Health Care". In David R. Henderson (ed.). *Concise Encyclopedia of Economics* (2nd ed.). Indianapolis: Library of Economics and Liberty. ISBN 978-0865976658. OCLC 237794267.

- Starr, Paul, *The Social Transformation of American Medicine*, Basic Books, 1982. ISBN 0-465-07934-2

- Reid, T.R. (2009). *The Healing of America: A Global Quest for Better, Cheaper and Fairer Health Care*. Penguin Books. ISBN 978-1-59420-234-6.

2.3.9 External links

- Healthcare reform in the United States at DMOZ

2.4 Medicare (Canada)

Medicare is an U.S. term which could be used to describe the Canadian Health Care system (French: *assurance-maladie*). Canada's publicly funded single-payer system consists of 13 provincial and territorial socialized health insurance plans that provides universal health care coverage to all Canadian citizens. It is administered on a provincial or territorial basis, within the guidelines set by the federal government. [1] The formal terminology for the insurance system is provided by the *Canada Health Act* and the health insurance legislation of the individual provinces and territories.

Under the terms of the Canada Health Act, all "insured persons" (basically, legal residents of Canada, including permanent residents) are entitled to receive "insured services" without copayment. Such services are defined as medically necessary services if provided in hospital, or by 'practitioners' (usually physicians).[2] Approximately 70% of expenditures for health care in Canada come from public sources, with the rest paid privately (both through private insurance, and through out-of-pocket payments). The extent of public financing varies considerably across services. For example, approximately 99% of physician services, and 90% of hospital care, are paid by publicly funded sources, whereas almost all dental care is paid for privately.[3] Most physicians are self-employed private entities which enjoy coverage under each province's respective healthcare plans.

Services of non-physicians working within hospitals are covered; but provinces can, but are not forced to, cover services by non-physicians if provided outside hospitals. Changing the site of treatment may thus change coverage. For example, pharmaceuticals, nursing care, and physical therapy must be covered for inpatients, but there is considerable variation from province to province in the extent to which they are covered for patients discharged to the community (e.g., after day surgery). The need to modernize coverage was pointed out in 2002 by both the Romanow Commission and by the Kirby committee of the Canadian Senate (see External links below). Similarly, the extent to which non-physician providers of primary care are funded varies; Quebec offers primary health care teams through its CLSC system.

2.4.1 History

Main article: Health Care in Canada – the beginning of coverage

The first implementation of public hospital care in Canada came at the provincial level in Saskatchewan in 1947 and in Alberta in 1950, under provincial governments led by the Co-operative Commonwealth Federation and the Social Credit party respectively.[4] The first implementation of nationalized public health care -at the federal level- came about with the Hospital Insurance and Diagnostic Services Act (HIDS), which was passed by the Liberal majority government of Louis St. Laurent in 1957,[5] and was adopted by all provinces by 1961. Lester B. Pearson's government subsequently expanded this policy to universal health care with the Medical Care Act in 1966.[6]

Some have argued that these developments towards public national health care came as a result of the adoption of a publicly funded health plan in 1961-1962 in Saskatchewan government. The fight for a publicly funded system was originally led by Premier Tommy Douglas and implemented by Woodrow Stanley Lloyd, who became pre-

mier of the province when Douglas resigned to become the leader of the new federal New Democratic Party. Although Saskatchewan is often credited with the birth of public health care funding in Canada, the federal legislation itself was actually drafted (and first proposed to parliament) by Allan MacEachen, a Liberal MP from Cape Breton.[7]

In 1984, the Canada Health Act was passed, amalgamating the 1966 Medical Care Act and the 1957 Hospital Insurance and Diagnostic Services Act. The Canada Health Act affirmed and clarified five founding principles: (a) *public administration* on a non-profit basis by a public authority; (b) *comprehensiveness* – provincial health plans must insure all services that are medically necessary; (c) *universality* – a guarantee that all residents in Canada must have access to public healthcare and insured services on uniform terms and conditions; (d) *portability* – residents must be covered while temporarily absent from their province of residence or from Canada; and (e) *accessibility* – insured persons must have reasonable and uniform access to insured health services, free of financial or other barriers. These five conditions prevent provinces from radical innovation, but many small differences do exist between the provinces.[8]

2.4.2 Eligibility

Although in theory all Canadians should qualify for coverage, each province or territory operates its own health insurance program, and provinces and territories have enacted qualification rules which effectively exclude many Canadians from coverage. For example, to qualify for enrollment in Ontario, one must, among other requirements, "be physically present in Ontario for 153 days in any 12-month period; and be physically present in Ontario for at least 153 days of the first 183 days immediately after establishing residency in the province."[9] While there are exceptions for students studying out of province, and for mobile workers, many Canadians who regularly travel from one province to another for other reasons, as well as those who often travel outside Canada, cannot qualify for enrollment in any province. Proof-of-residency provisions requiring presentation of documents such as utility bills and bank statements also operate to exclude migrants.

2.4.3 Funding

According to Canada's constitution, the provinces have responsibility for health care, education and welfare. However, the federal Canada Health Act sets standards for all the provinces. The Canada Health Act requires coverage for all medically necessary care provided in hospitals or by physicians; this explicitly includes diagnostic, treatment and preventive services. Coverage is universal for qualifying

Canadian residents, regardless of income level.

Funding for the health care is transferred from the general revenues of the Canadian federal government to the 10 provinces and 3 territories through the Canada Health Transfer. Some provinces also charge annual health care premiums. These are, in effect, taxes (since they are not tied to service use, nor to provincial health expenditures). The system is accordingly classified by the OECD as a tax-supported system, as opposed to the social insurance approaches used in many European countries. Boards in each province regulate the cost, which is then reimbursed by the federal government. Currently, patients do not pay out of pocket costs to visit their doctor.

2.4.4 Delivery

Canada uses a mix of public and private organizations to deliver health care in what is termed a publicly funded, privately delivered system. Hospitals and acute care facilities, including long term complex care, is typically directly funded. Health care organizations bill the provincial health authorities, with few exceptions.[10] Hospitals are largely non-profit organizations, historically often linked to religious or charitable organizations. In some provinces, individual hospital boards have been eliminated and combined into quasi-private regional health authorities, subject to varying degrees of provincial control.

Private services are provided by diagnostic laboratories, occupational and physical therapy centres, and other allied professionals. Non-medically necessary services, such as optional plastic surgery, are also often delivered by for-profit investor-owned corporations. In some cases patients pay directly and are reimbursed by the health care system, and in other cases a hospital or physician may order services and seek reimbursement from the provincial government.

With rare exceptions, medical doctors are small for-profit independent businesses. Historically, they have practiced in small solo or group practices and billed the government Canadian Health Care system on a fee for service basis. Unlike the practice in fully socialized countries, hospital-based physicians are not all hospital employees, and some directly bill the provincial insurance plans on a fee-for-service basis. Since 2000, physicians have been allowed to incorporate for tax reasons (dates of authorization vary province to province).

Efforts to achieve *primary health care reform* have increasingly encouraged physicians to work in multidisciplinary teams, and be paid through blended funding models, including elements of capitation and other 'alternative funding formulas'. Similarly, some hospitals (particularly teaching hospitals and rural/remote hospitals) have also experimented with alternatives to fee-for-service.

In summary, the system is known as a "public system" due to its public financing, but is not a nationalized system such as the UK's NHS: most health care services are provided privately.[11]

An additional complexity is that, because health care is deemed to be under provincial jurisdiction, there is not a "Canadian health care system". Most providers are private, and may or may not coordinate their care. Publicly funded insurance is organized at the level of the province/territory; each manages its own insurance system, including issuing its own healthcare identification cards (a list of the provincial medical care insurance programs is given at the end of this entry). Once care moves beyond the services required by the Canada Health Act—for which universal comprehensive coverage applies—there is inconsistency from province to province in the extent of publicly funded coverage, particularly for such items as outpatient drug coverage and rehabilitation, as well as vision care, mental health, and long-term care, with a substantial portion of such services being paid for privately, either through private insurance, or out-of-pocket.[12][13] Eligibility for these additional programs may be based on various combinations of such factors as age (e.g., children, seniors), income, enrollment in a home care program, or diagnosis (e.g., HIV/AIDS, cancer, cystic fibrosis).

Drug coverage

Unlike a number of other countries with universal health insurance systems, Canada lacks a universal pharmaceutical subsidy scheme, with co-payment, cost ceilings, and special subsidy groups varying by private insurer and by province.[14][15] Each province may provide its own prescription drug benefit plan, although the Canada Health Act requires only coverage for pharmaceuticals delivered to hospital inpatients.[16] Provincial prescription drug benefit plans differ across provinces. Some provinces cover only those in particular age groups (usually, seniors) and/or those on social assistance. Others are more universal. Quebec achieves universal coverage through a combination of private and public plans. Co-payments also vary.[17] Provinces maintain their own provincial formularies, although the Common Drug Review provides evidence-based formulary listing recommendations to the provincial ministries. Note that there is ongoing controversy in Canada, as in other countries, about inclusion of expensive drugs and discrepancies in their availability, as well as in what if any provisions are made for allowing medications not yet approved to be administered under "exceptional drug" provisions.[18] Drug costs are contentious. Their prices are controlled by the Patented Medicine Prices Review Board (PMPRB).[19]

The PMPRB's pricing formula ensures that Canada pays prices based on the average of those charged to selected countries; they are neither the highest, nor the lowest.

Dental care, eye care, and other services

Dental care is not required to be covered by the government insurance plans. In Quebec, children under the age of 10 receive almost full coverage, and many oral surgeries are covered for everyone.[20] Canadians rely on their employers or individual private insurance, pay cash themselves for dental treatments, or receive no care. In some jurisdictions, public health units have been involved in providing targeted programs to address the need of the young, the elderly or those who are on welfare. The Canadian Association of Public Health Dentistry tracks programs, and has been advocating for extending coverage to those currently unable to receive dental care.[21]

The range of services for vision care coverage also varies widely among the provinces. Generally, "medically required" vision care is covered if provided by physicians (cataract surgery, diabetic vision care, some laser eye surgeries required as a result of disease, but not if the purpose is to replace the need for eyeglasses). Similarly, the standard vision test may or may not be covered. Some provinces allow a limited number of tests (e.g., no more than once within a two-year period). Others, including Ontario, Alberta, Saskatchewan, and British Columbia, do not, although different provisions may apply to particular subgroups (e.g., diabetics, children).

Naturopathic services are covered in some cases, but homeopathic services are generally not covered. Chiropractic is partially covered in some provinces. Cosmetic procedures are not typically covered. Psychiatric services (provided by physicians) are covered, fee-for-service psychology services outside of hospitals or community based mental health clinics are usually not. Physical therapy, occupational therapy, speech therapy, nursing, and chiropractic services are often not covered unless within hospitals. Some provinces, including Ontario include some rehabilitation services for those in the home care program, those recently discharged from hospitals (e.g., after a hip replacement), or those in particular age categories. Again, considerable variation exists, and provinces can (and do) alter their coverage decisions.

2.4.5   Inter-provincial Imbalances

The fact that health insurance plans are administered by the provinces and territories in a country where large numbers of residents of certain provinces work in other provinces may lead to inequitable inter-provincial outcomes with respect to revenues and expenditures. For example, many residents of the Atlantic provinces work in the oil and gas industry in the western province of Alberta. For most of the year these workers may be contributing significant tax revenue to Alberta (e.g. through fuel, tobacco and alcohol taxes) while their health insurance costs are borne by their home province in Atlantic Canada.

Another considerable inter-provincial imbalance is a person who is insured by Quebec and obtains healthcare in another province or territory. Quebec does not have any physician payment agreements with any other provinces or territories of Canada. As a result, someone that sees a physician outside Quebec, even in another part of Canada, must either pay the cost themselves and submit a request to the Régie de l'Assurance Maladie du Québec (RAMQ Medicare) for reimbursement (even then, expenses are often denied), or take out a third party insurance plan. The same situation also applies to a resident of any other part of Canada visiting Quebec, only they submit any claims to their respective provincial healthplan. All provinces and territories of Canada, however, do have reciprocal hospital agreements, so hospital admissions, for example, are covered throughout Canada.[22]

2.4.6   Opinions on Canadian Health Care

Polling data in the last few years have consistently cited Canadian Health Care as among the most important political issues in the minds of Canadian voters. Along with peacekeeping, Canadian Health Care was found, based on a CBC poll, to be among the foremost defining characteristics of Canada. [23]

It has increasingly become a source of controversy in Canadian politics. As a recent report from the Health Council of Canada has noted "Herein lies one of the puzzles of Canadian health care: Canadians increasingly view the health care system as unsustainable and under threat, even as their own experiences with the system are mostly positive."[24]

As analysts have noted, the root of the concern may be traced to successful cost control efforts in the mid 1990s, where public health expenditure per capita, in inflation-adjusted dollars, actually fell.[25] These efforts arose from efforts by the federal government to deal with its deficit through various austerity measures, which led to cuts in their transfers to the provinces, and in turn to squeezing hospital budgets and physician reimbursements. The number of physicians being trained was reduced. The result was seen in increased wait times, particularly for elective procedures. More recently, government has been reinvesting in health care, but public confidence has been slow to recover.

A number of studies have compared Canada with other

countries, and concluded that each system has its own strengths and weaknesses.[26][27] The World Health Organization, ranked Canada in 2000 as 30th worldwide in performance. However, the basis for these rankings has been highly contentious. As Deber noted, "The measure of "overall healthsystem performance" derives from adjusting "goal attainment" for educational attainment. Although goal attainment is in theory based on five measures (level and distribution of health, level and distribution of "responsiveness" and "fairness of financial contribution"), the actual values assigned to most countries, including Canada, were never directly measured. The scores do not incorporate any information about the actual workings of the system, other than as reflected in life expectancy. The primary reason for Canada's relatively low standing rests on the relatively high educational level of its population, particularly as compared to France, rather than on any features of its health system."[28] Other countries had similar complaints, and the WHO has not repeated this ranking.

2.4.7 2003 Accord

In 2003, the prime minister and the provincial premiers agreed upon priority areas for reinvestment. The 2003 First Ministers' Accord on Health Care Renewal[29] reaffirmed their commitment to the principles of the Canada Health Act. They indicated the following principles:

"Drawing from this foundation, First Ministers view this Accord as a covenant which will help to ensure that:

- all Canadians have timely access to health services on the basis of need, not ability to pay, regardless of where they live or move in Canada;

- the health care services available to Canadians are of high quality, effective, patient-centred and safe; and

- our health care system is sustainable and affordable and will be here for Canadians and their children in the future."

The accord set the following priority areas: primary health care, home care, catastrophic drug coverage, access to diagnostic/medical equipment and information technology and an electronic health record. The extent of progress in meeting reform goals has varied across these areas.

2.4.8 Evaluating claims about the system

Evaluating the accuracy of claims about the system is hampered by several factors. The highly decentralized nature of health care delivery means that good data is not always available. It is often difficult to distinguish compelling but atypical anecdotes from systemic problems. Considerable effort is being made to develop and implement comparable indicators to allow better assessment of progress. However, the Health Council of Canada—with a mandate to monitor and report on health reform—complained in 2007 that progress has stalled.[30]

The debate about health care has also become heavily ideological. The Fraser Institute, a right leaning think tank supporting "competitive market solutions for public policy problems" is a frequent critic of publicaly funded Canadian Health Care. It publishes yearly reports about wait times which are then used to argue that the system is both failing and unsustainable.[31] Others criticize their methodology, which is based on physician perceptions rather than actual waits.[32] Other complaints come from the political left, who object to 'privatization' (by which they usually mean a heavier involvement of for-profit providers). (See, for example, the Canadian Health Coalition web page.)[33] There are frequent debates in the media and on line between advocates and opponents of Canadian healthcare.

Wait times and access

Common complaints relate to access, usually to elective surgery (especially hip and knee replacement and cataract surgery) and diagnostic imaging. These have been the primary targets of health care reinvestment, and it appears that considerable progress has been made for certain services, although the implications for procedures not on the target list are unclear.[34][35][36] Canadian physicians have been heavily involved, particularly in developing appropriateness criteria to ensure timely access for necessary care.[37] It is estimated to have cost Canada's economy $14.8 billion in 2007 to have patients waiting longer than needed for medical procedures.[38] Barua and Esmail completed a study in October 2013, Waiting Your Turn, Wait Times for Health Care in Canada. The authors surveyed both private and publicly funded outpatient health care offices and found the amount of wait time between general practitioner and specialists. The second segment was determining wait times between consultation and time of procedure. They studied each province and found where the longest and shortest wait times were. Barua and Esmail found that the wait times for health services have increased 95% from 1993-2013. Esmail and Barua also compared the wait times in 2012 to the wait times in 2013. A few provinces wait times decreased but mostly provinces wait times increased slightly. The number of procedures overall that people in 2013 waited for was 928,120. This is a 6.6% increase from 2012.[39]

Health human resources

A related issue is the volume, and distribution, of health human resources.[40] There are ongoing issues about the distribution of physicians, with the pendulum swinging from arguing that there were too many, to arguing that there were too few. As Ben Chan found, the major factor driving the drop in physician numbers was changes in training programs.[41] Combined with such factors as changes in the hours worked by each physician, and a decrease in the proportion of doctors choosing to go into family practice, there were shortages in some areas, particularly for general practitioners (GP) / family doctors. One response has been to encourage 'primary care reform', including greater use of multidisciplinary health care teams.[42] There are also ongoing issues regarding nurses. (See Nursing Health Services Research Unit, which links to some reports.[43] CIHI also gives data about nursing.)

Delisting

Delisting is the term used in Canada when a province decides that a medical procedure will no longer be covered by the health care system in that province.

While health care coverage is country wide, and is required to be portable and to have equal access, there are a few differences between what provinces will cover. In some cases, this has resulted in lost grants to the provinces; in other cases it has not.

An example of a delisted service is circumcision in Ontario. It is still possible to have a boy circumcised in Ontario by a doctor but the parents must pay the cost.

The issue of delisting services is becoming increasingly a political battleground in Canadian health care. In an effort to save health care money some provinces are delisting some services; however, some delisted services are ones that could be considered "medically necessary". For example, except for seniors, children, and diabetics eye exams to check vision are no longer covered in Ontario.[44]

2.4.9 Parallel private debate

Some politicians and think tanks have proposed removing barriers to the existence of a parallel private healthcare system. Others note that such systems act to erode cost control and impede equity.[45] Though polling suggests support for such reforms has been increasing, it has yet to be adopted as official policy by any of the main federal political parties.

Under federal law, private clinics are not legally allowed to charge patients directly for services covered by the Canada Health Act, if they qualify for the public insurance. Regardless of this legal issue, many do offer such services. There are disputes as to whether surgical procedures can be performed. Two related issues have obstructed the growth of such clinics. One is regulatory — hospital-based quality assurance often failed to encompass them. This gap has been filled in most provinces, but sometimes only after celebrated incidents in which patients died in unregulated clinics, including one physician who performed cosmetic surgery in an Ontario hotel room. The second is economic — there may be no way for physicians to recoup the additional costs of running a surgical facility from their fees. Here, provinces can choose to offer 'facility fees' to these clinics, but doing so has often been contentious, particularly if hospitals felt that these costs would be better devoted to allowing them to increase their operating room time.

Note that uninsured persons can pay for care (including medical tourism), and that insured persons can still pay for uninsured services. These are both niche markets.

Opponents of Canadian health care often raise issues such as long wait times, a 'brain-drain' drawing qualified professionals away from Canada to other jurisdictions where working in the health care field is more profitable, and impairment of the Canadian health care system due to budget cuts. Fox News ran a story in 2007 reporting that during a period of above average numbers of births, at least 40 Canadian mothers of premature babies had to travel to the U.S. for treatment due to insufficient capacity for premature babies in British Columbia neonatal units. Nonetheless, Canada's health care system covered the health care costs of those mothers affected.[46]

In 2003, the Government in Canada spent $2,998 USD per capita on healthcare as compared to $5,711 USD per capita in the United States, while almost every Canadian citizen is fully covered.[47] In the United States, 11.9% of adults lack public or private health coverage,[48] despite higher proportional spending along with large private investment.

The lack of competition has given healthcare unions a monopoly on essential services, thus ensuring a very strong bargaining position. Nova Scotia is currently debating healthcare legislation aimed at removing the threat of striking healthcare workers and replacing it with binding arbitration.[49]

2.4.10 Proposed reforms

One proposed solution for improving the Canadian healthcare system is to increase funding. Proponents of this approach point to the rise of neo-conservative economic policies in Canada and the associated reduction in welfare state expenditure (particularly in the provinces) from the 1980s onwards as the cause of degradation in the system. While some say evidence clearly indicate an overall percentage increase on healthcare spending, the net spending has been drastically decreasing on top of inflation.

Other critics of healthcare state that increased funding will not solve systemic problems in the healthcare system including a rising cost of medical technology, infrastructure, and wages. These critics say that Canada's proximity to the United States causes a "brain drain" or migration of Canadian-trained doctors and nurses (as well as other professionals) to the United States, where private hospitals can pay much higher wages and income tax rates are lower (partially because health care is not covered through taxation). Some of these critics argue that increased privatization of healthcare would improve Canada's health infrastructure. Others[50] argue vehemently against it. For example, large resources are required to train and educate doctors. Since the number of available doctors is therefore limited, doctors working for a private system would not be working under the public system creating little to no net increase in available services.

Critics of greater privatization state that healthcare should be kept public, (public in funding only, as most services are provided by the private sector including doctors who in most cases are private corporations) in part because it separates Canadians from Americans by mandating equality and fairness in health care. This is in contrast to other states where doctors are on a per capita based salary. In this sense the Canadian Healthcare system is merely a publicly funded one where services are provided by a mixture of public and private entities, which most Canadians appreciate and desire. Changing the system to eliminate the balance between public and private service providers to a completely public system is one such alternative.

2.4.11 Ontario's reform experiments

Since the early 1990s, Ontario has implemented several systematic reforms to reduce health care costs. Similar reforms have been implemented in other provinces.

User premiums

Currently in Ontario, people with an annual taxable income above $20,000 must pay an annual health care premium ranging from $60–$900.[51] Funding for health care in Ontario also comes in part from a dedicated Employer Health Tax (EHT) that ranges from 0.98%−1.95% of employer payroll.[52] Eligible employers are exempted from EHT on the first $400,000 of payroll. British Columbia and Quebec charge similar premiums.

Medical clinics

Ontario has increased the number of 24-hour drop-in medical clinic networks to reduce costs associated with treating off-hours emergencies in hospital emergency rooms.

Many family doctor practices have created their own clinics, offering 24-hour service for their patients if needed. Each doctor in the practice takes a turn at being "on call" on a rotating basis. Patients who have family doctors belonging to these practices are able to have a doctor come to their home in extreme situations. There is no additional charge for these services as they are billed to the Province, the same as an office visit.

Hospitals in some major Canadian cities, such as London, Ontario, have restructured their emergency services to share emergency treatment among several hospitals. One hospital may provide full emergency room care, while another sees patients who have broken limbs, minor injuries and yet another sees patients suffering cold, flu, etc.

In 2007, the first nurse practitioner-led office to relieve waiting times caused by a shortage of primary practitioners was opened in Sudbury, Ontario.[53][54]

Alternatives to fee-for-visit or service

Ontario has also attempted to move the system away from bill for service or visit and toward preventive and community-based approaches to healthcare. The Ontario government in the early 1990s helped develop many community health care centres, often in low-income areas, which provide both medical and social support which combines health care with programs such as collective kitchens, Internet access, anti-poverty groups and groups to help people quit smoking.

While funding has decreased for these centres, and they have had to cut back, they have had a lower cost than the traditional fee-for-service approach. Many of these centres are filled to capacity in terms of general doctors, and there are often fairly long waiting lists and the centres also utilize nurse practitioners, who reduce the workload on the doctors and increase efficiency.

Midwives and hospital birthing reforms

Ontario and Quebec have recently licensed midwives, providing another option for childbirth which can reduce costs for uncomplicated births. Midwives remain close to hospital facilities in case the need for emergency care emerges. These births often cost much less than the traditional hospital delivery. Hospitals have also reformed their approach to birthing by adding private birthing areas, often with a hot tub (which is good for relieving pain without medication).

Privatization

Currently, privately owned and operated hospitals that allow patients to pay out-of-pocket for services cannot obtain public funding in Canada, as they contravene the "equal accessibility" tenets of the Canada Health Act. Some politicians and medical professionals have proposed allowing public funding for these hospitals. Workers' Compensation Boards, the Canadian Forces, the RCMP, federally incarcerated prisoners, and medical care for which an insurance company has liability (e.g., motor vehicle accidents) all pay for health care outside of the public systems in all provinces.[2][55]

In Quebec, a recent legal change has allowed this reform to occur. In June 2005, the Supreme Court of Canada overturned a Quebec law preventing people from buying private health insurance to pay for medical services available through the publicly funded system and this ruling does not apply outside the province. See: Chaoulli v. Quebec (Attorney General).[56]

In November 2005, the Quebec government announced that it would allow residents to purchase private medical insurance to comply with this ruling.

Private insurance from companies such as Blue Cross, Green Shield and Manulife have been available for many years to cover services not covered by the Canadian health care system, such as dental care and some eye care. Private insurance is provided by many employers as a benefit.

The Canadian Medical Association (CMA) released a report[57] in July 2007 endorsing private healthcare as a means to improve an ailing healthcare system. Dr. Brian Day, who acted as President of the CMA in 2007/2008, is the owner of the largest private healthcare hospital in Canada and a proponent of mixed public and private healthcare in Canada.

Canadian Health Practitioner standards

It is generally accepted that physicians arriving in Canada from other countries must meet Canadian Health Practitioner standards. So there is concern that doctors from other countries are not trained or educated to meet Canadian standards. Consequently, doctors who want to practice in Canada must meet the same educational and medical qualifications as Canadian-trained practitioners. Others suggest that the Canadian Medical Association, the Ontario Medical Association, and the regulatory bodies (the provincial Colleges of Physicians and Surgeons) have created too much red tape to allow qualified doctors to practise in

Canada.[58] Canada's health system is ranked 30th in the world, suggesting the logic of the doctor shortage defies the statistics.[59] In fact according to a report by Keith Leslie of the Canadian Press in the Chronicle Journal, Nov 21, 2005, over 10,000 trained doctors are working in the United States, a country ranked 37th in the world. It would suggest money or the perception of better working conditions, or both, are resulting in an exodus of Canadian doctors (and nurses) to the USA.[60]

It is important to recognize that many consider the doctor shortage in Canada to be a very severe problem affecting all sectors of health care. It may relate in part to the details of how doctors are paid; a detail often misunderstood. In Canada, almost all doctors receive a fee per-visit, not per-service. It has been suggested that this type of "fee-for-visit" payment system can encourage complexity, volume visits, repeat visits, referrals, and testing.[61][62]

One consequence of the shortage in Canada is that a great many patients are left without family doctors, and trained specialists, making early intervention very difficult. As the article in the Toronto Star specially isolates, it is not so much a problem of a doctor shortage but of a shortage of 'licensed doctors'. Michael Urbanski states that Canada already has a hidden reserve of foreign-trained MDs eager to begin medical practice. "However, what's crucial to understanding the issue of doctor shortage in Ontario is that while the Liberal government is planning to go "poaching" for other countries' doctors, there are an estimated 4,000 internationally trained doctors right here in Ontario working at low-wage jobs."[63]

A CBC report [6](August 21, 2006) on the health care system reports the following:

> Dr. Albert Schumacher,[64] former president of the Canadian Medical Association estimates that 75 per cent of health-care services are delivered privately, but funded publicly. "Frontline practitioners whether they're GPs or specialists by and large are not salaried. They're small hardware stores. Same thing with labs and radiology clinics ...The situation we are seeing now are more services around not being funded publicly but people having to pay for them, or their insurance companies. We have sort of a passive privatization.

In a report by Keith Leslie of the Canadian Press in the Chronicle Journal, Nov 21, 2005, commenting on an Ontario Medical Association Report, prepared by the human resources committee states "The year 2005 finds the province in the midst of a deepening physician resources crisis". The report continues to report, "the government should make it easier for doctors from other provinces to work in Ontario and .... ". Here we have signs of inter-provincial competition affecting the doctor shortage in one province over another.[60] Essentially, privatized healthcare is not a choice of interest for lower income Canadians, it is most likely to be unaffordable and unfair to those who suffer on a social standard.

2.4.12 Provincial insurance plans

Though the Canada Health Act provides national guidelines for healthcare, the provinces have exclusive jurisdiction over health under the constitution and are free to ignore these guidelines, although if they ignore the guidelines, the federal government may deny federal funding for healthcare. All provinces currently abide by the Canada Health Act in order to receive this funding; however the Alberta legislature has considered proposals to ignore the Act to allow them to implement reforms not allowed under the Act.

The federal government has no direct role in the delivery of medicine in the provinces and territories so each province and territory has its own independent public health insurance program. Under the Canada Health Act, each province and territory must provide services to members of plans in other provinces and territories.

List of provincial programs

2.4.13 See also

- Father of medicare

- Ontario Health Insurance Plan

- Medicare (Australia)

- Medicare (United States)

- National Health Service (UK)

- Canada Health Act

- Canada Health Transfer

- Canada Health and Social Transfer

- Indian Health Transfer Policy (Canada)

- Health care in Canada

- Canada's Health Care providers, 2007

- First Nations Health Authority

- Canadian Institute for Health Information

- Canadian and American health care systems compared

- Royal Commission on the Future of Health Care in Canada

- Saskatchewan doctors' strike of 1962

- Health Evidence Network of Canada

2.4.14 References

[1] Government of Canada, Health Canada. "Canada's Health Care System – Health Canada" (landing page). Retrieved 2011-07-11.

[2] Government of Canada, Health Canada. "Canada Health Act – Health Care System – Health Canada" (landing page). Retrieved 2011-07-11.

[3] Canadian Institute for Health Information (September 27, 2005). "CIHI exploring the 70–30 split". Retrieved 2007-12-21.

[4] Quinlan, Don (2008). *The Canadian Challenge*. Canada: Oxford University Press. ISBN 978-0-19-542647-2.

[5] J. Gilbert Turner. "The Hospital Insurance and Diagnostic Services Act: Its Impact on Hospital Administration". PMC 1829926.

[6] Lillian E. Forman (January 2009). *Health Care Reform*. ABDO. p. 2002. ISBN 978-1-60453-532-7. Retrieved 6 June 2011.

[7] "Civilization.ca – History of Canadian Medicare – 1958–1968 – Allan J. MacEachen". Retrieved 2012-04-19.

[8] "Benefits Canada". Retrieved May 16, 2014.

[9] Ministry of Health; Long-Term Care (2011-11-28). "Ontario Health Insurance Plan (OHIP) – Eligibility". Queen's Printer for Ontario. Retrieved 2012-02-15.

[10] Raisa Deber (August 2002). "Delivering Health Care Services: Public, Not-For-Profit or Private" (PDF). Retrieved 2008-08-07.

[11] "CBC Health Care Private versus Public". Cbc.ca. 2006-12-01. Retrieved 2011-06-06.

[12] "Neil MacKinnon. Commentary: Provincial drug plans. 2004" (PDF). Retrieved 2011-06-06.

[13] "Mark Kaplan. Myths and Realities of Canadian Medicare. Fall 2004" (PDF). Intl.pdx.edu. Retrieved 2011-06-06.

[14] Morgan SG, Law M, Daw JR, Abraham L, Martin D (2015). "Estimated cost of universal public coverage of prescription drugs in Canada". *CMAJ*. **187**: 491–7. doi:10.1503/cmaj.141564. PMC 4401594. PMID 25780047.

[15] http://www.academia.edu/17685108/From_the_city_
to_the_bush_increases_in_patient_co-payments_for_
medicines_have_impacted_on_medicine_use_across_
Australia

[16] "Prescription Drug Coverage in Canada". Drugcoverage.ca.
Retrieved 2011-06-06.

[17] "Valérie Paris and Elizabeth Docteur. Pharmaceutical Pricing and Reimbursement Policies in Canada. OECD Health
Working Papers 24, 2006." (PDF). Retrieved 2011-06-06.

[18] "on rejected claims". Drugcoverage.ca. Retrieved 2011-06-
06.

[19] "PMPRB Home page. Accessed Dec 26, 2007". Pmprb-
cepmb.gc.ca. Retrieved 2011-06-06.

[20] "RAMQ – Health Insurance – Dental Services - Services
Covered". Ramq.gouv.qc.ca. 2011-04-14. Retrieved 2011-
06-06.

[21] "Canadian Association of Public Health Dentistry home
page". Caphd-acsdp.org. Retrieved 2011-06-06.

[22] "AHCIP coverage within Canada". Retrieved 2012-09-25.

[23] http://www.cbc.ca/news/canada/
maple-leaf-best-defines-canada-survey-finds-1.722322

[24] Stuart N. Soroka. Canadian Perceptions of the Health Care
System. 2007. ISBN 0-9739726-8-8

[25] CIHI National Health Expenditures in Canada 1975–2007

[26] "Schoen et al., Toward Higher-Performance Health Systems:
Adults' Health Care Experiences in Seven Countries, 2007".
Commonwealthfund.org. 2007-11-01. Retrieved 2011-06-
06.

[27] "OECD Health Data 2007. How Does Canada Compare?"
(PDF). Retrieved 2011-06-06.

[28] "R. Deber. Why Did the World Health Organization Rate
Canada's Health System as 30th? Some Thoughts on League
Tables. Longwoods Review 2(1) 2004". Longwoods.com.
2003-06-20. Retrieved 2011-06-06.

[29] "Home page on the accord". Hc-sc.gc.ca. Retrieved 2011-
06-06.

[30] "Health Council of Canada. Health Care Renewal in
Canada: Measuring UP? 2007". Healthcouncilcanada.ca.
Retrieved 2011-06-06.

[31] "Fraser Institute press release, October 2007". Fraserinsti-
tute.org. Retrieved 2011-06-06.

[32] "CHSRF Mythbusters: A parallel private system would relieve waiting times in the public system. 2005" (PDF).
Chsrf.ca. 2010-12-13. Retrieved 2011-06-06.

[33] "Canadian Health Coalition. Home Page. Accessed Dec 26,
2007". Healthcoalition.ca. 2011-05-24. Retrieved 2011-
06-06.

[34] "Health Council of Canada. Wading through wait times.
2007". Healthcouncilcanada.ca. Retrieved 2011-06-06.

[35] "Health Canada home page on wait times, with links to major
studies. 2007". Hc-sc.gc.ca. 2007-05-25. Retrieved 2011-
06-06.

[36] CIHI Waiting for Health Care in Canada: What We Know
and What we Don't Know. 2006.

[37] "Home page of Wait Time Alliance accessed December 26,
2007". Waittimealliance.ca. Retrieved 2011-06-06.

[38] "Patient wait times costing economy $14.8B". CTV.ca.
2008-01-15. Retrieved 2011-06-06.

[39] Barua, B., & Esmail, N. (October, 2013). Waiting Times
Wait Times for Health Care in Canada. Fraser Institute . Retrieved October 21, 2014, from http://www.fraserinstitute.
org/uploadedFiles/fraser-ca/Content/research-news/
research/publications/waiting-your-turn-2013.pdf

[40] CIHI Canada's Health Care Providers accessed Dec 26,
2007

[41] CIHI report, From Perceived Surplus to Perceived Shortage: What Happened to Canada's Physician Workforce in
the 1990s? 2002

[42] "Health Canada Primary Health Care home page, accessed
Dec 26, 2007". Hc-sc.gc.ca. 2004-10-01. Retrieved 2011-
06-06.

[43] "NHRSU home page. Accessed Dec 26, 2007". Nhsru.com.
Retrieved 2011-06-06.

[44] "Ontario Ministry of Health and Long Term Care – Public
Information – Ontario Health Insurance Plan - Health Ser-
vices". Retrieved July 2012. Check date values in: |access-
date= (help)

[45] "I. Dhalla. Private Health Insurance: An International
Overview and Considerations for Canada. Longwoods Review vol 5(3) 2007". Longwoods.com. Retrieved 2011-06-
06.

[46] "Canada's Expectant Moms Heading to U.S. to Deliver".
Fox News. 2007-10-10.

[47] Health Care Spending in the United States and OECD Countries, January 2007 Retrieved October 19th, 2008.

[48] https://web.archive.org/web/20160315000410/http:
//money.cnn.com/2015/04/13/news/economy/
obamacare-uninsured-gallup/

[49] Province of Nova Scotia (2011-03-21). "Dispute Resolution
in Healthcare and Community Services Collective Bargaining". Retrieved 2011-07-11.

[50] "Privatizing Health Care is Not the Answer". Cmaj.ca.
doi:10.1503/cmaj.081177. Retrieved 2011-06-06.

[51] "Ontario Health Premium Rate Chart". Ontario Ministry Of Finance.

[52] "Employer Health Tax". Ontario Ministry Of Finance.

[53] "First Nurse Practitioner-Led Clinic Opens Doors in Sudbury". *REGISTERED NURSES' ASSOCIATION OF ONTARIO.* CNW Group. 2007-08-31. Retrieved 2007-09-02.

[54] "1st nurse practitioner-governed clinic opens in Sudbury". *CBC News.* CBC. 2007-08-31. Retrieved 2007-09-02.

[55] B.C. Canadian Taxpayers Federation Archived November 8, 2007, at the Wayback Machine.

[56] *Chaoulli v. Quebec (Attorney General), 2005 SCC 35*, 2005-06-09, retrieved 2011-07-11

[57] "Doctors' group prescribes private health care". Canada.com. 2007-07-30. Retrieved 2011-06-06.

[58] "Red tape is strangling foreign-trained physicians CANADIAN MEDICAL ASSOCIATION JOURNAL". Cmaj.ca. 2000-04-04. Retrieved 2011-06-06.

[59] "Universal Health Care – Canada ranks 30th". Cthealth.server101.com. 2000-06-20. Retrieved 2011-06-06.

[60] Ont. Medi Scare – Chronicle Journal, Thunder Bay, November 21, 2005 – Physician shortage puts stability of healthcare system at risk. OMA

[61] "Improving health care for Canadians". Epe.lac-bac.gc.ca. Retrieved 2011-06-06.

[62] "Health Care Costs Nobody Talks About". Web.archive.org. 2007-04-08. Archived from the original on 2007-04-08. Retrieved 2011-06-06.

[63] "What doctor shortage? - Toronto Star, August 19, 2004". Triec.ca. Retrieved 2011-06-06.

[64] "Private verses Public – Dr. Albert Schumacher". Cbc.ca. 2006-12-01. Retrieved 2011-06-06.

2.4.15 External links

- Canada Health Act

- Canadian Health Coalition (Canadian lobby group supporting public medicare)

- Medicare: A People's Issue

- Maple Leaf Web: The Charter & Public Health Care in Canada

- CBC Digital Archives – The Birth of Medicare

- Building on Values: The Future of Health Care in Canada (*The Romanow Report*, PDF) archived at Collections Canada

- Health Canada page linking to key Federal reports and commissions and their background material, including Romanow Report and Kirby Commission

- Pharmaceutical Pricing and Reimbursement Policies in Canada. OECD Health Working Papers 24, 2006

- Marchildon's backgrounder on Canadian healthcare for WHO 2005

- Benjamin Isitt and Melissa Moroz, "The Hospital Employees' Union Strike and the Privatization of Medicare in British Columbia, Canada," International Labor and Working-Class History, 71 (Spring 2007): 91-111

2.5 National Health Service

"NHS" redirects here. For other uses, see NHS (disambiguation).
For the individual national healthcare services of England, Scotland, Wales and Northern Ireland, see National Health Service (England), NHS Scotland, NHS Wales, and Health and Social Care in Northern Ireland.

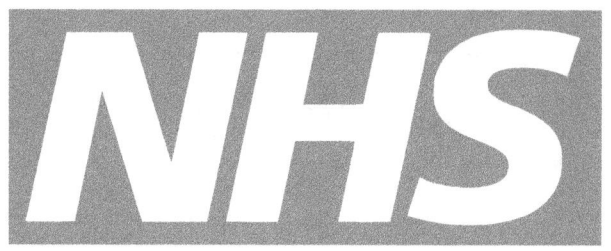

NHS logo in England

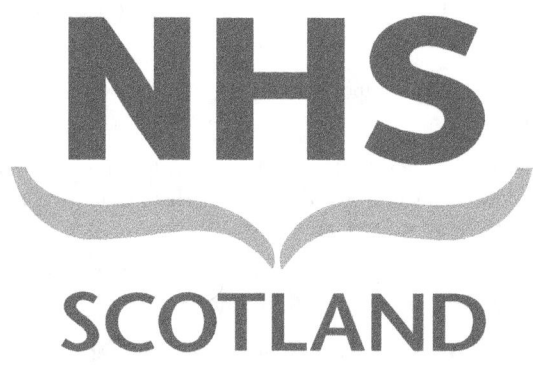

NHS Scotland logo

The **National Health Service** (**NHS**) is the name of the public health services of England, Scotland and Wales, and

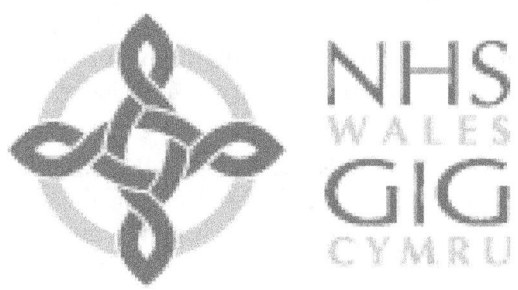

NHS Wales logo

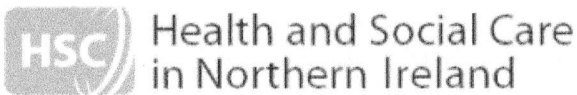

Logo of Health and Social Care in Northern Ireland, the equivalent in Northern Ireland

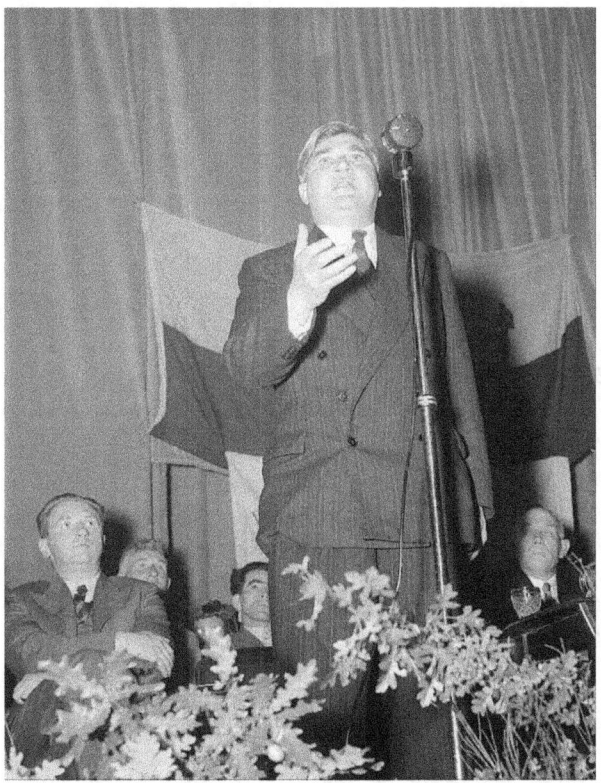

Aneurin Bevan, who spearheaded the establishment of the National Health Services

is commonly used to refer to those of Northern Ireland. They were established together as one of the major social reforms following the Second World War on the founding principles of being comprehensive, universal and free at the point of delivery.[1] Today, each provides a comprehensive range of health services, the vast majority of which are free for people ordinarily resident in the United Kingdom.[2]

Taken together, the four National Health Services in 2015-16 employed around 1.6 million people with a combined budget of £136.7 billion. UK residents are not charged for most medical treatment, with exceptions such as a fixed charge for prescriptions; dental treatment is administered differently, with standard charges for most procedures. For non-residents, the NHS is free at the time of use, for general practitioner (GP) and emergency treatment not including admission to hospital.

2.5.1 History

Further information: History of the National Health Service

The NHS began on the 'Appointed Day' of 5 July 1948. This put into practice Westminster legislation for England and Wales from 1946 and Scotland from 1947, and the Northern Ireland Parliament's 1947 Public Health Services Act.[3] Calls for a "unified medical service" can be dated back to the Minority Report of the Royal Commission on the Poor Law in 1909,[4] but it was following the 1942 Beveridge Report's recommendation to create "comprehensive health and rehabilitation services for prevention and cure of disease" that cross-party consensus emerged on introducing a National Health Service of some description.[5] When Clement Attlee's Labour Party won the 1945 election he appointed Aneurin Bevan as Health Minister. Bevan then embarked upon what the official historian of the NHS, Charles Webster, called an "audacious campaign" to take charge of the form the NHS finally took.[6]

Three years after the founding of the NHS, Bevan resigned from the Labour government in opposition to the introduction of charges for the provision of dentures and glasses.[7] The following year, Winston Churchill's Conservative government introduced prescription charges. These charges were the first of many controversies over reforms to the NHS throughout its history.[8]

Each of the UK's four nations have their own separate NHS, each with its own history. NHS Scotland and Health and Social Care in Northern Ireland (HSC) were separate from the foundation of the NHS, whereas the NHS in Wales was originally combined with England until devolved to the Secretary of State for Wales in 1969 and then to the Welsh Executive and Assembly under devolution in 1999,[9] the same year as responsibility for the Scottish NHS was transferred from the Secretary of State for Scotland to the new Scottish Government and Parliament.

From its earliest days, the cultural history of the NHS has shown its place in British society reflected and debated in film, TV, cartoons and literature.

2.5.2 Structure

Each of the UK's health service systems operates independently, and is politically accountable to the relevant government: the Scottish Government, Welsh Government, the Northern Ireland Executive, and the UK Government which is responsible for England's NHS. NHS Wales was originally part of the same structure as England until powers over the NHS in Wales were firstly transferred to the Secretary of State for Wales in 1969 and thereafter, in 1999, to the Welsh Assembly (now the Welsh Government) as part of Welsh devolution. However, some functions might be routinely performed by one health service on behalf of another. For example, Northern Ireland has no high-security psychiatric hospitals and thus depends on using hospitals in Great Britain, routinely Carstairs State Mental Hospital in Scotland for male patients and Rampton Secure Hospital in England for female patients.[10] Similarly, patients in North Wales use specialist facilities in Manchester and Liverpool which are much closer than facilities in Cardiff, and more routine services at the Countess of Chester Hospital NHS Foundation Trust. There have been issues about cross-border payments.[11]

Taken together, the four National Health Services in 2015-16 employed around 1.6 million people with a combined budget of £136.7 billion.[12] In 2014 the total health sector workforce across the UK was 2,165,043. This broke down into 1,789,586 in England, 198,368 in Scotland, 110,292 in Wales and 66,797 in Northern Ireland.[13]

2.5.3 Eligibility for treatment

UK residents are not charged for most medical treatment, with exceptions such as a fixed charge for prescriptions; dental treatment is administered differently, with standard charges for most procedures. The NHS is free at the time of use, for general practitioner (GP) and emergency treatment not including admission to hospital, to non-residents.[14] People with the right to medical care in European Economic Area (EEA) nations are also entitled to free treatment by using the European Health Insurance Card. Those from other countries with which the UK has reciprocal arrangements also qualify for free treatment.[15][16] Since 6 April 2015, non-EEA nationals who are subject to immigration control must have the immigration status of indefinite leave to remain at the time of treatment and be properly settled, to be considered ordinarily resident. People not ordinarily resident in the UK are in general not entitled to free hospital treatment, with some exceptions such as refugees.[2][17]

People not ordinarily resident may be subject to an interview to establish their eligibility, which must be resolved before non-emergency treatment can commence. Patients who do not qualify for free treatment are asked to pay in advance, or to sign a written undertaking to pay, except for emergency treatment.

The provision of free treatment to non-UK-residents, formerly interpreted liberally, has been increasingly restricted, with new overseas visitor hospital charging regulations introduced in 2015.[18]

People from outside the EEA coming to the UK for a temporary stay of more than six months may be required to pay an immigration health surcharge at the time of visa application, and will then be entitled to NHS treatment on the same basis as a resident. As of 2016 the surcharge was £200 per year, with exemptions and reductions in some cases.[19]

2.5.4 Funding

The systems are 98.8% funded from general taxation and National Insurance contributions, plus small amounts from patient charges for some services.[20] About 10% of GDP is spent on health and most is spent in the public sector.[21]

The money to pay for the NHS comes directly from taxation. The 2008/9 budget roughly equates to a contribution of £1,980 for every man, woman and child in the UK.[22]

When the NHS was launched in 1948 it had a budget of £437million (roughly £9billion at today's value).[23] In 2008/9 it received over 10 times that amount (more than £100billion). In 1955/6 health spending was 11.2% of the public services budget. In 2015/6 it was 29.7%.[24]

This equates to an average rise in spending over the full 60-year period of about 4% a year once inflation has been taken into account. Under the Blair government investment levels increased to around 6% a year on average. Since 2010 spending growth has been constrained to just over 1% a year.[24]

Some 60% of the NHS budget is used to pay staff. A further 20% pays for drugs and other supplies, with the remaining 20% split between buildings, equipment, training costs, medical equipment, catering and cleaning. Nearly 80% of the total budget is distributed by local trusts in line with the particular health priorities in their areas.

70% of people say they would willingly pay an extra penny in the pound in income tax if the money were ringfenced and guaranteed for the NHS.[25]

There was concern that the Chancellor's 2016 Autumn Statement did not include extra funding for the NHS.[26] See Autumn Statement for more.

Investment and efficiency

The Organisation for Economic Cooperation and Development (OECD) stated in a 2015 study that the UK had one of the worst healthcare systems among the nations looked at and that people were dying needlessly due to lack of investment in the NHS.[27] It has been suggested that while the UK government and people are focused on Brexit, problems with the NHS are being neglected.[28] A wide range of medical professionals consider hospital conditions in winter 2017 to have been the worst ever and worse than during corresponding periods in 2016. Hospitals are overcrowded with patients on trolleys in corridors due to lack of beds in wards.[29] The Royal College of Nursing reported nurses claiming current conditions are the worst they have experienced. The Royal College of Physicians (RCP) asked for urgent investment to deal with "over-full hospitals with too few qualified staff". Prof Jane Dacre of the RCP, said: "Our members tell me it is the worst it has ever been in terms of patients coming in during a 24-hour period and numbers of patients coming in when there are no beds to put them in. And there are patients within the hospital who can no longer get home because of the difficulties there are in placing people in social care. Our members fear that patients' lives are at risk because they can't get round to see patients who aren't in the emergency and accident department or are waiting for results to come back." The Royal College of Radiologists also calls for increased investment.[30] Trusts are told to make a surplus when that is not feasible, then lose funds for being in deficit.[31]

There were 30,000 more deaths than expected in England and Wales in 2015. Peer reviewed research by the London School of Hygiene & Tropical Medicine, Oxford University and Blackburn with Darwen council was published in the Journal of the Royal Society of Medicine.[32][33] The research claims the increase happened during "severe cuts" to the NHS and social care, which compromised their performance. Relevant NHS performance data was studied showing almost all targets were missed. Researchers concluded: "The evidence points to a major failure of the health system, possibly exacerbated by failings in social care." The percentage rise in mortality was the largest in nearly 50 years and the excess was the largest in the post war period. The increase was mainly due to older people dying and older people depend more on medical and social care. There was a spike in January which it is feared could become normal. Prof Martin McKee of the London School of Hygiene & Tropical Medicine, said, "The impact of cuts resulting from the imposition of austerity on the NHS has been profound. Expenditure has failed to keep pace with demand and the situation has been exacerbated by dramatic reductions in the welfare budget of £16.7 billion and in social care spending. (...) The possibility that the cuts to health and

social care are implicated in almost 30,000 excess deaths is one that needs further exploration. Given the relentless nature of the cuts, and potential link to rising mortality, we ask why is the search for a cause not being pursued with more urgency?" Prof Danny Dorling of Oxford University said, "It may sound obvious that more elderly people will have died earlier as a result of government cutbacks, but to date the number of deaths has not been estimated and the government have not admitted responsibility." Researchers noted that the rise in deaths coincided with a rise in waiting times in A&E departments, though there were not exceptional numbers of patients in A&E. Ambulances also took longer to respond and more operations were cancelled for non-clinical reasons. More staff were absent and more posts remained unfilled. £16.7bn was cut from welfare spending and 17% was cut from spending on older people since 2009 though the numbers of old people rose nearly 9%. Both factors compounded the problems that health service austerity caused. Report co-author, Dominic Harrison of Blackburn with Darwen council, warned the research "raises a red flag that is telling us that the health and care system may have reached the limits of its capacity to safely and effectively care for the population that funds it. Our analysis suggests that the most likely cause of that failure, when all other possible explanations have been excluded, is insufficient resources and capacity". [32][33]

Intensive care beds are sometimes 100% occupied despite 85% occupancy being considered the maximum safe occupancy rate. There is a shortage of intensive care beds and of qualified staff to deal with patients in intensive care. Dr Carl Waldmann of the Faculty of Intensive Care Medicine (FICM) said, "Intensive care is at its limits in terms of capacity and struggles to maintain adequate staffing levels." Life saving operations are being postponed due to a lack of available post-operative intensive care. Patients who need intensive care do not always get it because beds or skilled staff are not available. Patients who should be in intensive care have to wait in A&E, sometimes for many hours. Hospitals struggle to manage and patients are put at risk. Jonathan Ashworth said, "The truth is problems are getting worse and more widespread than in previous years with even life-saving cardiac, abdominal or neurosurgery operations being cancelled. Theresa May needs to get a grip of the crisis and explain what action she's going to take to make sure that hospitals can get in place the number of staff they need to keep patients safe."[34]

Pathology laboratories that diagnose cancer are struggling to cope with rising demand. Many of the staff are nearing retiring age and young graduates are not joining the profession to replace them. Cancer Research UK claims similar problems exist with other diagnostic services like scans and endoscopies. Because the UK population is growing and aging more people need cancer diagnosis. Still services are not growing to meet rising demand. The 'Cancer Research UK' report also advises the Royal College of Pathologists to update guidance and study how to attract staff to train for pathology. UK cancer survival rates are below those of other European nations and earlier diagnosis would help deal with this. If nothing is done the problem will worsen.[35][36] In winter 2017 cancer operations are being cancelled, sometimes at short notice due to insufficient beds. This is stressful for patients and leads to fears that a cancer will get worse.[37]

Waiting times for routine knee and hip operations are excessively long and long waits lead to a worse outcome. Waiting times also increased for other routine operations. Waiting times more than doubled in England between 2012 and 2016 and rose significantly in Scotland, Wales and Northern Ireland. Richard Murray of the King's Fund think tank, expects numbers on waiting lists to continue rising and exceed 4 million by spring.[38] Hospital leaders and experts in health say increased waiting times result inevitably from NHS budgets increasing less than patient demand. Emergency admissions are rising, delayed transfer of care further reduces bed availability, something must give, patients waiting for routine surgery lose out.[39]

An editorial in *The Independent* stated "The National Health Service is in trouble. Statistics on ambulance response times, accident and emergency waiting times and delayed discharges, published [in 2016], are all markedly worse than over the previous year. Ambulances reached critically ill patients within the target of eight minutes less than 70% of the time in the year to June, down from 75% the previous year. The proportion of patients at accident and emergency seen within four hours fell from 92 per cent to 86 per cent. The number of days lost to delayed discharges rose by a quarter from 91,000 to 115,000." The editorial argued further that if the efficiency of the NHS does not improve, this could affect the popularity of the current government.[40] Further almost half of hospital authorities are reducing the number of beds while a third of A&E's are due to close because of increasing hospital deficits. Total NHS deficits reached £2.4bn in 2015, the largest recorded deficit in NHS history.[41] BMA chairman, Mark Porter, said: "The UK already has the second lowest number of hospital beds per head in Europe and these figures paint an even bleaker picture of an NHS that is at breaking point. (...) The delays that vulnerable patients are facing, particularly those with mental health issues, have almost become the norm and this is unacceptable. Failures within the social care system are also having a considerable knock-on effect on an already stretched and underfunded NHS. (...) In the short term we need to see bed plans that are workable and focused on the quality of care and patient experiences, rather than financial targets. But in the long term we need politicians to take their heads out of the sand and provide a sustainable solution to the funding and capacity challenges that are overwhelming the health service."[42]

Chris Hopson of NHS Providers said, "Despite doing everything they possibly can, NHS trusts are £300m behind the target of reducing the provider sector deficit to £580m by the end of March. This is largely because of winter pressures. Trusts spent more than they planned and they lost income from cancelled operations – both were needed to create the extra bed capacity to meet record emergency winter demand. This shows the danger of planning with no margin for unexpected extra demand. We can't expect to run NHS finances on wafer thin margins year after year and keep getting away with it."[43]

Bob Kerslake maintains that the NHS is struggling from day to day to maintain services despite inadequate funding. Kerslake maintains the NHS needs increased funding of at least 4% per year to deal with medical advances and an aging population, he wrote "The hardest thing for governments to do is to listen and act on inconvenient advice. It is also the most important."[44]

There are calls for an extra 10bn annually to be spent on the Health Service to match health spending in other advanced European nations. Dr Mark Porter of the BMA wrote, "Our members report that services are truly at breaking point, with unprecedented rising patient demand met only with financial restraint and directives for the NHS and social care to make huge, unachievable savings through sustainability and transformation plans (STPs) across England. We are not calling for more than other comparable nations, we are simply calling for you to match the average spending of other leading European economies. Based on our analysis of the figures available, this would, in 2015, have equated to an increase of £10.3bn for NHS funding; an increase which is desperately needed." Porter also wrote, "The crisis currently facing the NHS and social care is well known and becoming increasingly severe – the government cannot remain a bystander any longer. An entire system under such strain is not due to frontline financial mismanagement, or individual chief executives' poor decision making, it is due to the conscious underinvestment in our health service."[45]

Denis Campbell wrote in, *The Guardian* "A poll of 96 MPs of all parties by the Royal College of Emergency Medicine, which represents A&E doctors, has found that only 33% of them believe A&E departments have enough money and staff to provide safe care. More than six in 10 MPs believe A&E departments need more money, said the college."[46]

Mental health services

The Public Accounts Committee claims that plans to improve mental health services have a doubtful future due to uncertainties over funding. Only a quarter of patients needing mental health services get them. Mental health services were found hard to navigate and with quality varying. Meg Hillier said, "Many people can make a full recovery from mental health problems if they receive appropriate treatment at an early stage. This is good for them and has wider benefits for the economy and society in general. It is therefore crucial that mental health is given equal priority to physical health and that service provision reflects this. (...) If [the government] is serious about achieving its aims it must also plan to secure skilled staff in sufficient numbers."[47] Nine former health secretaries claim the government broke promises on mental health.[48] A Guardian article cited widespread distrust that government promises to increase mental health funding were being met.[49] Polling suggests the British public overwhelmingly support increased funding for mental health care.[50]

Mental health services for young people are inadequate according to a poll of nurses working in that area. Shortage of resources and staff are seen as a problem and nurses have insufficient time to talk to young patients or to show patients they matter. Sarah Brennan of YoungMinds said new money promised by the government will only reach a third of those who need it. Nurses fear the need to ration care puts young people at risk of self harm and suicide.[51] Numbers of young people admitted to hospital for self-harm are increasing.[52] The NSPCC claims children needing help following abuse are not getting it and children need to reach rock bottom, regularly self-harming or feeling suicidal before getting help. A leaked government report showed sick children were taken "almost anywhere in the country" to be treated. Suicides are increasing.[50] 54% of parents with children in psychiatric hospitals claim they did not improve and 24% say they got worse. Parents cannot visit as often as they would like because children are too far away. Parents are frequently not consulted over children's medication and frequently feel unable to challenge decisions over their child's treatment. Just over half parents were not confident their child was getting appropriate treatment. In the worst cases children deteriorated in inappropriate places while parents tried desperately to get the child home. Sarah Brennan finds it alarming that so many parents are dissatisfied. There are calls for a charter of rights for young patients. Patients and their families should be involved in treatment decisions. Patients should be treated with dignity and respect, restraints and seclusion should not be over used. Patients should be treated as near home as possible. Mark Lever of the National Autistic Society wants families fully involved in decisions about care decisions for their loved ones. He said, "Our joint survey with YoungMinds suggests that many parents of children and young people in mental health inpatient units feel powerless."[53]

When patients with mental health issues are in hospital with physical illness, hospital staff do not know how to treat them, leading to worse outcomes.[54]

Staffing

According to the General Medical Council, many doctors experience low morale which can put patients at risk.[55] The GMC criticised the amount of funding that the NHS receives, saying that years of constraint coupled with social care pressures were leaving services struggling to cope with rising demand. GP consultations average 10 minutes and are the shortest in Europe. Many patients need more complex care than can be delivered in 10 minutes and the aging population means the numbers of patients needing longer consultations is increasing. Plans to transfer some work now done in hospitals to GP's will increase the numbers of patients needing complex care that GP's cannot deliver under the present system and patient care may suffer. Extra funding for GP's is in the pipeline but will not become available till after hospital work has been transferred to GP's and patient care may be compromised during the time between transferring services from hospitals and providing extra funding.[56][57]

According to MP Dr Dan Poulter, pressure to deal with patients prevents doctors getting necessary training and there are too few middle grade doctors in paediatrics, obstetrics and gynaecology.[55] 38% of GP's plan to leave within five years.[58] Junior hospital doctors reportedly face burnout and exhaustion, often work unpaid beyond their shift, and skip meals or fail to get adequate hydration during shifts. Their physical and mental health frequently suffers. "We are exhausted, frustrated and burned out. I see lapses in safety daily and, even if somebody cared, there is no money or staff to do anything about it," a trainee anaesthetist stated. Another stated, "I have reached a point where my physical and mental health have been seriously adversely affected, and I wonder whether I'm suffering from burnout." Unpaid overtime is common. Due to understaffing junior doctors must work extra shifts to cover for gaps in rotas. The family life of doctors suffers. Many doctors are considering leaving the profession to do alternative work with a better work-life balance, while others are considering emigrating to countries where doctors' work is less demanding. Doctors reportedly have insufficient time to train and improve skills, which will cause problems for them and for patients in the future.[59] According to the Royal College of Physicians (RCP), the Health Service budget has not kept pace with rising demand for services and either funding must increase or care must be cut.[60] GP's are overstretched and some patients must wait three weeks for problems which do not appear urgent like lumps or bleeding. There is concern over this because such problems can be life-threatening. There is also concern that chronic disease management may get insufficient attention because overstretched GP's are too busy dealing with acute illnesses. Maintaining GP services is considered important because if GP's fail patients are likely to overwhelm hospitals instead.[61] Pressuring doctors to remain open 7 days a week will add to the difficulties of recruiting and retaining GP's.[62]

4 million people were left without emergency cover during 2016 due to a shortage of doctors. Some patients needing emergency treatment were sent to A&E which is also under pressure, others were seen by less qualified staff. Many doctors have expressed concern for patient safety due to this. The Royal College of GPs wants the government to make out-of-hours work more attractive for family doctors.[63]

There is apprehension that the numbers of medical students fell since 2010 despite patient numbers increasing.[64] The RCP wants NHS efficiency targets overhauled, wants government goals to be realistic and wants investment in 'long-term sustainability' of the NHS. The RCP warns further that government's promise of 5,000 more GP's should not come 'at the expense of other specialties'. Prompt action is needed to counter funding and staff shortages and staff feel like 'collateral damage' when struggling over rising demand and budget shortages. Efficiency improvements can help but it is unclear for how long. Dr Andrew Goddard of the RCP said that providing more expensive treatments for increasing numbers of patients would fail. "As doctors, we see the problems this creates on a daily basis, be it at the front door of the hospital, in A&E or in out-patients. Patients can see it too and realise that the NHS is no longer the envy of the world and isn't fit for our changing world. There are some big decisions that society has to make and the political parties have to stop blaming each other for where we are and work together to build a health and social care system that is fit for the UK in the 21st century." The RCP maintains the NHS is living beyond its means which cannot be sustained long term. More 'training places' are needed from medical school onwards to counter staff shortages. 2 in 5 NHS doctors are from overseas, the RCP fears uncertainties over Brexit and immigration regulations render their position unpredictable.[64] Many doctors from other nations in the EEA have said that they feel unwelcome after Brexit and are considering leaving.[65]

The RCP reports 70% of doctors in training have a permanent gap in their work rota and 96% reported gaps in nursing rotas. Hospitals record 40% of consultant posts remain vacant. Close to 50% of consultants state they were asked to do more junior work and over 10% of junior doctors said patients were not guaranteed treatment with appropriately experienced doctors. The RCP maintains this makes the government's goal of a 7-day week unachievable.[64][66]

Staff pay

Nurses' pay has not kept pace with inflation and their real pay has fallen while people wanting to become nurses lack training bursaries. Unfilled nursing vacancies rose sixfold since 2010.[48] In 2013 over half of the 600 nurses responding to an online poll by the Nursing Times believed their ward or unit is sometimes or always dangerously understaffed. Three-quarters had witnessed poor patient care and thirty percent said poor patient care happened regularly. A spokesperson for the Royal College of Nursing commented that in the worst cases this can cause unnecessary deaths and called for clear national guidelines for safe staffing levels and said one registered nurse to eight patients was considered risky while there should be one nurse to five patients. A spokesperson for Patient Concern, a patient campaigning group, commented that the work expected of nurses was rising continually while staffing levels did not rise.[67] The Royal College of Nursing (RCN) said nurses from Scotland to London were seriously concerned about the quality of care they could provide.[30] 43% of A&E staff have suffered physical assaults and lack of staff increases the risk that patients will be violent.[68]

2.5.5 Sustainability and transformation plans

Consultation will start over cost saving, streamlining and reduction of some services in the National Health Service. The streamlining will lead to ward closures including psychiatric ward closures and reduction in the number of beds in many areas among other changes. There is concern that hospital beds are being closed without increased community provision.[69] See Sustainability and transformation plans in England for more.

Effect of Brexit

The plan to exit the European Community will affect physicians from EU countries, about 11% of the physician workforce.[70] In this scenario many of these feel unwelcome and are considering leaving the UK if the Brexit would be enacted, as they have doubts that they and their families can live in the country.[70] A survey suggests 60% are considering leaving.[71]

2.5.6 Outsourcing and privatisation

Although the NHS routinely outsources the equipment and products that it uses and dentistry, eye care, pharmacy and most GP practices are provided by the private sector, the outsourcing of hospital health care has always been controversial.[72]

According to a BMA survey over two thirds of doctors are fairly uncomfortable or very uncomfortable about the independent sector providing NHS services. The BMA believes it is important the independent sector is held to the same standards as the NHS when giving NHS care. The BMA recommends: data collection, thorough impact analysis before independent providers are accepted to ensure existing NHS services are not disrupted, risk assessment to find out likely results if NHS staff are unwilling to transfer to the private sector, transparent reporting by the private sector of patient safety and performance, independent providers should be regulated like NHS providers, patients should be protected if independent providers terminate a contract early, transfers from independent providers to the NHS should be regularly reviewed to establish how much this costs the NHS, private sector contracts should be amended so private sector providers contribute to the cost of staff training financially or by providing training opportunities.[73]

2.5.7   Comparative performance

Although there have been increasing policy divergence between the four systems there is very little evidence linking these policy differences to a matching divergence of performance.[74] It has been suggested that this is because of the uniform professional culture. There are national terms and conditions of employment across the UK, regulation of clinicians is performed on a UK basis and the health trades unions operate across the UK. However, it does not help that, as Nick Timmins noted "Some of the key data needed to compare performance – including data on waiting times – is defined and collected differently in the four countries."[75][76]

For details see:

- National Health Service (England)

- Health and Social Care in Northern Ireland

- NHS Scotland

- NHS Wales

2.5.8   See also

- History of the National Health Service (England)

- History of NHS Scotland

- History of NHS Wales

- Healthcare in the United Kingdom

- Scottish Government Health and Social Care Directorates

- British Medical Association

- Royal College of General Practitioners

- Gibraltar Health Authority

- Health Service Executive (Republic of Ireland)

2.5.9   References

[1] Choices, NHS. "The principles and values of the NHS in England - NHS Choices". *www.nhs.uk*. Retrieved 2016-11-23.

[2] "NHS entitlements: migrant health guide - Detailed guidance". *UK Government*. Retrieved 6 June 2016.

[3] Ruth Barrington, *Health, Medicine & Politics in Ireland 1900-1970* (Institute of Public Administration: Dublin, 1987) pp. 188-189

[4] Brian Abel-Smith, *The Hospitals 1800-1948 (London, 1964), p.229*

[5] Beveridge, William (November 1942). "Social Insurance and Allied Services" (PDF). HM Stationery Office. Retrieved 3 March 2013.

[6] Charles Webster, The Health Services since the War, Volume 1: Problems of Health Care, The National Health Service Before 1957 (London: HMSO, 1988), p.399

[7] Kenneth O. Morgan, 'Aneurin Bevan' in Kevin Jeffreys (ed.), *Labour Forces: From Ernie Bevin to Gordon Brown* (I.B. Taurus: London & New York, 2002), pp. 91-92.

[8] Martin Powell and Robin Miller, 'Seventy Years of Privatizing the British National Health Service?', *Social Policy & Administration*, vol. 50, no. 1 (January 2016), pp. 99-118.

[9] Wales, NHS. "NHS Wales | 1960's". *www.wales.nhs.uk*. Retrieved 2016-11-22.

[10] The Transfer of Mentally Disordered Patients – Guidance on the transfer of mentally disordered patients detained under the Mental Health (NI) Order 1986 to and from Hospitals in Great Britain – August 2011

[11] "Breakdown of cross-border agreements is costing English trusts millions". Health Service Journal. 14 February 2008. Retrieved 19 January 2016.

[12] "10 truths about Britain's health service". Guardian. 18 January 2016. Retrieved 19 January 2016.

[13] Cowper, Andy (23 May 2016). "Visible and valued: the way forward for the NHS's hidden army". Health Service Journal. Retrieved 28 July 2016.

[14] "Visiting or moving to England? - How to access NHS services (see "Hospital Services" section)". *NHS Choices.* 26 June 2015. Retrieved 6 June 2016.

[15] "NHS charges for people from abroad". Citizens Advice. Retrieved 2010-11-16.

[16] "Non-EEA country-by-country guide - Healthcare abroad". *NHS Choices.* 1 January 2016. Retrieved 6 June 2016.

[17] "Categories of exemption - Healthcare in England for visitors - NHS Choices". *NHS England.* 18 August 2015. Retrieved 6 June 2016.

[18] "Guidance on overseas visitors hospital charging regulations - Publications - GOV.UK". *UK Government.* 6 April 2016. Retrieved 6 June 2016. Links to many relevant documents: Guidance on implementing the overseas visitor hospital charging regulations 2015; Ways in which people can be lawfully resident in the UK; Summary of changes made to the way the NHS charges overseas visitors for NHS hospital care; Biometric residence permits: overseas applicant and sponsor information; Information sharing with the Home Office: guidance for overseas patients; Overseas chargeable patients, NHS debt and immigration rules: guidance on administration and data sharing; Ordinary residence tool; and documents on Equality analysis.

[19] "Moving from outside the EEA - Access to healthcare in England - NHS Choices". *Nhs.uk.* 18 August 2015. Retrieved 6 June 2016.

[20] "How the NHS is funded". *TheKing'sFund.* 15 January 2016. Retrieved 6 June 2016.

[21] "Health care spending compared to other countries".

[22] NHS Choices The NHS in England: The NHS: About the NHS: Overview. Retrieved 22 June 2010.

[23] "The NHS in England". NHS choices. 28 January 2013. Retrieved 27 July 2014.

[24] "10 charts that show why the NHS is in trouble". BBC News. 8 February 2017. Retrieved 10 February 2017.

[25] People may be ready to pay extra penny on tax for NHS, Tim Farron says *The Guardian*

[26] NHS completely absent from 72-page Autumn Statement document *The Independent*

[27] Four charts showing the NHS is underfunded and understaffed *The Independent*

[28] The NHS needs a rethink. Its priorities no longer make sense *The Guardian*

[29] 'Deeply worrying' waits for hospital beds *BBC*

[30] NHS conditions worst ever, say leading nurses *BBC*

[31] NHS crisis: the one act of self-sacrifice that could rescue our health service *The Guardian*

[32] Health cuts most likely cause of rise in mortality study claims *The Guardian*

[33] New analysis links 30,000 excess deaths in 2015 to cuts in health and social care

[34] NHS intensive care 'at its limits' because of staff shortages *The Guardian*

[35] UK's pathology services at tipping point

[36] NHS cancer testing service 'at breaking point' *BBC*

[37] NHS in crisis as cancer operations cancelled due to lack of beds *The Guardian*

[38] Hospital operation 'long waiters' rise by 163% *BBC*

[39] Growing waiting times threat to NHS *BBC*

[40] "After Brexit, turning around the NHS is Theresa May's most urgent task". *The Independent.* 11 August 2016. Retrieved 8 October 2016.

[41] NHS completely absent from 72-page Autumn Statement document *The Independent*

[42] NHS at breaking point, according to British Medical Association *The Guardian*

[43] NHS trusts post 'unsustainable' £886m third-quarter deficit *The Guardian*

[44] May's inconvenient truth: the NHS cannot carry on as it is *The Guardian*

[45] BMA calls for extra £10bn a year for NHS in Hammond's budget *The Guardian*

[46] NHS forced to provide 4,500 extra beds a day

[47] Stone, Jon (20 September 2016). "NHS budget pressures will leave mental health services underfunded, spending watchdog warns". *The Independent.* Retrieved 8 October 2016.

[48] 2016 was the worst year in NHS history – we must fight for its survival *The Guardian*

[49] NHS mental health funding is still lagging behind, says report *The Guardian*

[50] 'This isn't acceptable': outcry at state of NHS mental health care funding *The Guardian*

[51] Young people's mental health care is 'inadequate' according to specialist nurses *BBC*

[52] Self-harm hospital admissions of children show 'frightening rise' *BBC*

[53] Children in UK mental health hospitals 'not improving', parents say *The Guardian*

[54] Mentally ill patients face 'double whammy' of poor hospital care *The Guardian*

[55] Doctors' low morale 'puts patients at risk' *BBC*

[56] NHS Health Check: Short GP consultations crazy, say GPs *BBC*

[57] GP consultations too short for complex cases, says doctors' leader *The Guardian*

[58] Proposals for seven-day NHS are immoral, says leading GP *The Guardian*

[59] Two-thirds of young hospital doctors under serious stress, survey reveals *The Guardian*

[60] "Underfunded, underdoctored, overstretched: The NHS in 2016". 21 September 2016.

[61] Senior GP Helen Stokes-Lampard voices fears for services *BBC*

[62] Why our healthcare crisis won't be over anytime soon *New Statesman*

[63] Doctor shortage left 4m patients without cover last year *The Guardian*

[64] "NHS is underfunded, underdoctored and in crisis, doctors warn - GPonline".

[65] Thousands of doctors trained in Europe 'may quit UK after Brexit' *The Guardian*

[66] "Starved NHS 'at point of no return' and 'no longer envy of the world'".

[67] Wards dangerously understaffed, say nurses in survey *BBC*

[68] The hidden crisis in the National Health Service *New Statesman*

[69] NHS plans closures and radical cuts to combat growing deficit in health budget *The Guardian*

[70] mamk (February 23, 2017). "Brexit gelungenn, Patient tot" (in German). Der Spiegel. Retrieved February 23, 2017.

[71] Poll shows 60% of European doctors are considering leaving UK *The Guardian*

[72] "Is the NHS being privatised?". The King's Fund. 19 March 2015. Retrieved 11 October 2016.

[73] Privatisation and independent sector provision of NHS healthcare *BMA*

[74] Bevan, Gwyn; Mays, Nicholas (11 April 2014). "The four health systems of the UK: How do they compare?". Nuffield Trust. Retrieved 2 February 2016.

[75] "Outcomes in EHCI 2015" (PDF). Health Consumer Powerhouse. 26 January 2016. Retrieved 27 January 2016.

[76] Timmins, Nick. "The four UK health systems: Learning from each other,". *Kings Fund*. Retrieved 2 February 2016.

2.5.10   Further reading

- Brady, Robert A. *Crisis in Britain. Plans and Achievements of the Labour Government* (1950) pp 352–41 excerpt

- Gorsky, Martin. "The British National Health Service 1948–2008: A Review of the Historiography," *Social History of Medicine,* Dec 2008, Vol. 21 Issue 3, pp 437–460

- Hacker, Jacob S. "The Historical Logic of National Health Insurance: Structure and Sequence in the Development of British, Canadian, and U.S. Medical Policy," *Studies in American Political Development,* April 1998, Vol. 12 Issue 1, pp 57–130.

- Loudon, Irvine, John Horder and Charles Webster. *General Practice under the National Health Service 1948-1997* (1998) online

- Rintala, Marvin. *Creating the National Health Service: Aneurin Bevan and the Medical Lords* (2003) online.

- Rivett G C From *Cradle to Grave – the first 50 (65) years of the NHS.* King's Fund, London, 1998 now updated to 2014 and available at www.nhshistory.co.uk

- Stewart, John. "The Political Economy of the British National Health Service, 1945–1975: Opportunities and Constraints," *Medical History,* Oct 2008, Vol. 52 Issue 4, pp 453–470

- Valier, Helen K. "The Manchester Royal Infirmary, 1945–97: a microcosm of the National Health Service," *Bulletin of the John Rylands University Library of Manchester,* 2005, Vol. 87 Issue 1, pp 167–192

- Webster, Charles. "Conflict and Consensus: Explaining the British Health Service," *Twentieth Century British History,* April 1990, Vol. 1 Issue 2, pp 115–151

- Webster, Charles. *Health Services since the War. 'Vol. 1:' Problems of Health Care. The National Health Service before 1957* (1988) 479pp online

2.5.11   External links

- NHS Choices official website for England's NHS

- Health and Social Care in Northern Ireland official website for Health & Personal Social Services in Northern Ireland

- NHS Scotland official website for NHS Scotland

- Health in Wales official website for NHS Wales

- Birth of the national Health Service *BBC* archive collection of programmes and documents

2.6 PAMI

This article is about the public health insurance agency in Argentina. For Egyptian Pharaoh, see Pami.
For the journal, see IEEE Transactions on Pattern Analysis and Machine Intelligence.

PAMI (Spanish: *Programa de Atención Médica Integral*; English: Comprehensive Medical Attention Program) is a public health insurance agency in Argentina managed by the Ministry of Health.

2.6.1 Overview

Administered under the aegis of the *Instituto Nacional de Servicios Sociales para Jubilados y Pensionados* (National Institute of Social Services for Retirees and Pensioners, or INSSJP), PAMI serves senior citizens, the indigent, and veterans of the 1982 Falklands War.

PAMI maintains 36 regional offices and 550 local offices for its over 4 million enrollees. The agency provides free medicine to 650,000 pensioners and retirees, 87% of whom earn the minimum pension of around us$300 a month.[1][2] Another 13% receive a benefit of the high cost of their treatment, in cases where this exceeds a retiree's income. The agency covers 100% of the cost of drugs to treat cancer, AIDS, and other chronic medical conditions. Medications for hypertension, which affects nearly nine of out of ten seniors in Argentina, are covered with an 80% discount, including prescription drugs for cholesterol and cardiovascular disease.[1] The agency covers over 2,000 stent insertions annually,[3] as well as over 6,000 pacemaker implants (70% of those provided in Argentina).[1]

PAMI covers around 25 million doctor's visits and nearly 2 million prescriptions annually.[3] Surgical procedures covered by the agency in 2009 included over 55,000 for cataracts, 50,000 intraocular lenses, 20,000 hip and knee surgeries, and 700 organ transplants.[1] Other benefits include kinesiology, legal aid, mental health, and funeral expense assistance.[4] Benefits represent 10% of the total pension payments issued by ANSES, the national social security agency. The real market value of the medical services, medicine, and other services provided by PAMI, however, amount to 30% of retirees' income. the total expenditure on drugs for PAMI in 2010 was almost us$750 million; were retirees to pay the market price of these drugs, their cost would have approximated us$3 billion. Private health insurance is widely available in Argentina. The cost of premiums for those over age 60 would be unaffordable to most retirees, however, as these average around us$150 per person per month.[1]

2.6.2 History

Historically, health expenses in Argentina were met on an out-of-pocket basis, or through a number of mutual aid societies and health care co-operatives established by guilds, as well as by immigrant associations. Health care co-operatives developed into employer and trade union sponsored *obras sociales* beginning in 1910. They expanded rapidly during the administration of President Juan Perón from 1946 to 1955, when unionization was fostered.[5] Health coverage for senior citizens remained sparse, however, and those who could retain their *obra social* generally received less adequate care than younger enrollees.[3]

PAMI was thus established to absorb the growing number of seniors on the initiative of Social Welfare Minister Francisco Manrique, and was signed into law by President Alejandro Lanusse via Decree 19.032, on May 13, 1971.[3] The insurer functioned only in Buenos Aires at its outset, though by 1976, it had opened offices in all the nation's provinces. PAMI established a network of affiliated general practitioners,[3] and negotiated rates and prices with other *obras sociales*, health care federations such as the Argentine Medical Association, and with local governments.[6] It also financed other needs affecting seniors, notably a mortgage loan program benefiting thousands whose homes were slated for demolition in 1978, during the construction of new freeways in Buenos Aires by Mayor Osvaldo Cacciatore.[3]

The prolonged economic downturn of the 1980s affected the agency's finances, however. President Raúl Alfonsín placed PAMI under Federal intervention in March 1988, and appointed the former Governor of Buenos Aires, Dr. Alejandro Armendáriz, as head of the Crisis Management Commission. The agency's finances were stabilized by September, and the crisis commission was dissolved in favor of a panel presided by Argentina's two leading senior citizens' advocacy groups. PAMI was restored to solvency while adding spousal benefits and vacation subsidies for beneficiaries.[7] Accordingly, Alfonsín signed Law 23.660 on January 5, 1989, which made affiliation in PAMI mandatory for all registered employees, and enacted a 6% payroll tax to that effect.[5][8]

The agency's financial crisis was compounded by a series of administrative crises during the subsequent administration of President Carlos Menem. Menem's third appointee to the post, Matilde Menéndez, and most of her board of advisers would be indicted for fraud stemming from contracts signed during her 1992—94 tenure.[9] The 1995 recession cut its revenues from us$3.1 billion to us$2.4 billion, and led to an us$1.2 billion debt.[10] Alejandro Bramer Markovic was appointed in 1996 with a mandate to eliminate waste, fraud, and abuse at the insurer, only to resign the following year amid accusations of excessive spending on outside auditing services.[11] His successor, Víctor Alderete, remained at the post until the end of Menem's presidency in 1999. His tenure, however, was marked by subcontractor cost overruns, and he faced over 20 charges to that related to these.[12]

PAMI had entered a crisis stage. The agency's annual budget declined to us$900 million in 2003. Coverage, in addition, was managed through a system consisting of 72 intermediaries whose costs reached 50% of the agency's benefits spending, and the resulting deficits at PAMI prompted a reduction in prescription drug coverage to 40% by 2003. These developments led most retirees to opt out of the system, and membership declined from four million in 1992[5] to 900,000 by 2003, or fewer than one fourth of Argentine seniors.[1]

The administrations of Presidents Néstor and Cristina Kirchner prioritized the agency in their budget policy, and from 2003 to 2010, budgets for PAMI increased from 2.6 billion pesos to 15.6 billion pesos, or 500%. Its related social assistance programs were expanded, and 800,000 seniors received nutritional, rent, and other assistance from PAMI. The agency's chronic deficits were reversed, and by 2010, it maintained a reserve fund of around us$1.75 billion. Its enrollment also recovered, and services were provided to a total of 3.7 million patients in 2009, or 89% of the agency's members.[1]

2.6.3 References

[1] "El presupuesto del PAMI aumentó 500 % desde el 2003". *El Libertador*.

[2] "La jubilación mínima subirá a $1.227 en marzo". *InfoBae*.

[3] "El PAMI sufrió hasta ahora 13 intervenciones". *Clarín*.

[4] "Centros de Atención". PAMI.

[5] *Argentina: From Insolvency to Growth*. The World Bank. 1993.

[6] "Historia del PAMI". Portal Geriátrico.

[7] "Alejandro Armendáriz". Municipalidad de Saladillo.

[8] "Ley N° 23.660". Información Legislativa.

[9] "Procesan a ex directores del PAMI". *La Nación*.

[10] "PAMI: admiten que se paga de más en los contratos". *Clarín*.

[11] "PAMI: gastó $ 3.290.000 en auditorías en cinco meses". *La Nación*.

[12] "El PAMI, signado por los escándalos". *La Nación*.

2.6.4 External links

- Official website

2.7 Political positions of Dennis Kucinich

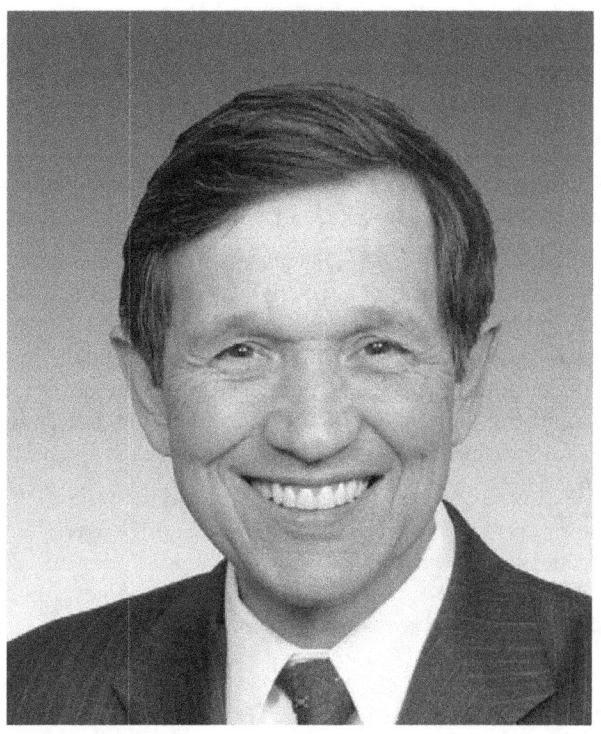

Rep. Kucinich (D-OH)

Dennis John Kucinich (born October 8, 1946) is an American politician, a former representative of Ohio's 10th congressional district (since 1997), a former Mayor of Cleveland (1978–1979), and twice a candidate for President of the United States.[1]

Kucinich is often regarded as one of the most liberal members of the United States House of Representatives.[2][3][4] Describing his views in the 2008 Democratic Party presidential primaries, he said, "I'm from the universal-healthcare wing of the Democratic Party. I'm from the Roe v. Wade-litmus-test wing of the Democratic Party. I'm from the abolish-the-death-penalty wing of the Democratic Party."[5] Dennis Kucinich has also gained reputation as a pacifist. On *The Daily Show with Jon Stewart* he said as he ran for president in 2004 he wanted to end the idea that war is inevitable.[6] He has authored a bill to create a Department of Peace.[7]

2.7.1 Social issues

Abortion

Prior to 2002, Kucinich's voting record was strongly pro-life, but he currently maintains a pro-choice stance on abortion. In 1996, he was quoted as saying that "life begins at conception", and he has also voted in favor on banning partial birth abortion and preventing the transport of minors to undergo abortion procedures. However, since then he has been a strong supporter of abortion rights. He said in a 2003 interview that he had a "journey" regarding the abortion issue which "caused me to break from a voting record that had not been pro-choice."[8]

Kucinich said that, as President, he would not appoint anyone to the U.S. Supreme Court who would vote to repeal the decision of *Roe v. Wade*.[9]

Kucinich supports a woman's right to abort, having stated that "there are circumstances in which a woman and her doctor should be allowed to make this most difficult decision without government intervention." However, he advocates minimizing the number of abortions by use of prevention techniques, including providing sexual education and health care.[10]

He is currently rated 100% by NARAL's Congressional Record on Choice, indicating a pro-choice voting record. Prior to 2003, Kucinich's NARAL rating had never been above 25% in his previous six years in Congress.[11]

Animal rights

Kucinich identifies himself as a vegan, and he is a long-time advocate of the ethical treatment of animals. He has stated that "As a necessary component of the living world, we must extend compassion to one another and to every living thing.".[12]

Civil liberties

The American Civil Liberties Union gave Kucinich a 100% rating on civil liberties for the 2006-2007 legislative session. In addition he has been given an 89% lifetime rating by the ACLU.[13]

Kucinich supports same-sex marriage and opposes the definition of marriage as "between a man and a woman".[14] Rather, he feels that all citizens deserve equal treatment under the law, and should be allowed to choose for themselves whom they want to marry. He has also voted for the expansion of hate crime laws in the United States and against banning LGBT adoption in Washington, D.C.[15]

Kucinich has opposed the USA PATRIOT Act since its inception. He voted against the act in 2001, and against its renewal in 2006. He voted for an amendment to the constitution outlawing flag burning and desecration, however he has since taken up the opposite stance and voted against a similar amendment in 2005.[16]

In 2007, Kucinich voted to require the Department of Defense to present a detailed plan for transferring prisoners out of the Guantanamo Bay detention camp.[16]

D.C. statehood

Kucinich supports giving rights of state to the District of Columbia, including its own executive, legislative and judicial powers and eliminating all federal government committees and/or subcommittees that have oversight or appropriation power over the DC government.

Kucinich supports giving DC an equal and proportional voting delegation in Congress.[17]

Death penalty

Kucinich strongly opposes the death penalty. He states that because human judgments are "fallible and often wrong," we do not have the moral authority to take human life. He advocates elimination of the federal death penalty "even if unpopular" and has introduced a national moratorium on executions. He has contended that 98% of those executed have been poor.[18]

Kucinich has introduced legislation that would abolish the death penalty under federal law.[19]

Drinking age and alcohol education

About the legal drinking age, Kucinich said, "We have to have confidence in young Americans... a president who reaches out to them and talks about drinking responsibly is much better than a president who tells them 'thou shalt not' because young people will do what they do. But they're looking for leadership from a President. I'm ready to provide that leadership. Of course they should be able to drink at age 18, and they should be able to vote at age 16."

Drugs

Kucinich supports marijuana decriminalization for recreational and medical users. He supports penalties for those who provide the drug to minors and endanger others through irresponsible use. He likens the ban on marijuana use to the failed Prohibition policy, which outlawed alcohol.[20]

He has stated that the "war on drugs" has failed, and that "Prison should be for people who hurt other people, not themselves."[21]

Environmental issues

Kucinich had a 100% rating during 2005 and 2006 from the League of Conservation Voters, indicating pro-environment votes.[22] He has stated that clean water is "a basic human right".[23]

He proposed a Works Green Administration modeled after Franklin D. Roosevelt's Works Progress Administration during the 2008 presidential election. The initiative would "involve millions of Americans in new energy projects including retrofitting homes with wind and solar micro technologies."[24] Kucinich has been critical of organizations like the World Trade Organization and the North American Free Trade Agreement for their environmental records.[25] In the House of Representatives Kucinich said after the BP oil spill "When we look at the oil disaster in the Gulf of Mexico we learn how far we must journey to reconcile with nature. The false doctrine of subduing the natural world has put us in danger of extinction, because it ultimately attacks the precondition of human existence, and because it separates us from understanding the essential interconnectedness of all life. So were lulled into distancing ourselves from the oil disaster, from its effects on the natural world, from its effects on future generations...Only when we truly understand the deep significance of the Deepwater Horizon disaster will we be prepared to take a new direction, not only with our energy policy, but with our way of life."[26]

Education

Kucinich supports universal education including free access to high quality to pre-kindergarten education beginning at age 3 for any families who want it and tuition-free colleges for many students.[27] He has called the right to high quality free education as one of America's most treasured values.

Gun ownership

Kucinich is graded "F" by the National Rifle Association, indicating a pro-gun control voting record. He also received a 100% lifetime rating from the Brady Campaign to Prevent Gun Violence.[28] In 2007 he introduced legislation that would have banned handguns.[29]

Health care

Kucinich believes that health care is a "right in a democratic society".[30] He is a critic of the for-profit health insurance and pharmaceutical industries in the United States, and is concerned about the large number of uninsured and underinsured in the United States.[5] He contends that if the overhead related to the for-profit insurance system, such as "stock options, executive salaries, [and] advertising", were used for medically necessary care, he says, there would be enough money in the system to cover all people at no extra cost.[30]

To this end, Kucinich prefers a national health insurance program for health care reform in the United States. He is a cosponsor of HR 676, a bill to do this by extending the national insurance program for the elderly, Medicare, to all American citizens.[31] He also supports the lifting of the prohibitions on the reimportation of prescription drugs from Canada and on Medicare negotiating prescription drug prices with drug companies.[32]

Kucinich Amendment In July 2009, the House Education and Labor Committee approved an amendment authored by Kucinich to its version of the unsuccessful America's Affordable Health Choices Act of 2009 by a vote of 27-19, with 14 Democrats and 13 Republicans voting for it.[33] The amendment empowers the Secretary of Health and Human Services to waive the federal law that pre-empts state law on employee-related health care, the Employee Retirement Income Security Act, in response to state requests.[34] It has been speculated that the amendment's bipartisan support was for its appeal to states' rights in supporting progressive legislation.[33] In the past, states attempting to enact single-payer reforms have been successfully sued and stopped under ERISA.[34] It has also been speculated that this law's passage would open up vital new avenues for promoting, and actually implementing a single-payer system for the United States, as newly unbound states would show single-payer's success, just as Saskatchewan did for Canada.[33] However, the Kucinich Amendment was stripped from the merged House bill. Speaker Nancy Pelosi said that it would have violated President Obama's promise that Americans who liked their health insurance could keep it.[35]

Kucinich's healthcare vote On November 7, 2009, Kucinich voted with 38 other Democrats (mostly Blue Dogs) and 176 Republicans against the Affordable Health-care for America Act because he believed the bill "incentivizes the perpetuation, indeed the strengthening, of the for-profit health insurance industry, the very source of the problem."[36] In his press release for why he voted as he had, Kucinich continues, "In H.R. 3962, the government is requiring at least 21 million Americans to buy private health insurance from the very industry that causes costs to be so high, which will result in at least $70 billion in new annual revenue, much of which is coming from taxpayers. This inevitably will lead to even more costs, more subsidies, and higher profits for insurance companies — a bailout under a blue cross.... The 'robust public option' which would have offered a modicum of competition to a monopolistic industry was whittled down from an initial potential enrollment of 129 million Americans to 6 million. An amendment which would have protected the rights of states to pursue single-payer health care was stripped from the bill at the request of the Administration.... America will someday come to recognize the broad social and economic benefits of a not-for-profit, single-payer health care system, which is good for the American people and good for America's businesses, with of course the notable exceptions being insurance and pharmaceuticals."[36] Unlike many, if not all, of his fellow democrats who voted against the bill, Kucinich has not been the target of scorn from liberal media outlets, but has instead been well received as being a man of conviction to his goal of a single-payer system.[37] When the bill comes out of conference committee, Kucinich will have the opportunity to vote for final passage of the bill, or vote 'no' as he previously had. The bill has been differed from conference committee due to a perceived time constraint, so the House and Senate are now playing political ping-pong to create the final bill.[38] However, he changed his vote to a yes in March 2010.[39]

Immigration

Kucinich has said that "Welcoming immigrants to our shores is one of our country's vital traditions." He supports immigration reform and giving resident undocumented workers "a clear road map to legal status".[40] In 2001, Kucinich was a co-sponsor of H.R. 500, which would have given legal status to all those living in the U.S. for at least five years.[41]

2.7.2 Foreign policy

Israel and Palestine

Kucinich spoke in the House of Representatives opposing H. Res. 34 which would recognize Israel's right to defend itself as he claims the resolution was incomplete in examining the conflict. He said "The Israeli Army evacuated 100 Palestinians to a house, and then bombed the house, killing 30 people. They don't have bomb shelters in Gaza. Emergency workers have been blocked by the Israeli Army from reaching hundreds of injured persons. Today's *Washington Post* headline documents that. We all want peace, but we're not going to get peace until we recognize that there are two parties to this dispute and that we have to also review Israel's conduct as well. That path to peace has to begin with stopping the war, having a cease-fire, constructing a truce, ending the blockade, getting humanitarian assistance through to all the people, rebuilding the infrastructure of the Palestinians, rebuilding their economic possibilities, bringing Hamas and Israel together for talks, using that as the basis to the path for peace in the Middle East."[42]

Venezuela

Kucinich was the only member in the House of Representatives to condemn US interference in Venezuela's internal affairs in a letter signed by Jesse Jackson, Howard Zinn, Edward Asner, Saul Landau, Naomi Klein, Doug Henwood, and others. The letter also praising Hugo Chavez's Bolivarian Revolution said "The world knows that you are achieving something remarkable in Venezuela: you are investing your country's vast oil wealth in ways that benefit everyone, not just small minority of well-connected elites. Over the last year your government's literacy campaign taught one million Venezuelans to read. And today, millions of others are benefiting from the governments investment in job training, small businesses and health care...We are committed to doing what we can, as U.S. citizens, to heal those relationships and encourage Congress and the White House to see Venezuela not only as a model democracy but also as a model of how a country's oil wealth can be used to benefit all of its people."[43]

Afghanistan

Kucinich voted in favor of going to war against Afghanistan after the 9/11 attacks, but has since been an opponent of the ongoing War in Afghanistan citing costs, corruption of the Karzai government, deaths of NATO troops, deaths of innocent Afghan civilians, and the fact that occupation is fueling insurgency as a reason for withdrawal of military forces. He has led the opposition against the war by demanding withdrawal under the War Powers Act. Kucinich has called Obama's classification of the War in Afghanistan as a just war a beginning of an Orwellian journey to a world where war is peace and also said "Wars in Afghanistan and Pakistan are based on flawed doctrines of counter-insurgency. War is often not just; sometimes it is just war. And our ability to rethink the terms of our existence, to explore the possibility of peace without war, may well determine whether we end war, or war ends us."[44]

Cuba

Kucinich favors normalizing relations with Cuba. He advocates a full repeal of the Helms-Burton Act and the immediate lifting of the trade embargo and travel restrictions. He claims that America's "aggressive rhetoric and actions" have not helped US interests, but have hurt the Cuban people.[45]

Iran

Kucinich believes that the US should engage in direct diplomacy with Iran. He has claimed that the Bush administration was purposely escalating tensions with Iran and preparing to use military force without Congressional authorization.[46] After a December 3, 2007 National Intelligence Estimate report indicated that Iran was not developing nuclear weapons, Kucinich stated that it was clear that there was "no threat to the international community from Iran right now, or in the near future."[47]

Iraq war

Kucinich voted against the authorization of military force against Iraq in 2002. He has also voted consistently against funding the war.[48]

Kucinich cited the war as one of his primary reasons for entering the 2008 presidential race. He said that the 2006 mid-term elections were a message that Americans were unhappy with the situation in Iraq. "Instead of heeding those concerns and responding with a strong and immediate change in policies and direction," Kucinich said, "the Democratic congressional leadership seems inclined to continue funding the perpetuation of the war."[49]

The "Kucinich Plan" for Iraq includes an immediate withdrawal of all US troops and contractors, as well as the closing of military bases, to be replaced with a UN peacekeeping force. He would also work towards rebuilding the Iraqi infrastructure and economy, and "repair[ing] our relationship with Iraqis and with the world".[50]

Military intervention in Libya

Kucinich objected to the 2011 Military intervention in Libya missile strikes and questioned whether they weren't impeachable offenses. Kucinich also questioned why Democratic leaders didn't object when President Barack Obama told them of his plan for US participation in enforcing the Libyan no-fly zone. He said Obama's action in Libya was "a grave decision that cannot be made by the president alone", and claimed that failing to first seek approval of Congress was in violation of the Constitution.[51][52]

Military intervention in Syria

Kucinich objected to a prospective United States war with Russia in Syria in October 2016.[53]

2.7.3   Economic issues

Trade

Kucinich opposes participation in North American Free Trade Agreement (NAFTA) and the World Trade Organization (WTO). He says that "one of my first acts as president will be to cancel NAFTA and the WTO."[54] Kucinich has consistently opposed free trade on the grounds that it costs American jobs and enables abusive working conditions in other countries.[55]

Farm policy

"Something is wrong when profits of agribusiness corporations skyrocket, but farmers must find off-farm jobs or sell their farms to survive," says Kucinich on his website. Kucinich has been an opponent of market led agrarian reform and has advocated canceling NAFTA and the WTO and replacing them with bilateral agreements that benefit farmers, empowering farmers by providing incentives to join collective bargaining units, breaking apart agribusiness monopolies through enforcing anti-trust laws, shifting towards local food systems such as a farm-to-school program, reducing environmental impacts through safeguarding family farms from factory farm pollution, and restoring family farms in the United States.[56] Kucinich has also said he gives "strong and unwavering support to our organic family farmers.[57]

Social Security

Kucinich has been opposed to the privatization of social security. On the topic of retirement he said "I see a new vision for American seniors. I see a country where all citizens can retire with full benefits at age 65, where social security will never become privatized, and where retirement years won't land in the hands of the stock market."[58]

Tax policy

Kucinich introduced the Progressive Tax Act of 2003, which was designed to repeal what he called the "unfair Bush tax cuts" for wealthy Americans and corporate tax loopholes.[59][60] He also favors simplifying the tax code and a Payroll Tax Credit and a Family Credit.

2.7.4 See also

- Dennis Kucinich presidential campaign, 2008
- United States presidential election, 2008

2.7.5 References

[1] Dennis Kucinich Dropping Out Of Presidential Race Newsday.com. Accessed 24-January 2008

[2] Klein, Joe (2009-08-20). "The GOP Has Become a Party of Nihilists". Time magazine. Retrieved 2009-08-20.

[3] Hechtkopf, Kevin (2009-08-18). "Artist Behind Obama "Joker" Picture Revealed". CBS News. Retrieved 2009-08-20.

[4] March, William (2003-11-29). "Kucinich Hit Stage As Cleveland Mayor". The Tampa Tribune. p. 15.

[5] Curry, Tom (2008-07-14). "Kucinich spices up the race". MSNBC. Retrieved 2009-08-20.

[6]

[7]

[8] David Enrich, Kucinich's Continued Evolution National Review, June 9, 2003

[9] Dennis Kucinich at November 2007 Democratic Presidential Debate

[10] Issues - Reproductive Rights Kucinich.us

[11] Congressional Record on Choice by State NARAL.org

[12] Issues - Animal Rights Kucinich.us

[13] Tom Head Congressional Scorecard ACLU.org

[14] Tom Diemer and Sabrina Eaton, Kucinich supports marriage for same-sex couples, Cleveland Plain Dealer, July 16, 2003

[15] 2008 Presidential Candidates' Positions TheTaskForce.org

[16] Representative Dennis J. Kucinich, VoteSmart.org

[17] Issues - D.C. Statehood Kucinich.us

[18] Issues - Death Penalty Kucinich.us

[19] H.R.4923 - Federal Death Penalty Abolition Act OpenCongress.org

[20] Issues - Marijuana Decriminalization Kucinich.us

[21] Issues - Drug War Kucinich.us

[22] Representative Dennis J. Kucinich, LCV.org

[23] Dennis Kucinich: The Candidates in Print Time.com

[24]

[25]

[26]

[27] http://education.kucinich.us/

[28] Interest Group Ratings - Gun Issues VoteSmart.org

[29] "Kucinich Offers Comprehensive Plan to Address Violence in America" (Press release). April 18, 2007. Archived from the original on December 12, 2012.

[30] Martin, Michel (2009-05-12). "White House Looks For Ways To Lower Health Care Costs". National Public Radio. Retrieved 2009-08-20.

[31] Kucinich, Dennis (2009-07-15). "Healthcare: Change the Debate Support a Real Public Option". kucinich.us. Retrieved 2009-08-20.

[32] "Kucinich: Eliminate Medicare Part D drug program". McKnight's Long-Term Care News & Assisted Living. 2008-08-11. Retrieved 2009-08-20.

[33] Nichols, John (2009-07-17). "A Real Win for Single-Payer Advocates". The Beat. The Nation. Retrieved 2009-08-18.

[34] "Kucinich Amendment Grants ERISA Waiver for Single Payer States.". Center for Policy Analysis. Archived from the original on August 18, 2009. Retrieved 2009-08-18.

[35] Grim, Ryan (2009-11-06). "Pelosi: Single-Payer Amendment Breaks Obama's Health Care Promise". The Huffington Post. Common Dreams NewsCenter.

[36] http://kucinich.house.gov/NEWS/DocumentSingle.aspx?DocumentID=153995

[37] Stranahan, Lee (2009-11-08). "Kucinich's Brave Health Vote vs. Obama's Failed Promise". Huffington Post.

[38] http://www.huffingtonpost.com/.../dems-will-bypass-conferen_n_410403.html

[39] http://www.cleveland.com/open/index.ssf/2010/03/rep_dennis_kucinichs_health_ca.html

[40] Issues - Immigrants' Rights Kucinich.us

[41] H.R. 500 [107th]: U.S. Employee, Family Unity, and Legalization Act GovTrack.us

[42]

[43]

[44]

[45] Issues - Cuban Embargo Kucinich.us

[46] Dennis J. Kucinich, Collision Course With Iran TheNation.com, Feb. 26, 2007

[47] Kucinich Slams Bush Over Iran Report All Headline News, Dec. 3, 2007

[48] Use of Military Force Against Iraq VoteSmart.org

[49] Zachary A. Goldfarb and Peter Slevin, Unhappy With Democrats Over Iraq, Kucinich Plans Another Bid for White House, Washington Post, December 12, 2006

[50] The Kucinich Plan for Iraq Kucinich.us

[51] Liberal Democrats in uproar over Libya action; *Politico*; March 19, 2011

[52] Dennis Kucinich: Obama's Libya Attack An Impeachable Offense; Talking Points Memo; March 21, 2011

[53] Kucinich, Dennis (October 26, 2016). "Why Is the Foreign Policy Establishment Spoiling for More War? Look at Their Donors.". *The Nation*. Retrieved October 27, 2016. The American people are fed up with war, but a concerted effort is being made through fearmongering, propaganda, and lies to prepare our country for a dangerous confrontation, with Russia in Syria. [...] I'm fed up with the DC policy elite who cash in on war while presenting themselves as experts, at the cost of other people's lives, our national fortune, and the sacred honor of our country.

[54] Campaign for America's Future June 20, 2007 Speech

[55] The Candidates on Trade Council on Foreign Relations

[56]

[57]

[58]

[59] Tax Reform House.gov

[60] H.R.3655 Library of Congress

2.8　Public health insurance option

The **public health insurance option**, also known as the **public insurance option** or the **public option**, is a proposal to create a government-run health insurance agency which would compete with other private health insurance companies within the United States. The public option is not the same as publicly funded health care, but was proposed as an alternative health insurance plan offered by the government. The public option was initially proposed for the Patient Protection and Affordable Care Act, but was removed after Sen. Joe Lieberman (I-CT) threatened a filibuster.[1][2]

2.8.1　History

Debate in 2009-10

The public option was featured in three bills considered by the United States House of Representatives in 2009: the proposed Affordable Health Care for America Act (H.R. 3962), which was passed by the House in 2009, its predecessor, the proposed America's Affordable Health Choices Act (H.R. 3200), and a third bill, the Public Option Act, also referred to as the "Medicare You Can Buy Into Act", (H.R. 4789). In the first two bills, the public option took the form of a Qualified Health Benefit Plan competing with similar private insurance plans in an internet-based exchange or marketplace, enabling citizens and small businesses to purchase health insurance meeting a minimum federal standard. The Public Option Act, in contrast, would have allowed all citizens and permanent residents to buy into a public option by participating in the public Medicare program. Persons covered by other employer plans or by state insurance plans such as Medicare would have not been eligible to obtain coverage from the exchange. The federal government's health insurance plan would have been financed entirely by premiums without subsidy from the Federal government,[3] although some plans called for government seed money to get the programs started.[4]

President Barack Obama promoted the idea of the public option while running for election in 2008.[5] Following his election, Obama downplayed the need for a public health insurance option, including calling it a "sliver" of health care reform,[6] but still campaigned for the option up until the health care reform was passed.[7]

Ultimately, the public option was removed from the final bill. While the United States House of Representatives passed a public option in their version of the bill, the public option was voted down in the Senate Finance Committee[8] and the public option was never included in the final Senate bill, instead opting for state-directed health insurance exchanges.[9] Critics of the removal of the public option accused President Obama of making an agreement to drop the public option from the final plan,[10] but the record showed that the agreement was based on vote counts than backroom deals, as substantiated by the final vote in the Senate.[11]

Since 2010

In January 2013, Representative Jan Schakowsky and 44 other U.S. House of Representatives Democrats introduced H.R. 261, the "Public Option Deficit Reduction Act" which would amend the Affordable Care Act to create a public option. The bill would set up a government-run health insurance plan with premiums 5% to 7% percent lower than private insurance. The Congressional Budget Office estimated it would reduce the United States public debt by $104 billion over 10 years.[12] Representative Schakowsky reintroduced the bill as H.R. 265 in January 2015, where it gained 35 cosponsors.[13]

In the run-up to the 2016 Democratic National Convention, the Democratic Platform Committee approved a plank supporting the addition of a public option onto the Affordable Care Act.[14] The decision was seen as a compromise measure between the Hillary Clinton campaign who during the 2016 presidential primaries advocated for keeping and reforming the ACA, and the Bernie Sanders campaign who advocated for repealing and replacing the ACA with a single-payer Medicare for All program. The Clinton campaign stated shortly before the plank was added that as president Clinton would "pursue efforts to give Americans in every state in the country the choice of a public-option insurance plan", while Bernie Sanders applauded the decision to "see that all Americans have the right to choose a public option in their health care exchange, which will lower the cost of healthcare".[15][16] The call was echoed by President Obama, who in an article for the American Medical Association stated that Congress "should revisit a public plan to compete alongside private insurers in areas of the country where competition is limited."[17]

2.8.2 Rationale

See also: Health care reform debate in the United States

The purpose behind the public option was to make more affordable health insurance for uninsured citizens who are either unable to afford the rates of or are rejected by private health insurers. Supporters argued that a government insurance company could successfully lower its rates by using greater leverage than private industry when negotiating with hospitals and doctors,[18] as well as paying the employees of the public option insurance company salaries as opposed to

paying based on individual medical procedures.[19]

Supporters of a public plan, such as *Washington Post* columnist E. J. Dionne, argue that many places in the United States have monopolies in which one company, or a small set of companies, control the local market for health insurance. Economist and *New York Times* columnist Paul Krugman also wrote that local insurance monopolies exist in many of the smaller states, accusing those who oppose the idea of a public insurance plan as defenders of local monopolies. He also argued that traditional ideas of beneficial market competition do not apply to the insurance industry given that insurers mainly compete by risk selection, claiming that "[t]he most successful companies are those that do the best job of denying coverage to those who need it most."[20]

Economist and former US Secretary of Labor Robert Reich argued that only a "big, national, public option" can force insurance companies to cooperate, share information, and reduce costs while accusing insurance and pharmaceutical companies of leading the campaign against the public option.[21][22]

Many Democratic politicians were publicly in favor of the public option for a variety of reasons. President Obama continued campaigning for the public option during the debate. In a public rally in Cincinnati on September 7, 2009, President Obama said: "I continue to believe that a public option within the basket of insurance choices would help improve quality and bring down costs."[23] The President also addressed a Joint Session of Congress on September 9, 2009, reiterating his call for a public insurance option, saying that he had "no interest in putting insurance companies out of business" while saying that the public option would "have to be self-sufficient" and succeed by reducing overhead costs and profit motives.[24] Democratic Representative Sheila Jackson-Lee, who represents the 18th congressional district in Houston, believed that a "vigorous public option" would be included in the final bill and would "benefit the state of Texas."[25]

Alternative plans

See also: Single-payer health care § Proposals for a single-payer system in the United States, and Patient Protection and Affordable Care Act

The final bill, the Patient Protection and Affordable Care Act, included provisions to open health insurance exchanges in each state by October 1, 2013. As the Act requires Americans to purchase health insurance, the federal government will offer subsidies to Americans with income levels up to four times the federal poverty level.[26]

An alternative proposal is to subsidize private, non-profit health insurance cooperatives to get them to become large and established enough to possibly provide cost savings[27][28] Democratic politicians such as Howard Dean were critical of abandoning a public option in favor of co-ops, raising questions about the ability of the cooperatives to compete with existing private insurers.[6] Paul Krugman also questioned the ability of cooperatives to compete.[29]

While politically difficult, some politicians and observers have argued for a single-payer system.[30] A bill, the United States National Health Care Act, was first proposed by Representative John Conyers in 2003[31] and has been perennially proposed since, including during the debate on the public option and the Patient Protection and Affordable Care Act.[32] President Obama has come out against a single-payer reform at this time, stating in the joint session of Congress that "it makes more sense to build on what works and fix what doesn't, rather than try to build an entirely new system from scratch."[33] Obama had previously expressed that he is a proponent of a single payer universal health care program during an AFL-CIO conference in 2003.[34]

A number of alternatives to the public option were proposed in the Senate. Instead of creating a network of statewide public plans, Senator Olympia Snowe proposed a "trigger" in which a plan would be put into place at some point in the future in states that do not have more than a certain number of private insurance competitors. Senator Tom Carper has proposed an "opt-in" system in which state governments choose for themselves whether or not to institute a public plan. Senator Chuck Schumer has proposed an "opt-out" system in which state governments would initially be part of the network but could choose to avoid offering a public plan.[35]

In January 2013, Representative Jan Schakowsky and 44 other U.S. House of Representatives Democrats introduced H.R. 261, the "Public Option Deficit Reduction Act" which would amend the 2010 Affordable Care Act to create a public option. The bill would set up a government-run health insurance plan with premiums 5% to 7% percent lower than private insurance, with the Congressional Budget Office estimating a reduction in the United States public debt by $104 billion over 10 years.[12]

2.8.3 Opposition and criticism

See also: Health care reform debate in the United States

Both before and after passage in the House, significant controversy surrounded the Stupak–Pitts Amendment, added to the bill to prohibit coverage of abortions – with limited exceptions – in the public option or in any of the health insurance exchange's private plans sold to customers receiving federal subsidies. In mid-November, it was reported that 40 House Democrats would not support a final bill containing the Amendment's provisions.[36] The Amendment was abandoned after a deal was struck between Representative Bart Stupak and his voting bloc would vote for the bill as written in exchange for the signing of Executive Order 13535.

Republican House Minority Whip Eric Cantor has argued that a public plan would compete unfairly with private insurers and drive many of them out of business.[37]

Michael F. Cannon, a senior fellow of the libertarian CATO Institute, has argued that the federal government can hide inefficiencies in its administration and draw away consumers from private insurance even if the government offers an inferior product. A study by the Congressional Budget Office found that profits accounted for only about 4 or 5 percent of private health insurance premiums, and Cannon argued that the lack of a profit motive reduces incentives to eliminate wasteful administrative costs.[38]

Dr. Robert E. Moffit of the Heritage Foundation has argued that a public plan in competition in private plans would likely be used as a "dumping ground" for families and individuals with higher than average health risks. This, in his view, would lead to costs that business should pay being passed onto the taxpayer.[39]

Marcia Angell, M. D., Senior Lecturer in the Department of Social Medicine at Harvard Medical School and former Editor-in-Chief of the New England Journal of Medicine, believes that the result of a public option would be more "under-55's" opting to pay the fine rather than purchase insurance under a public option scenario, instead advocating lowering the Medicare age to 55.[40]

The chief executive of Aetna, Ron Williams, argued against the public option based on issues of fairness. On the *News Hour with Jim Lehrer*, Williams noted that a public option creates a situation where "you have in essence a player in the industry who is a participant in the market, but also is a regulator and a referee in the game". He said, "we think that those two roles really don't work well."[41]

2.8.4 Public opinion

Further information: Public opinion on health care reform in the United States

Public polling consistently showed majority support for a public option. A July 2009 survey by the Quinnipiac University Polling Institute found that 28% of Americans would like to purchase a public plan while 53% would prefer to have a private plan. It also stated that 69% would support its creation in the first place.[42] Survey USA estimated that the majority of Americans (77%) feel that it is either "Quite Important" or "Extremely Important" to "give people a choice of both a public plan administered by the federal government and a private plan for their health insurance" in August 2009.[43] A Rasmussen Reports poll taken on August 17–18 stated that 57% of Americans did not support the current health care bill being considered by Congress that did not include a public option,[44] a change from their findings in July 2009.[45] A NBC News/*Wall Street Journal* poll, conducted August 15–17, found that 47% of Americans opposed the idea of a public option and 43% expressed support.[46] A Pew Research Center report published on October 8, 2009 stated that 55% of Americans favor a government health insurance plan to compete with private plans. The results were very similar to their polling from July, which found 52% support.[47] An October 2009 *Washington Post*/ABC poll showed 57% support,[48] a *USA Today*/Gallup survey described by a *USA Today* article on October 27 found that 50% of Americans supported a government plan proposal,[49] and a poll from November 10 and 11 by Angus Reid Public Opinion found that 52% of Americans supported a public plan.[50] On October 27, journalist Ray Suarez of *The News Hour with Jim Lehrer* noted that "public opinion researchers say the tide has been shifting over the last several weeks, and now is not spectacularly, but solidly in favor of a public option."[51]

Between October 28 and November 13, 2009, Democratic Senator Dick Durbin's campaign organization polled Americans to rank their support for various forms of the "public option" currently under consideration by Congress for inclusion in the final health care reform bill. The 83,954 respondents assigned rankings of 0 to 10. A full national option had the most support, with an 8.56 average, while no public option was least favored, with a 1.10 average.[52]

Physician reaction

A survey designed and conducted by Drs. Salomeh Keyhani and Alex Federman of Mount Sinai School of Medicine done over the summer of 2009 found that 73% of doctors supported a public option.[53] A survey reported by the *New England Journal of Medicine* in September, based on a random sample of 6,000 physicians from the American Medical Association, stated that "it seems clear that the majority of U.S. physicians support using both public and private insurance options to expand coverage."[54]

Conversely, an IBD/TIPP poll of 1,376 physicians showed that 45% of doctors "would consider leaving or taking early retirement" if Congress passes the health care plan wanted by the White House and Democrats. This poll also found that 65% of physicians oppose the White House and Demo-

cratic version of health reform.[55] Statistician and polling expert Nate Silver has criticized that IBD/TIPP poll for what he calls its unusual methodology and bias and for the fact that it was incomplete when published as responses were still coming in.[56]

2.8.5 See also

- Health care compared
- Health care reform in the United States
- Publicly funded health care
- SustiNet

2.8.6 Notes

[1] Lieberman: I'll block vote on Reid plan, By Manu Raju, Politico.com, 10/27/09

[2] Helen A. Halpin, Peter Harbage (June 2010). "The Origins And Demise Of The Public Option". *Health Aff*. **29** (6): 1117–1124. doi:10.1377/hlthaff.2010.0363. PMID 20530340.

[3] Why We Need a Public Health-Care Plan Robert Reich *The Wall Street Journal*

[4] e.g. House Bill H.R.3962 Section 322 (b)2(B) "AMORTIZATION OF START-UP FUNDING- The Secretary shall provide for the repayment of the startup funding provided under subparagraph (A) to the Treasury in an amortized manner over the 10-year period beginning with Y1". The Senate HLP Committee bill contains a similar clause in § 3106 "A Health Benefit Plan Start-up Fund will be created to provide loans for initial operations, which the plan will be required to pay back no later than 10 years after the payment is made."

[5] Wangsness, Lisa (June 21, 2009). "Health debate shifting to public vs. private". Boston Globe. Retrieved September 21, 2009.

[6] Kranish, Michael (August 19, 2009). "Health co-ops' fans like cost and care: But successful models still rare nationwide". The Boston Globe.

[7] Obama, Congress easing debate on public option - Beaver County Times

[8] CNN: Senate panel votes down public option for health care bill. September 29, 2009.

[9] Bankrate: Key details of health reform bills.

[10] David D. Kirkpatrick, August 12, 2009, "Obama is taking an active role in talks on health care plan," New York Times, http://www.nytimes.com/2009/08/13/health/policy/13health.html

[11] *Washington Post*: Obama never secretly killed the public option. It's a myth.. November 17, 2011.

[12] "House Dems push again for creation of government-run health insurance option" *The Hill*, January 16, 2013

[13] "Cosponsors: H.R.265 — 114th Congress (2015-2016)" *Congress.gov*, August 5, 2016

[14] Alex Seitz-Wald, Democrats Advance Most Progressive Platform in Party History, NBC News (July 10, 2016).

[15] *Hillary Clinton: The Briefing*: Hillary Clinton's Commitment: Universal, Quality, Affordable Health Care for Everyone in America. July 9, 2016.

[16] *Truth Out*: Sanders Cites Democratic Platform, Public Option as Basis for Endorsing Clinton. July 13, 2016.

[17] *NPR*: Obama Renews Call For A 'Public Option' In Federal Health Law. July 11, 2016.

[18] Gauvey Herbert, David (January 2, 2011) "Public Option", *National Journal*.

[19] *Washington Post*: 8 Questions About Health-Care Reform.

[20] Paul Krugman (2009-06-22). "Competition, redefined". The New York Times. Retrieved 2009-10-10.

[21] "Robert Reich Public Option Video".

[22] "How Pharma and Insurance Intend to Kill the Public Option, And What Obama and the Rest of Us Must Do". Archived from the original on 2009-06-11.

[23] "Obama: Public option should be part of reform". MSNBC.com. 2009-09-07.

[24] Weiner, Rachel (September 9, 2009). "Obama Health Care Speech: FULL VIDEO, TEXT". *Huffington Post*.

[25] *Houston Chronicle*: Jackson Lee predicts "vigorous public option" on health care. July 31, 2009

[26] CNN: The marketing of Obamacare exchanges begins. June 21, 2013.

[27] Kranish, Michael (August 19, 2009). "Health co-ops' fans like cost and care: But successful models still rare nationwide". The Boston Globe.

[28] Are health care co-ops the answer for reforming the system? - Kansas City Star

[29] *New York Times*: Baucus and the Threshold, Paul Krugman, September 17, 2009

[30] Colliver, Victoria (May 30, 2009). "Health care activists lament single-payer snub". San Francisco Chronicle. Retrieved October 10, 2009.

[31] H.R. 676

[32] "House Reps Introduce Medicare-for-All Bill" *Becker's Hospital Review*, Feb. 14, 2013

[33] Remarks by the President to a joint session of Congress on health care

[34] Obama on single payer health insurance - Youtube

[35] Ezra Klein. "A guide to the public option compromises in the Senate". The Washington Post.

[36] Alec MacGillis, "Health-care reform and abortion coverage: Questions and answers", Washington Post, November 14, 2009.

[37] Molly Hooper, "Cantor: Public option poll 'skewed'", Blog Briefing Room, 10/21/09

[38] Michael F. Cannon (August 6, 2009). "Fannie Med? Why a "Public Option" Is Hazardous to Your Health" (PDF). CATO Institute. Retrieved October 10, 2009.

[39] "Government as "Competitor": The Latest Prescription for Government Control of Health Care". Heritage Foundation. August 14, 2008.

[40] *The Huffington Post*: "Is the House Health Care Bill Better than Nothing?" Marcia Angell, M. D., November 9, 2009.

[41] "Aetna CEO: Public Insurance Option 'Wrong Way to Go'". News Hour with Jim Lehrer. August 18, 2009.

[42] "U.S. Voters Back Public Insurance 2-1, But Won't Use It". Quinnipiac University. July 1, 2009. Retrieved September 4, 2009.

[43] "News Poll #15699 "Health Care Data Gathered Using NBC News Wall Street Journal Questions" on 8/19/09". SurveyUSA. August 20, 2009.

[44] "57% oppose reforming healthcare without including the public option". Rasmussen Reports.

[45] "50% Oppose Government Health Insurance Company". Rasmussen Reports. July 17, 2009. Retrieved August 28, 2009.

[46] Murray, Mark (August 18, 2009). "NBC poll: Plurality opposes public option". MSNBC.com. Retrieved August 27, 2009.

[47] "Mixed Views of Economic Policies and Health Care Reform Persist". Pew Research Center. October 8, 2009. Retrieved October 9, 2009.

[48] *Washington Post*: Public option gains support. October 20, 2009.

[49] Fritze, John (October 27, 2009). "Dems Advance opt-out 'public option'". USA Today.

[50] Connelly, Joel (November 20, 2009). "New Poll: Voters back, but also fear, health reform". *Seattle Post-Intelligencer*.

[51] Archived October 31, 2009, at the Wayback Machine.

[52] Dick Durbin Public Option Poll Results GetActive Software, Inc., 16-Nov-2009

[53] Shapiro, Joseph (September 14, 2009). "Poll Finds Most Doctors Support Public Option". National Public Radio. Retrieved October 10, 2009.

[54] Salomeh Keyhani, M.D., M.P.H., and Alex Federman, M.D., M.P.H. "Doctors on Coverage — Physicians' Views on a New Public Insurance Option and Medicare Expansion" NEJM • September 14th, 2009.

[55] "45% Of Doctors Would Consider Quitting If Congress Passes Health Care Overhaul". Investors.com. 2009-09-15. Retrieved 2016-01-18.

[56] IBD/TIPP doctors poll is not trustworthy

2.9 Public health system in India

The **public health system in India** comprises a set of state-owned health care facilities funded and controlled by the government of India. Some of these are controlled by agencies of the central government while some are controlled by the governments of the states of India. The governmental ministry which controls the central government interests in these institutions is the *Ministry of Health & Family Welfare*. Governmental spending on health care in India is exclusively this system, hence most of the treatments in these institutions are either fully or partially subsidised.

2.9.1 Facilities

The facilities are:

- **All India Institutes of Medical Sciences** owned and controlled by the central government. These are referral hospitals with specialized facilities. All India institutes presently functional are All India Institute of Medical Sciences, New Delhi, AIIMS Bhopal,[1] AIIMS Bhubaneshwar, AIIMS Jodhpur, AIIMS Raipur, and AIIMS Rishikesh.

- Regional Cancer Centres are cancer care hospitals and research institutes controlled jointly by the central and the respective state governments.

- **Government Medical Colleges** owned and controlled by the respective state governments. These are referral hospitals.

- **District Hospitals** or **General Hospitals**: Controlled by the respective state governments and serving the respective districts (administrative divisions in India).

- **Taluk hospitals**: Taluk level hospitals controlled by the respective state governments and serving the respective taluks (administrative divisions in India, and smaller than districts).

- Community Health Centre CHCs: Community Health Centres are available is basic health unit in the urban areas.

- Primary Health Centres: The basic units with the most basic facilities, and especially serving rural India, generally at the level of a panchayat.[2]

- Sub-centers - The most basic units of health in villages; first point of contact between villagers and public health care system in India.

2.9.2 References

[1] AIIMS Bhopal.

[2] Ministry of Health & Family Welfare. 'Indian Public Health Standards'. (PDF)

2.10 Public hospital

A **public hospital** or **government hospital** is a hospital which is owned by a government and receives government funding. In some countries, this type of hospital provides medical care free of charge, the cost of which is covered by government reimbursement.

2.10.1 Australia

In Australia, public hospitals are operated and funded by each individual state's health department. The federal government also contributes funding. Services in public hospitals for all Australian citizens and permanent residents are fully subsidized by the federal government's Medicare Universal Healthcare program. Hospitals in Australia treat all Australian citizens and permanent residents regardless of their age, income, or social status.

Emergency Departments are almost exclusively found in public hospitals. Private hospitals rarely operate emergency departments, and patients treated at these private facilities are billed for care. Some costs, however (pathology, X-ray) may qualify for billing under Medicare.

Where patients hold private health insurance, after initial treatment by a public hospital's emergency department, the patient has the option of being transferred to a private hospital.

2.10.2 Brazil

The Brazilian health system is a mix composed by public hospitals, non-profit philanthropic hospitals, and private hospitals. The majority of low- and-medium income population uses services provided by a public hospitals run by either State or by the municipality. Since the inception of 1988 Federal Constitution, health care is a universal right for everyone living in Brazil: citizens, permanent residents, and foreigner. For that reason, Brazilian government created a national public health insurance system called SUS (Sistema Unico de Saude, Unified Health System) where all public funded hospitals (public and philanthropic entities)receive payments based on number of patients and procedures performed. Also, hospitals and health clinics are built by government in all three levels.

In general, all patients are supposed to have a global coverage including emergency care, preventive medicine, complex procedures, diagnostic procedures (blood exams, x-rays, CT-scan, etc.), surgeries (excluding cosmetic procedures), and medicines need to treat their condition. Because of the limitation in the budget, those services are often unavailable in most part of the country, in exception in large metropolis like São Paulo, Rio de Janeiro, and Belo Horizonte. Even in those metropolis, the access to some complex health care may take months if not completely ignored. However, patients that sued the government were able to get their treatment covered by the SUS, even with experimental therapeutics.

Recently, new legislation mandate that no private hospitals should refuse accept poor or uninsured patients in case of life threat emergencies. Cost of emergency care in this case is also paid by SUS.

2.10.3 Canada

In Canada all hospitals are funded through Medicare, Canada's publicly funded universal health insurance system.[1] Hospitals in Canada treat all Canadian citizens and permanent residents regardless of their age, income, or social status.

2.10.4 Norway

In Norway, all public hospitals are funded from the national budget[2] and run by four Regional Health Authorities (RHA) owned by the Ministry of Health and Care Services. In addition to the public hospitals, a few privately owned health clinics are operating. The four Regional Health Authorities are: Northern Norway Regional Health Authority, Central Norway Regional Health Authority, Western Norway Regional Health Authority, and South-eastern Norway

Regional Health Authority.[3][4] All citizens are eligible for treatment free of charge in the public hospital system. According to The Patients' Rights Act,[5] all citizens have the right to Free Hospital Choices.[6]

2.10.5 South Africa

South Africa has private and public hospitals. Public hospitals are funded by the Department of Health. The majority of the patients use public hospitals in which patients pay a nominal fee, roughly $3–5. The patients point of entry usually is through primary health care (Clinics) usually run by nurses. The next level of care would be district hospitals which have General Practitioners and basic radiographs. The next level of care would be Regional hospitals which have general practitioners, specialists and ICU's, and CT SCANS. The highest level of care is Tertiary which includes super specialists, MRI scans, and nuclear medicine scans.

Private patients either have healthcare insurance, known as medical aid, or have to pay the full amount privately if uninsured.

2.10.6 United Kingdom

In the UK public hospitals provide health care free at the point of use for the patient. Private health care is used by less than 8 percent of the population. The UK system is known as the National Health Service (NHS) and has been funded from general taxation since 1948.

2.10.7 United States

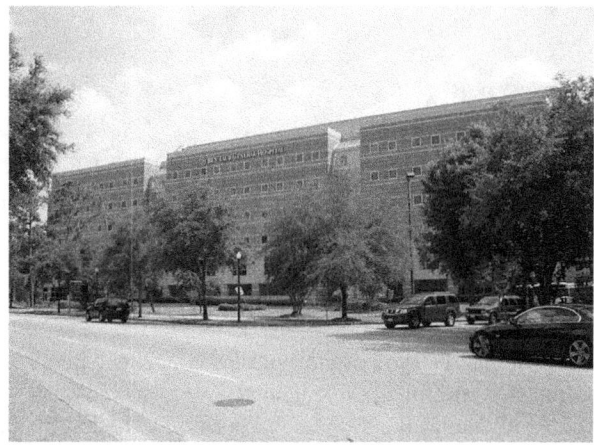

Ben Taub General Hospital in Houston, Texas

In the United States, two thirds of all urban hospitals are non-profit. The remaining third is split between for-profit and public. The urban public hospitals are often associated with medical schools.[7] The largest public hospital system in America is the New York City Health and Hospitals Corporation, which is associated with the New York University School of Medicine.

In the U.S., public hospitals receive significant funding from local, state, and/or federal governments. In addition, they may charge Medicaid, Medicare, and private insurers for the care of patients. Public hospitals, especially in urban areas, have a high concentration of uncompensated care and graduate medical education as compared to all other American hospitals. Public hospitals in America are closing at a much faster rate than hospitals overall. The number of public hospitals in major suburbs declined 27% (134 to 98) from 1996 to 2002. It is thought that the increase in uninsured has drained public hospitals to near bankruptcy.[8] Non-profit rural hospitals were disproportionately represented with high numbers of patients with uncompensated care. Public and non-profit rural hospitals form a large part of the health care safety net for the uninsured and poor underinsured in the U.S.[9]

For-profit hospitals were more likely to provide profitable medical services and less likely to provide medical services that were relatively unprofitable. Government or public hospitals were more likely to offer relatively unprofitable medical services. Not-for-profit hospitals often fell in the middle between public and for-profit hospitals in the types of medical services they provided. For-profit hospitals were quicker to respond to changes in profitability of medical services than the other two types of hospitals.[10]

In 2009, at non-profit hospitals, the average CEO made $600,000 annually. The range was from $100,000 to $3 million.[11]

2.10.8 India

In India, public hospitals (called Government Hospitals) provide health care free at the point of use for any Indian citizen. These are usually individual state funded. However, hospitals funded by the central (federal) government also exist. State hospitals are run by the state (local) government and may be dispensaries, peripheral health centers, rural hospital, district hospitals or medical college hospitals (hospitals with affiliated medical college). In many states (like Tamil Nadu) the hospital bill is entirely funded by the state government with patient not having to pay anything for treatment. However, other hospitals will charge nominal amounts for admission to special rooms and for medical and surgical consumables. The fees in public hospitals for these rooms is up to 900 rupees.

2.10.9 See also

- The Waiting Room (documentary)
- Private hospital

2.10.10 References

[1] Government of Canada, Health Canada. "Canada's Health Care System (Medicare) - Health Canada" (landing page). Retrieved 2011-07-11.

[2] "Norwegian National Budget Web Portal". Retrieved 2012-06-19.

[3] "Norway's Regional Health Authorities info". Retrieved 2012-06-19.

[4] "South-Eastern Norway Regional Health Authority info". Retrieved 2012-06-19.

[5] "The Act of 2 July 1999 No. 63 relating to Patients' Rights (the Patients' Rights Act)" (PDF). Retrieved 2012-06-19.

[6] "Free Hospital Choice Norway". Retrieved 2012-06-19.

[7] (Horwitz, 2005)

[8] Higgins, M. (17 August 2005). "Public hospitals decline swiftly". The Washington Times. Retrieved 2007-05-14.

[9] Fisherman L (July–August 1997). "What Types Of Hospitals Form The Safety Net? -- Despite public financial support, safety-net hospitals are in a worse financial position than other hospitals are." (PDF). *Health Affairs*. **16** (4): 215–222. doi:10.1377/hlthaff.16.4.215. Retrieved 2007-05-14.

[10] Horwitz J.R. (2005). "Making Profits And Providing Care: Comparing Nonprofit, For-Profit, And Government Hospitals" (Abstract). *Health Affairs*. **24** (3): 790–801. doi:10.1377/hlthaff.24.3.790. PMID 15886174. Retrieved 2007-05-14.

[11] Tanner, Lindsey (16 October 2013). "Nonprofit hospital CEO average pay: $600K". *Florida Today*. Melbourne, Florida. pp. 7B. Retrieved 16 October 2013.

2.11 Social insurance

Social insurance is any government-sponsored program with the following four characteristics:

- the benefits, eligibility requirements and other aspects of the program are defined by statute;
- explicit provision is made to account for the income and expenses (often through a trust fund);

- it is funded by taxes or premiums paid by (or on behalf of) participants (but additional sources of funding may be provided as well); and

- the program serves a defined population, and participation is either compulsory or so heavily subsidized that most eligible individuals choose to participate.[1]

Social insurance has also been defined as a program whose risks are transferred to and pooled by an often government organisation legally required to provide certain benefits.[2]

In the US, programs that meet these definitions include Social Security, Medicare, the Pension Benefit Guaranty Corporation program, the Railroad Retirement Board program and state-sponsored unemployment insurance programs.[1] The Canada Pension Plan (CPP) is also a social insurance program.

2.11.1   Similarities to private insurance

Typical similarities between social insurance programs and private insurance programs include:

- Wide pooling of risks;

- Specific definitions of the benefits provided;

- Specific definitions of eligibility rules and the amount of coverage provided;

- Specific premium, contribution or tax rates required to meet the expected costs of the system.[3]

2.11.2   Differences from private insurance

Typical differences between private insurance programs and social insurance programs include:

- Private insurance programs are generally designed with greater emphasis on equity between individual purchasers of coverage, and social insurance programs generally place a greater emphasis on the social adequacy of benefits for all participants.[3]

- Participation in private insurance programs is often voluntary; if the purchase of insurance is mandatory, individuals usually have a choice of insurers. Participation in social insurance programs is generally mandatory; if participation is voluntary, the cost is heavily subsidised enough to ensure essentially universal participation.[3]

- The right to benefits in a private insurance program is contractual, based on an insurance contract. The insurer generally does not have a unilateral right to change or terminate coverage before the end of the contract period (except in such cases as nonpayment of premiums). Social insurance programs are not generally based on a contract but on a statute, and the right to benefits is thus statutory rather than contractual. The provisions of the program can be changed if the statute is modified.[3]

- Individually purchased private insurance generally must be fully funded. Full funding is a desirable goal for private pension plans as well, but is often not achieved. Social insurance programs are often not fully funded, and some argue that full funding is not economically desirable.[3] Most international systems of social insurance are funded on an ongoing basis without reference to future liabilities. That is seen as a matter of solidarity between generations and between the sick and the healthy as a part of the social contract. The current generation of healthy working people pay something now to meet the health care and living costs of those who are currently temporarily incapacitated through sickness or who have ceased work through old age or disability. The main exception is in the United States, where the two largest programs, Medicare and Social Security programs, the administrators have historically collected more in social premiums than they have paid out as social benefits. The difference is retained in a trust fund. In both programs, US government actuaries periodically attempt to predict up to 70 years in advance the longevity of the fund and must estimate the future rates of contributions and pensions, the types of health care needs of the beneficiaries, and what that might cost. No other country in the world does so. Despite the US programs being in considerable surplus, the political argument is often that these programs are "going bankrupt" or that politicians have spent the money on other things.

2.11.3   Difference from welfare

See also: Welfare state

With social insurance, the beneficiary's contributions to the program are taken into account. A welfare program pays recipients based on need, not contributions. In the US, Medicare is social insurance, and Medicaid is welfare.

2.11.4   See also

- Generational accounting

- Right to health

- Social Insurance Number (Canada)

- Social security

- Social Security (United States)

- Social Security (Sweden)

- Social Security (Australia)

- Social Security Disability Insurance (United States)

- Social health insurance

- Social Protection

- Social Protection Floor

- Social safety net

- Social welfare provision

- Universal health care

- Welfare state

- Welfare culture

2.11.5 References

[1] "Social Insurance", Actuarial Standard of Practice No. 32, Actuarial Standards Board, January 1998.

[2] Margaret E. Lynch, Editor, *Health Insurance Terminology*, Health Insurance Association of America, 1992, ISBN 1-879143-13-5.

[3] Robert J. Myers, *Social Security*, Third Edition, Richard D. Irwin, Inc., 1985, ISBN 0-256-03307-2.

2.12 Socialized medicine

This article is about the term "Socialized medicine" as it is used in U.S. politics. For national health care systems generally, see Universal health care.

Socialized medicine is a term used to describe and discuss systems of universal health care: medical and hospital care for all at a nominal cost by means of government regulation of health care and subsidies derived from taxation.[1] Because of historically negative associations with socialism in American culture, the term is usually used pejoratively in American political discourse.[2][3][4][5][6] The term was first widely used in the United States by advocates of the American Medical Association in opposition to President Harry S. Truman's 1947 health-care initiative.[7][8][9]

2.12.1 Background

The original meaning was confined to systems in which the government operates health care facilities and employs health care professionals.[10][11][12][13] This narrower usage would apply to the British National Health Service hospital trusts and health systems that operate in other countries as diverse as Finland, Spain, Israel, and Cuba. The United States Veterans Health Administration and the medical departments of the U.S. Army, Navy, and Air Force, would also fall under this narrow definition. When used in that way, the narrow definition permits a clear distinction from single payer health insurance systems, in which the government finances health care but is not involved in care delivery.[14][15]

More recently, American conservative critics of health care reform have attempted to broaden the term by applying it to any publicly funded system. Canada's Medicare system and most of the UK's NHS general practitioner and dental services, which are systems where health care is delivered by private business with partial or total government funding, fit the broader definition, as do the health care systems of most of Western Europe. In the United States, Medicare, Medicaid, and the US military's TRICARE fall under that definition. In specific regard to military benefits of a (currently) volunteer military, such care is an owed benefit to a specific group as part of an economic exchange, which muddies the definition yet further.

Most industrialized countries and many developing countries operate some form of publicly funded health care with universal coverage as the goal. According to the Institute of Medicine and others, the United States is the only wealthy, industrialized nation that does not provide universal health care.[16][17]

Jonathan Oberlander, a professor of health policy at the University of North Carolina, maintains that the term is merely a political pejorative that has been defined to mean different levels of government involvement in health care, depending on what the speaker was arguing against at the time.[10]

The term is often used by conservatives in the U.S. to imply that the privately run health care system would become controlled by the government, thereby associating it with socialism, which has negative connotations to some people in American political culture.[18] As such, its usage is controversial,[4][5][6][10] and at odds with the views of conservatives in other countries prepared to defend socialized medicine such as Margaret Thatcher.[19]

2.12.2   History of term

When the term "socialized medicine" first appeared in the United States in the early 1900s, it bore no negative connotations. Otto P. Geier, chairman of the Preventive Medicine Section of the American Medical Association, was quoted in *The New York Times* in 1917 as praising socialized medicine as a way to "discover disease in its incipiency," help end "venereal diseases, alcoholism, tuberculosis," and "make a fundamental contribution to social welfare."[20] However, by the 1930s, the term socialized medicine was routinely used negatively by conservative opponents of publicly funded health care who wished to imply it represented socialism, and by extension, communism.[21] Universal health care and national health insurance were first proposed by U.S. President Theodore Roosevelt.[22][23][24] President Franklin D. Roosevelt later championed it, as did Harry S. Truman as part of his Fair Deal[25] and many others. Truman announced before describing his proposal that: "This is not socialized medicine".[21]

Government involvement in health care was ardently opposed by the AMA which distributed posters to doctors with slogans such as "Socialized medicine ... will undermine the democratic form of government."[26] According to T.R. Reid (*The Healing of America*, 2009):

> The term ["socialized medicine"] was popularized by the public relations firm Whitaker and Baxter working for the American Medical Association in 1947 to disparage President Truman's proposal for a national health care system. It was a label, at the dawn of the cold war, meant to suggest that anybody advocating universal access to health care must be a communist. And the phrase has retained its political power for six decades.[8][9]

The AMA conducted a nationwide campaign called Operation Coffee Cup during the late 1950s and early 1960s in opposition to the Democrats' plans to extend Social Security to include health insurance for the elderly, later known as Medicare. As part of the plan, doctors' wives would organize coffee meetings in an attempt to convince acquaintances to write letters to Congress opposing the program.[27] In 1961, Ronald Reagan recorded a disc entitled *Ronald Reagan Speaks Out Against Socialized Medicine* warning its audience the "dangers" that socialized medicine could bring. The recording was widely played at Operation Coffee Cup meetings.[27] Other pressure groups began to extend the definition from state managed health care to any form of state finance in health care. President Dwight Eisenhower opposed plans to expand government role in healthcare during his time in office.[21]

In more recent times, the term was brought up again by Republicans in the 2008 U.S. presidential election.[28] In July 2007, one month after the release of Michael Moore's film *Sicko*, Rudy Giuliani, the front-runner for the 2008 Republican presidential nomination, attacked the health care plans of Democratic presidential candidates as socialized medicine that was European and socialist,[29][30] Giuliani claimed that he had a better chance of surviving prostate cancer in the US than he would have had in England[31] and went on to repeat the claim in campaign speeches for three months[32][33][34][35][36][37] before making them in a radio advertisement.[38] After the radio ad began running, the use of the statistic was widely criticized by FactCheck.org,[39] PolitiFact.com,[40] by *The Washington Post*,[41] and others who consulted leading cancer experts and found that Giuliani's cancer survival statistics to be false, misleading or "flat wrong," the numbers having been reported to have been obtained from an opinion article by Giuliani health care advisor David Gratzer, a Canadian psychiatrist in the Manhattan Institute's *City Journal* where Gratzer was a senior fellow.[42] *The Times* reported that the British Health Secretary pleaded with Giuliani to stop using the NHS as a political football in American presidential politics. The article reported that not only the figures were five years out of date and wrong but also that US health experts disputed both the accuracy of Giuliani's figures and questioned whether it was fair to make a direct comparison.[43] The *St. Petersburg Times* said that Giuliani's tactic of "injecting a little fear" exploited cancer, which was "apparently not beneath a survivor with presidential aspirations."[44] Giuliani's repetition of the error even after it had been pointed out to him earned him more criticism and was awarded four "Pinnochios" by the *Washington Post* for recidivism.[45][46]

Health care professionals have tended to avoid the term because of its pejorative nature, but if they use it, they do not include publicly funded private medical schemes such as Medicaid.[3][47][48] Opponents of state involvement in health care tend to use the looser definition.[49]

The term is widely used by the American media and pressure groups. Some have even stretched use of the term to cover any regulation of health care, publicly financed or not.[50] The term is often used to criticize publicly provided health care outside the US, but rarely to describe similar health care programs there, such as the Veterans Administration clinics and hospitals, military health care,[51] or the single payer programs such as Medicaid and Medicare. Many conservatives use the term to evoke negative sentiment toward health care reform that would involve increasing government involvement in the US health care system.

Medical staff, academics and most professionals in the field and international bodies such as the World Health Organization tend to avoid use of the term. Outside the US, the terms most commonly used are universal health care or public health care. According to health economist Uwe Reinhardt, "strictly speaking, the term 'socialized medicine' should be reserved for health systems in which the government operates the production of health care and provides its financing."[52] Still others say the term has no meaning at all.[49]

In more recent times, the term has gained a more positive reappraisal. Documentary movie maker Michael Moore in his documentary *Sicko* pointed out that Americans do not talk about public libraries or the police or the fire department as being "socialized" and do not have negative opinions of these. Media personalities such as Oprah Winfrey have also weighed in behind the concept of public involvement in healthcare.[53] A 2008 poll indicates that Americans are sharply divided when asked about their views of the expression *socialized medicine*, with a large percentage of Democrats holding favorable views, while a large percentage of Republicans holding unfavorable views. Independents tend to somewhat favor it.[54]

2.12.3 History in United States

See also: Health care in the United States, Health care reform in the United States, and Health insurance in the United States

The Veterans Health Administration, the Military Health System,[55] and the Indian Health Service are examples of socialized medicine in the stricter sense of government administered care, but they are for limited populations.

Medicare and Medicaid are forms of publicly funded health care, which fits the looser definition of socialized medicine. Part B coverage (Medical) requires a monthly premium of $96.40 (and possibly higher) and the first $135 of costs per year also fall to the senior, not the government.[56]

A poll released in February 2008, conducted by the Harvard School of Public Health and Harris Interactive, indicated that Americans are currently divided in their opinions of socialized medicine, and this split correlates strongly with their political party affiliation.[57]

Two thirds of those polled said they understood the term "socialized medicine" very well or somewhat well. When offered descriptions of what such a system could mean, strong majorities believed that it means "the government makes sure everyone has health insurance" (79%) and "the government pays most of the cost of health care" (73%). One third (32%) felt that socialized medicine is a system in which "the government tells doctors what to do." The poll showed "striking differences" by party affiliation. Among Republicans polled, 70% said that socialized medicine would be worse than the current system. The

same percentage of Democrats (70%) said that a socialized medical system would be better than the current system. Independents were more evenly split, with 43% saying socialized medicine would be better and 38% worse.

According to Robert J. Blendon, professor of health policy and political analysis at the Harvard School of Public Health, "The phrase 'socialized medicine' really resonates as a pejorative with Republicans. However, that so many Democrats believe that socialized medicine would be an improvement is an indication of their dissatisfaction with our current system." Physicians' opinions have become more favorable toward "socialized medicine."[57]

A 2008 survey of doctors, published in *Annals of Internal Medicine*, shows that physicians support universal health care and national health insurance by almost 2 to 1.[58]

2.12.4 Political controversies in the United States

See also: Health care economics

Although the marginal scope of free or subsidized medicine provided is much discussed within the political body in most countries with socialized health care systems, there is little or no evidence of strong public pressure for the removal of subsidies or the privatization of health care in those countries. The political distaste for government involvement in health care in the U.S. is a unique counter to the trend found in other developed countries

In the United States, neither of the main parties favors a socialized system that puts the government in charge of hospitals or doctors, but they do have different approaches to financing and access. Democrats tend to be favorably inclined towards reform that involves more government control over health care financing and citizens' right of access to health care. Republicans are broadly in favor of the status quo, or a reform of the financing system that gives more power to the citizen, often through tax credits.

Supporters of government involvement in health care argue that government involvement ensures access, quality, and addresses market failures[59] specific to the health care markets. When the government covers the cost of health care, there is no need for individuals or their employers to pay for private insurance.

Opponents also claim that the absence of a market mechanism may slow innovation in treatment and research.

Both sides have also looked to more philosophical arguments, debating whether people have a fundamental right to have health care provided to them by their government.

Cost of care

Socialized medicine amongst industrialized countries tends to be more affordable than in systems where there is little government involvement. A 2003 study examined costs and outputs in the U.S. and other industrialized countries and broadly concluded that the U.S. spends so much because its health care system is more costly. It noted that "the United States spent considerably more on health care than any other country ... [yet] most measures of aggregate utilization such as physician visits per capita and hospital days per capita were below the OECD median. Since spending is a product of both the goods and services used and their prices, this implies that much higher prices are paid in the United States than in other countries.[60]". The researchers examined possible reasons and concluded that input costs were high (salaries, cost of pharmaceutical), and that the complex payment system in the U.S. added higher administrative costs. Comparison countries in Canada and Europe were much more willing to exert monopsony power to drive down prices, whilst the highly fragmented buy side of the U.S. health system was one factor that could explain the relatively high prices in the United States of America. The current fee-for-service payment system also stimulates expensive care by promoting procedures over visits through financially rewarding the former ($1,500 - for doing a 10-minute procedure) vs. the latter ($50 - for a 30-45 minute visit). This causes the proliferation of specialists (more expensive care) and creating, what Don Berwick refers to as, "the world's best healthcare system for rescue care".

Other studies have found no consistent and systematic relationship between the type of financing of health care and cost containment; the efficiency of operation of the health care system itself appears to depend much more on how providers are paid and how the delivery of care is organized than on the method used to raise these funds.[61]

Some supporters argue that government involvement in health care would reduce costs not just because of the exercise of monopsony power, e.g. in drug purchasing,[62] but also because it eliminates profit margins and administrative overhead associated with private insurance, and because it can make use of economies of scale in administration. In certain circumstances, a volume purchaser may be able to guarantee sufficient volume to reduce overall prices while providing greater profitability to the seller, such as in so-called "purchase commitment" programs.[63] Economist Arnold Kling attributes the present cost crisis mainly to the practice of what he calls "premium medicine", which overuses expensive forms of technology that is of marginal or no proven benefit.[64]

Milton Friedman has argued that government has weak incentives to reduce costs because "nobody spends somebody else's money as wisely or as frugally as he spends his own".[65] Others contend that health care consumption is not like other consumer consumption. Firstly there is a negative utility of consumption (consuming more health care does not make one better off) and secondly there is an information asymmetry between consumer and supplier.[66]

Paul Krugman and Robin Wells argue that all of the evidence indicates that public insurance of the kind available in several European countries achieves equal or better results at much lower cost, a conclusion that also applies within the United States. In terms of actual administrative costs, Medicare spent less than 2% of its resources on administration, while private insurance companies spent more than 13%.[67] The Cato Institute argues that the 2% Medicare cost figure ignores all costs shifted to doctors and hospitals, and alleges that Medicare is not very efficient at all when those costs are incorporated.[68] Some studies have found that the U.S. wastes more on bureaucracy (compared to the Canadian level), and that this excess administrative cost would be sufficient to provide health care to the uninsured population in the U.S.[69]

Notwithstanding the arguments about Medicare, there is overall less bureaucracy in socialized systems than in the present mixed U.S. system. Spending on administration in Finland is 2.1% of all health care costs, and in the UK the figure is 3.3% whereas the U.S. spends 7.3% of all expenditures on administration.[70]

Quality of care

Some in the U.S. claim that socialized medicine would reduce health care quality. The quantitative evidence for this claim is not clear. The WHO has used Disability Adjusted Life Expectancy (the number of years an average person can expect to live in good health) as a measure of a nation's health achievement, and has ranked its member nations by this measure.[71] The U.S. ranking was 24th, worse than similar industrial countries which have very high public funding of health such as Canada (ranked 5th), the UK (12th), Sweden (4th), France (3rd) and Japan (1st). But the U.S. ranking was better than some other European countries such as Ireland, Denmark and Portugal, which came 27th, 28th and 29th respectively. Finland, with its relatively high death rate from guns and renowned high suicide rate came above the U.S. in 20th place. The British have a Care Quality Commission that commissions independent surveys of the quality of care given in its health institutions and these are publicly accessible over the internet.[72] These determine whether health organizations are meeting public standards for quality set by government and allows regional comparisons. Whether these results indicate a better or worse situation to that in other countries such as the U.S. is hard to tell because these countries tend to lack a similar set of standards.

Taxation

Opponents claim that socialized medicine would require higher taxes but international comparisons do not support this; the ratio of public to private spending on health is lower in the U.S. than that of Canada, Australia, New Zealand, Japan, or any EU country, yet the per capita tax funding of health in those countries is already lower than that of the United States.[73]

Taxation is not necessarily an unpopular form of funding for health care. In England, a survey for the British Medical Association of the general public showed overwhelming support for the tax funding of health care. Nine out of ten people agreed or strongly agreed with a statement that the NHS should be funded from taxation with care being free at the point of use.[74]

An opinion piece in *The Wall Street Journal* by two conservative Republicans argues that government sponsored health care will legitimatize support for government services generally, and make an activist government acceptable. "Once a large number of citizens get their health care from the state, it dramatically alters their attachment to government. Every time a tax cut is proposed, the guardians of the new medical-welfare state will argue that tax cuts would come at the expense of health care -- an argument that would resonate with middle-class families entirely dependent on the government for access to doctors and hospitals."[75]

Innovation

Some in the U.S. argue that if government were to use its size to bargain down health care prices, this would undermine American leadership in medical innovation.[76][77] It is argued that the high level of spending in the U.S. health care system and its tolerance of waste is actually beneficial because it underpins American leadership in medical innovation, which is crucial not just for Americans, but for the entire world.[78]

Others point out that the American health care system spends more on state-of-the-art treatment for people who have good insurance, and spending is reduced on those lacking it[79] and question the costs and benefits of some medical innovations, noting, for example, that "rising spending on new medical technologies designed to address heart disease has not meant that more patients have survived."[80]

Access

One of the goals of socialized medicine systems is ensuring universal access to health care. Opponents of socialized medicine say that access for low-income individuals can be achieved by means other than socialized medicine, for example, income-related subsidies can function without public provision of either insurance or medical services.[81] Economist Milton Friedman said the role of the government in health care should be restricted to financing hard cases.[65] Universal coverage can also be achieved by making purchase of insurance compulsory. For example, European countries with socialized medicine in the broader sense, such as Germany and The Netherlands, operate in this way. A legal obligation to purchase health insurance is akin to a mandated health tax, and the use of public subsidies is a form of directed income redistribution via the tax system. Such systems give the consumer a free choice amongst competing insurers whilst achieving universality to a government directed minimum standard.

Compulsory health insurance or savings are not limited to so-called socialized medicine, however. Singapore's health care system, which is often referred to as a free-market or mixed system, makes use of a combination of compulsory participation and state price controls to achieve the same goals.[82]

Rationing (access, coverage, price, and time)

See also: Healthcare rationing in the United States

Part of the current debate about health care in the United States revolves around whether the Affordable Care Act as part of health care reform will result in a more systematic and logical allocation of health care. Opponents tend to believe that the law will eventually result in a government takeover of health care and ultimately to socialized medicine and rationing based not on being able to afford the care you want but on whether a third party other than the patient and the doctor decides whether the procedure or the cost is justifiable. Supporters of reform point out that health care rationing already exists in the United States through insurance companies either denying coverage for pre-existing conditions or applying differential pricing for this coverage, or issuing denial for reimbursement on the grounds that the insurance company believes the procedure is experimental or will not assist even though the doctor has recommended it.[83] A public insurance plan was not included in the Affordable Care Act but some argue that it would have added to health care access choices,[84][85] and others argue that the central issue is whether health care is rationed sensibly.[86][87]

Opponents of reform invoke the term socialized medicine because they say it will lead to health care rationing by denial of coverage, denial of access, and use of waiting lists, but often do so without acknowledging coverage denial, lack of access and waiting lists exist in the U.S. health care system currently[88] or that waiting lists in the U.S. are sometimes longer than the waiting lists in countries with socialized medicine.[89] Proponents of the reform proposal point out a public insurer is not akin to a socialized medicine system because it will have to negotiate rates with the medical industry just as other insurers do and cover its cost with premiums charged to policyholders just as other insurers do without any form of subsidy.

There is a frequent misunderstanding to think that waiting happens in places like the United Kingdom and Canada but does not happen in the United States. For instance it is not uncommon even for emergency cases in some U.S. hospitals to be boarded on beds in hallways for 48 hours or more due to lack of inpatient beds[90] and people in the U.S. rationed out by being unable to afford their care are simply never counted and may never receive the care they need, a factor that is often overlooked. Statistics about waiting times in national systems are an honest approach to the issue of those waiting for access to care. Everyone waiting for care is reflected in the data which, in the UK for example, are used to inform debate, decision-making and research within the government and the wider community.[91][92][93] Some people in the U.S. are rationed out of care by unaffordable care or denial of access by HMOs and insurers or simply because they cannot afford co-pays or deductibles even if they have insurance.[94] These people wait an indefinitely long period and may never get care they need, but actual numbers are simply unknown because they are not recorded in official statistics.[95]

Opponents of the current reform care proposals fear that U.S. comparative effective research (a plan introduced in the stimulus bill) will be used to curtail spending and ration treatments, which is one function of the National Institute for Health and Care Excellence (NICE), arguing that rationing by market pricing rather by government is the best way for care to be rationed. However, when defining any group scheme, the same rules must apply to everyone in the scheme so some coverage rules had to be established. Britain has a national budget for public funded health care, and recognizes there has to be a logical trade off between spending on expensive treatments for some against, for example, caring for sick children.[96] NICE is therefore applying the same market pricing principles to make the hard job of deciding between funding some treatments and not funding others on behalf of everyone in the insured pool. This rationing does not preclude choice of obtaining insurance coverage for excluded treatment as insured persons do having the choice to take out supplemental health insurance

for drugs and treatments that the NHS does not cover (at least one private insurer offers such a plan) or from meeting treatment costs out-of-pocket.

The debate in the U.S. over rationing has enraged some in the UK and statements made by politicians such as Sarah Palin and Chuck Grassley resulted in a mass Internet protest on websites such as Twitter and Facebook under the banner title "welovetheNHS" with positive stories of NHS experiences to counter the negative ones being expressed by these politicians and others and by certain media outlets such as *Investor's Business Daily* and Fox News.[97] In the UK, it is private health insurers that ration care (in the sense of not covering the most common services such as access to a primary care physician or excluding pre-existing conditions) rather than the NHS. Free access to a general practitioner is a core right in the NHS, but private insurers in the UK will not pay for payments to a private primary care physician.[98] Private insurers exclude many of the most common services as well as many of the most expensive treatments, whereas the vast majority of these are not excluded from the NHS but are obtainable at no cost to the patient. According to the Association of British Insurers (ABI), a typical policy will exclude the following: going to a general practitioner; going to accident and emergency; drug abuse; HIV/AIDS; normal pregnancy; gender reassignment; mobility aids, such as wheelchairs; organ transplant; injuries arising from dangerous hobbies (often called hazardous pursuits); pre-existing conditions; dental services; outpatient drugs and dressings; deliberately self-inflicted injuries; infertility; cosmetic treatment; experimental or unproven treatment or drugs; and war risks. Chronic illnesses, such as diabetes and end stage renal disease requiring dialysis are also excluded from coverage.[98] Insurers do not cover these because they feel they do not need to since the NHS already provides coverage and to provide the choice of a private provider would make the insurance prohibitively expensive.[98] Thus in the UK there is cost shifting from the private sector to the public sector, which again is the *opposite* of the allegation of cost shifting in the U.S. from public providers such as Medicare and Medicaid to the private sector.

Palin had alleged that America will create rationing "death panels" to decide whether old people could live or die, again widely taken to be a reference to NICE. U.S. Senator Chuck Grassley alleged that he was told that Senator Edward Kennedy would have been refused the brain tumor treatment he was receiving in the United States had he instead lived a country with government run health care. This, he alleged, would have been due to rationing because of Kennedy's age (77 years) and the high cost of treatment.[99] The UK Department of Health said that Grassley's claims were "just wrong" and reiterated health service in Britain provides health care on the basis of clinical need regardless of age or ability to pay. The chairman of the British Medical Association, Hamish Meldrum, said he was dismayed by the "jaw-droppingly untruthful attacks" made by American critics. The chief executive of the National Institute for Health and Clinical Excellence (NICE), told *The Guardian* newspaper that "it is neither true, nor is it anything you could extrapolate from anything we've ever recommended" that Kennedy would be denied treatment by the NHS.[100] The business journal *Investor's Business Daily* recently claimed mathematician and astrophysicist Stephen Hawking, who has ALS and speaks with the aid of an American-accented voice synthesizer, would not have survived if he had been treated in the British National Health Service. Hawking is British and been treated throughout his life (67 years) by the NHS and issued a statement to the effect he owed his life to the quality of care he has received from the NHS.[100][101][102]

Some argue that countries with national health care may use waiting lists as a form of rationing compared to countries that ration by price, such as the United States, according to several commentators and healthcare experts.[84][103][104] *The Washington Post* columnist Ezra Klein compared 27% of Canadians reportedly waiting four months or more for elective surgery with 26% of Americans reporting that they did not fulfill a prescription due to cost (compared to only 6% of Canadians).[105][106] Britain's former age-based policy that once prevented the use of kidney dialysis as treatment for older patients with renal problems, even to those who can privately afford the costs, has been cited as another example.[84] A 1999 study in the *Journal of Public Economics* analyzed the British National Health Service and found that its waiting times function as an effective market disincentive, with a low elasticity of demand with respect to time.[104]

Supporters of private price rationing over waiting time rationing, such as *The Atlantic* columnist Megan McArdle, argue time rationing leaves patients worse off since their time (measured as an opportunity cost) is worth much more than the price they would pay.[86] Opponents also state categorizing patients based on factors such as social value to the community or age will not work in a heterogeneous society without a common ethical consensus such as the U.S.[84] Doug Bandow of the CATO Institute wrote that government decision making would "override the differences in preferences and circumstances" for individuals and that it is a matter of personal liberty to be able to buy as much or as little care as one wants.[107] Neither argument recognizes the fact that in most countries with socialized medicine, a parallel system of private health care allows people to pay extra to reduce their waiting time. The exception is that some provinces in Canada disallow the right to bypass queuing unless the matter is one in which the rights of the person under the constitution.

A 1999 article in the *British Medical Journal*, stated "there is much merit in using waiting lists as a rationing mechanism for elective health care if the waiting lists are managed efficiently and fairly."[103] Dr. Arthur Kellermann, associate dean for health policy at Emory University, stated rationing by ability to pay rather than by anticipated medical benefits in the U.S. makes its system more unproductive, with poor people avoiding preventive care and eventually using expensive emergency treatment.[85] Ethicist Daniel Callahan has written that U.S. culture overly emphasizes individual autonomy rather than communitarian morals and that stops beneficial rationing by social value, which benefits everyone.[84]

Some argue that waiting lists result in great pain and suffering, but again evidence for this is unclear. In a recent survey of patients admitted to hospital in the UK from a waiting list or by planned appointment, only 10% reported they felt they should have been admitted sooner than they were. 72% reported the admission was as timely as they felt necessary.[108] Medical facilities in the U.S. do not report waiting times in national statistics as is done in other countries and it is a myth to believe there is no waiting for care in the U.S. Some argue that wait times in the U.S. could actually be as long as or longer than in other countries with universal health care.[109]

There is considerable argument about whether any of the health bills currently before congress will introduce rationing. Howard Dean for example contested in an interview that they do not. However, *Politico* has pointed out that all health systems contain elements of rationing (such as coverage rules) and the public health care plan will therefore implicitly involve some element of rationing.[85][110]

Political interference and targeting

In the UK, where government employees or government-employed sub-contractors deliver most health care, political interference is quite hard to discern. Most supply-side decisions are in practice under the control of medical practitioners and of boards comprising the medical profession. There is some antipathy towards the target-setting by politicians in the UK. Even the NICE criteria for public funding of medical treatments were never set by politicians. Nevertheless, politicians have set targets, for instance to reduce waiting times and to improve choice. Academics have pointed out that the claims of success of the targeting are statistically flawed.[111]

The veracity and significance of the claims of targeting interfering with clinical priorities are often hard to judge. For example, some UK ambulance crews have complained that hospitals would deliberately leave patients with ambulance crews to prevent an accident and emergency department (A&E, or emergency room) target-time for treatment from starting to run. The Department of Health vehemently denied the claim, because the A&E time begins when the ambulance arrives at the hospital and not after the handover. It defended the A&E target by pointing out that the percentage of people waiting four hours or more in A&E had dropped from just under 25% in 2004 to less than 2% in 2008.[112] The original *Observer* article reported that in London, 14,700 ambulance turnarounds were longer than an hour and 332 were more than two hours when the target turnaround time is 15 minutes.[113] However, in the context of the total number of emergency ambulance attendances by the London Ambulance Service each year (approximately 865,000),[114] these represent just 1.6% and 0.03% of all ambulance calls. The proportion of these attributable to patients left with ambulance crews is not recorded. At least one junior doctor has complained that the four-hour A&E target is too high and leads to unwarranted actions that are not in the best interests of patients.[115]

Political targeting of waiting-times in Britain has had dramatic effects. The National Health Service reports that the median admission wait-time for elective inpatient treatment (non-urgent hospital treatment) in England at the end of August 2007, was just under 6 weeks, and 87.5% of patients were admitted within 13 weeks. Reported waiting times in England also overstate the true waiting-time. This is because the clock starts ticking when the patient has been referred to a specialist by the GP and it only stops when the medical procedure is completed. The 18-week maximum waiting period target thus includes all the time taken for the patient to attend the first appointment with the specialist, time for any tests called for by the specialist to determine precisely the root of the patient's problem and the best way to treat it. It excludes time for any intervening steps deemed necessary prior to treatment, such as recovery from some other illness or the losing of excessive weight.[116]

2.12.5 See also

- Health care compared - tabular comparisons of the U.S., Canada, and other countries not shown above.

- Publicly funded health care

- Social medicine

- Socialization (economics)

- Universal healthcare

2.12.6 References

[1] The American Heritage Medical Dictionary, Houghton Mifflin Harcourt Publishing Company

[2] Paul Burleigh Horton, Gerald R. Leslie, The Sociology of Social Problems, 1965, page 59 (cited as an example of a standard propaganda device).

[3] Rushefsky, Mark E.; Patel, Kant (2006). *Health Care Politics And Policy in America*. Armonk, N.Y.: M.E. Sharpe. p. 47. ISBN 0-7656-1478-2. ....socialized medicine, a pejorative term used to help polarize debate

[4] Dorothy Porter, Health, Civilization, and the State, Routledge, p. 252: "...what the Americans liked to call 'socialized medicine'..."

[5] Paul Wasserman, Don Hausrath, Weasel Words: The Dictionary of American Doublespeak, p. 60: "One of the terms to denigrate and attack any system under which complete medical aid would be provided to every citizen through public funding."

[6] Edward Conrad Smith, New Dictionary of American Politics, p. 350: "A somewhat loose term applied to..."

[7] W. Michael Byrd, Linda A. Clayton (2002) *An American Health Dilemma: Race, medicine, and health care in the United States, 1900-2000* pp 238 ff.

[8] T.R. Reid, (2009) *The Healing of America: A Global Quest for Better, Cheaper, and Fairer Health Care*

[9] http://abcnews.go.com/m/screen?id=8383452&pid=248

[10] Socialized Medicine Belittled on Campaign Trail from NPR.

[11] "The American Heritage Dictionary of the English Language: Fourth Edition".

[12] "The Columbia Encyclopedia, Sixth Edition".

[13] Jacob S. Hacker, "Socialized Medicine: Let's Try a Dose, We're Bound to Feel Better", Washington Post, March 23, 2008.

[14] "Single Payer article from AMSA" (PDF).

[15] "MedTerms medical dictionary".

[16] Insuring America's Health: Principles and Recommendations, Institute of Medicine at the National Academies of Science, 2004-01-14, accessed 2007-10-22

[17] The Case For Single Payer, Universal Health Care For The United States

[18] "Free to Choose: A Conversation with Milton Friedman" (PDF). Archived from the original (PDF) on May 30, 2008. Retrieved 2008-04-14.

[19] http://opinion.publicfinance.co.uk/2009/08/the-end-is-nye/

[20] "World at War is Facing a Shortage of Doctors" (PDF). *New York Times*. 1917-07-01. Retrieved 2009-04-02.

[21] Greenberg, David (2007-10-08). "Who's Afraid of Socialized Medicine? Two dangerous words that kill health-care reform". *Slate*. Retrieved 2008-02-27.

[22] National Health Care, HealthInsurance.info

[23] Chris Farrell, It's Time to Cure Health Care, BusinessWeek

[24] http://www.teachingamericanhistory.org/library/index.asp?document=607

[25] President Truman Addresses Congress on Proposed Health Program, Washington, D.C., Harry S. Truman Library and Museum

[26] Olivier Garceau, "Organized Medicine Enforces its 'Party Line'", Public Opinion Quarterly, September 1940, p. 416.

[27] Roger Lowenstein (2009-07-27). "A Question of Numbers". The New York Times.

[28] Meckler, Laura (January 25, 2008). "Tempering health-care goals; Democrats' proposals build on current system, reject single-payer". *The Wall Street Journal*. p. A5. Say something too kind about single-payer and there's a Republican around the corner ready to brand you a socialist"..."Say something too harsh and you will alienate many on the left wing of the party.

[29] Steinhauser, Paul (July 31, 2007). "Giuliani attacks Democratic health plans as 'socialist'". CNN.com. The American way is not single-payer, government-controlled anything. That's a European way of doing something; that's frankly a socialist way of doing something. That's why when you hear Democrats in particular talk about single-mandated health care, universal health care, what they're talking about is socialized medicine.

[30] Ramer, Holly (Associated Press) (July 31, 2007). "Giuliani offers health plan". USAToday.com. We've got to solve our health care problem with American principles, not the principles of socialism.

[31] Haberman, Shir (August 1, 2007). "Giuliani touts health plan". SeacoastOnline.com.

[32] Mayko, Michael P. (July 31, 2007). "Giuliani prescribes health care reform". ConnPost.com.

[33] March, William (September 18, 2007). "Giuliani breezes through state; He attends Tampa fundraising event". *The Tampa Tribune*. p. 5 (Metro).

[34] Hutchinson, Bill (September 18, 2007). "Giuliani fans greet 'the Mayor' in Tampa". *Sarasota Herald-Tribune*. p. BCE1.

[35] . (September 19, 2007). "Giuliani's warning over UK's NHS". BBC News Online.

[36] . (September 19, 2007). "Giuliani pays homage to Thatcher on UK visit". London: TimesOnline.co.uk.

[37] Cook, Emily (September 20, 2007). "Giuliani in blast at the NHS". Mirror.co.uk.

[38] Cillizza, Chris; Murray, Shailagh (October 28, 2007). "Giuliani's bid to woo New Hampshire independents centers on health care". *The Washington Post*. p. A02.

[39] Robertson, Lori; Henig, Jess (October 30, 2007). "A bogus cancer statistic". FactCheck.org.

[40] Greene, Lisa; August, Lissa (October 31, 2007). "A cancer ad gone wrong for Rudy". PolitiFact.com.

[41] Dobbs, Michael (October 30, 2007). "Rudy wrong on cancer survival chances". *The Fact Checker*. WashingtonPost.com.

[42] Lieberman, Trudy (November 21, 2007). "Rudy's unhealthy stats; Some good reporting holds Giuliani's phony cancer numbers at bay". Columbia Journalism Review.

[43] Baldwin, Tom (November 1, 2007). "Rudy Giuliani uses the NHS as 'political football to give Hillary Clinton a kicking". *The Times*. London. p. 2. "Doctors in the two countries have different philosophies for treating the disease with the US putting more emphasis on early diagnosis and surgery. An analysis of mortality rates suggests that about 25 out of 100,000 men are dying from prostate cancer each year in both Britain and the US.

[44] editorial (November 3, 2007). "Giuliani's dose of fear". *St. Petersburg Times*. p. 14A.

[45] Dobbs, Michael (November 7, 2007). "Four Pinocchios for recidivist Rudy". *The Fact Checker*. WashingtonPost.com.

[46] Robertson, Lori; Henig, Jess (November 8, 2007). "Bogus cancer stats, again". FactCheck.org.

[47] http://www.medterms.com/script/main/art.asp?articlekey=25520 Webster's New World Medical Dictionary, "Single-payer health care is distinct and different from socialized medicine in which doctors and hospitals work for and draw salaries from the government."

[48] http://www.pnhp.org/news/2006/june/kevin_drum_and_uwe_r.php Uwe Reinhardt, quoted in The Washington Monthly: " 'Socialism' is an arrangement under which the means of production are owned by the state. Government-run health insurance is not 'socialism,' and only an ignoramus would call it that. Rather, government-run health insurance is a form of 'social insurance,' that can be coupled with privately owned for-profit or not-for-profit health care delivery systems."

[49] "Dirty Words", Winston-Salem Journal, December 14, 2007, "Jonathan Oberlander, a professor of health policy at UNC Chapel Hill, explained that the term itself has no meaning. There is no definition of socialized medicine. It originated with an American Medical Association campaign against government-provided health care a century ago and has been used recently to describe even private-sector initiatives such as HMOs." See also Socialized Medicine Belittled on Campaign Trail, National Public Radio, Morning Edition, December 6, 2007: "The term socialized medicine,

technically, to most health policy analysts, actually doesn't mean anything at all," says Jonathan Oberlander, a professor of health policy at the University of North Carolina."

[50] "Socialized Medicine is Already Here".

[51] Timothy Noah (March 8, 2005). "The Triumph of Socialized Medicine". *Slate.*

[52] Dunlop, David W; Martins, Jo. M (June 1995). *Uwe Reinhardt, Germany's Health Care and Health Insurance System, p 163.* World Bank Publications. ISBN 978-0-8213-3253-5.

[53] http://www.alternet.org/blogs/video/63935/michael_moore_and_oprah_ask_audience:_why_should_us_health_care_be_for_profit/?comments=view&cID=741898&pID=741639 Video of Oprah Winfrey show on the issue of health care

[54] "Americans split on socialized medicine". *Harvard Gazette.* February 21, 2008.

[55] Phillip Boffey, "The Socialists Are Coming! The Socialists Are Coming!" Editorial on U.S. "socialized medicine" in the military, the Veterans Health Administration, and Medicare, *The New York Times,* September 28, 2007

[56] http://questions.medicare.gov/cgi-bin/medicare.cfg/php/enduser/std_adp.php?p_faqid=2100 Medicare rates

[57] "Poll Finds Americans Split by Political Party Over Whether Socialized Medicine Better or Worse Than Current System" (Press release). Harvard School of Public Health. 2007-02-14. Retrieved 2008-02-27.

[58] Doctors support universal health care: survey, Reuters, March 31, 2008 (first reported in Annals of Internal Medicine).

[59] Office of Health Economics (UK), The Economics of Health Care, Section 3.i, "Market Failure: an Overview," p. 38

[60] http://content.healthaffairs.org/cgi/content/full/22/3/89# T5 **It's The Prices, Stupid: Why The United States Is So Different From Other Countries** Gerard F. Anderson, Uwe E. Reinhardt, Peter S. Hussey and Varduhi Petrosyan *Health Affairs*

[61] Sherry A. Glied, "Health Care Financing, Efficiency, and Equity," National Bureau of Economic Research Working Paper No. 13881, March 2008

[62] Single-Payer FAQ | Physicians for a National Health Program

[63] ARPA: Purchase commitments: Big business bias or solution to the 'neglected diseases' dilemma?

[64] Arnold S. Relman, M.D., New England Journal of Medicine, Volume 355:1073-1074 September 7, 2006 (Review of "Crisis of Abundance").

[65] Milton Friedman, How to Cure Health Care

[66] http://healthcare-economist.com/2006/09/21/information-asymmetry-insurance-and-the-decision-to-hospitalize/ Blomqvist, Åke; Léger, Pierre Thomas (2005) "Information asymmetry, insurance and the decision to hospitalize" Journal of Health Economics, Vol 24(4), pp. 775-793.

[67] Paul Krugman and Robin Wells, "The Health Care Crisis and What to Do About It", The New York Review of Books, Volume 53, Number 5, March 23, 2006

[68] John Goodman (Winter 2005). "Five Myths of Socialized Medicine" (PDF). *Cato Institute.*

[69] Summary of New England Journal of Medicine Study, USA wastes more on health care bureaucracy than it would cost to provide health care to all of the uninsured, Medical News Today, 28 May 2004.

[70] http://www.commonwealthfund.org/usr_doc/Collins_universal_hlt_insurance_testimony_06-26-2007_figures.ppt?section=4039#320,14, Figure 14. Percentage of National Health Expenditures Spent on Health Administration and Insurance, 2003

[71] http://www.who.int/whr/2000/en/whr00_en.pdf WHO. World Health Report 2000

[72] http://www.nhssurveys.org

[73] http://hdr.undp.org/en/media/HDR_20072008_EN_Indicator_tables.pdf UN Human Development Report 2007/2008 Table 6 Page 247

[74] http://www.bma.org.uk/ap.nsf/AttachmentsByTitle/PDFnhssystreform2007/\protect\char"0024\relaxFILE/48751Surveynhsreform.pdf Survey of the general public's views on NHS system reform - in England: BMA June 2007

[75] Beware of the Big-Government Tipping Point, Peter Wehner and Paul Ryan, The Wall Street Journal, January 16, 2009

[76] Tyler Cowen, "Poor U.S. Scores in Health Care Don't Measure Nobels and Innovation", *The New York Times,* October 5, 2006.

[77] Julie Chan, "We're Number 37 in Health Care!"

[78] Kling, Arnold (June 30, 2007). "Two health-care documentaries". *The Washington Times.*

[79] Paul Krugman, Robin Wells, "The Health Care Crisis and What to Do About It"

[80] Maggie Mahar, The Mythology of Boomers Bankrupting Our Healthcare System, Health Beat, April 10, 2008.

[81] Patricia M. Danzon, "Health Care Industry", (The Concise Encyclopedia of Economics)

[82] John Tucci, "The Singapore health system – achieving positive health outcomes with low expenditure", Watson Wyatt Healthcare Market Review, October 2004.

[83] Man Dies After Insurance Co. Refuses To Cover Treatment ABC station KBMC report on case featured by Michael Moore in Sicko!

[84] Kant Patel; Mark E. Rushefsky (2006). *Health Care Politics and Policy in America*. 3rd Ed. M.E. Sharpe. pp. 360–361. ISBN 0-7656-1479-0.

[85] Horsley, Scott (July 1, 2009). "Doctors Say Health Care Rationing Already Exists". National Public Radio: *All Things Considered*. Retrieved September 7, 2009.

[86] "Rationing By Any Other Name". By Megan McArdle. *The Atlantic*. Published August 10, 2009.

[87] Leonhardt, David (June 17, 2009). "Health Care Rationing Rhetoric Overlooks Reality". *The New York Times*. Retrieved September 7, 2009.

[88] "95,000+ U.S. patients are currently waiting for an organ transplant; nearly 4,000 new patients are added to the waiting list each month. Every day, 17 people die while waiting for a transplant of a vital organ, such as a heart, liver, kidney, pancreas, lung or bone marrow. Because of the lack of available donors in this country, 3,916 kidney patients, 1,570 liver patients, 356 heart patients and 245 lung patients died in 2006 while waiting for life-saving organ transplants:National Kidney Foundation http://www.kidney.org/news/newsroom/fs_new/25factsorgdon&trans.cfm

[89] "Right now more than 8,000 people in the UK need an organ transplant that could save or improve their life. But each year around 400 people die while waiting for a transplant". National Kidney Federation. http://www.kidney.org.uk/donor.html. (Note: The UK population is about one sixth the size of the U.S. population).

[90] GIFFIN, ROBERT B.; SHARI M. ERICKSON; MEGAN MCHUGH; BENJAMIN WHEATLEY; SHEILA J. MADHANI; CANDACE TRENUM (June 2006). "THE FUTURE OF EMERGENCY CARE IN THE UNITED STATES HEALTH SYSTEM" (pdf). Institute of Medicine of the National Academies. Retrieved 2009-10-03. The number of patients visiting EDs has been growing rapidly. There were 113.9 million ED visits in 2003, for example, up from 90.3 million a decade earlier. At the same time, the number of facilities available to deal with these visits has been declining. Between 1993 and 2003, the total number of hospitals in the United States decreased by 703, the number of hospital beds dropped by 198,000, and the number of EDs fell by 425. The result has been serious overcrowding. If the beds in a hospital are filled, patients cannot be transferred from the ED to inpatient units. This can lead to the practice of "boarding" patients—holding them in the ED, often in beds in hallways, until an inpatient bed becomes available. It is not uncommon for patients in some busy EDs to be boarded for 48 hours or more.

[91] What does the Department of Health do? - Health Questions - NHS Direct

[92] Health Indicators

[93] http://www.18weeks.nhs.uk/endwaiting/documents/EWCL_patient_LON_280907.pdf Setting new standards for your care: 2007 NHS patient leaflet on the 18 week maximum wait time promise for Dec 2008.

[94] Singer, Peter (July 15, 2009). "Why we must Ration Health Care". *New York Times*. Retrieved May 23, 2010. But if the stories ... lead us to think badly of the British system of rationing health care, we should remind ourselves that the U.S. system also results in people going without life-saving treatment — it just does so less visibly. Pharmaceutical manufacturers often charge much more for drugs in the United States than they charge for the same drugs in Britain, where they know that a higher price would put the drug outside the cost-effectiveness limits set by NICE. American patients, even if they are covered by Medicare or Medicaid, often cannot afford the copayments for drugs. That's rationing too, by ability to pay.

[95] John P. Geyman (2003). "Myths as Barriers to Health Care Reform in the United States" (pdf). International Journal of Health Services. Retrieved 2008-06-12.

[96] https://www.nytimes.com/2008/12/03/health/03nice.html?_r=3&hp=&pagewanted=all Quote "Britain's National Health Service provides 95 percent of the nation's care from an annual budget, so paying for costly treatments means less money for, say, sick children." from NY Times article Dec 2, 2008

[97] http://www.mirror.co.uk/news/top-stories/2009/08/14/welove-thenhs-115875-21595748/The Mirror (UK newspaper) on public reaction and rage in UK to Palin, Grassley, IBD, and Fox (Hanan) interviews intended to denigrate the NHS

[98] "Are you buying private medical insurance? Take a look at this guide before you decide (Association of British Insurers, 2008)" (PDF). Association of British Insurers. 2008. Retrieved September 5, 2009.

[99] Audio of Senator Grassly repeating allegation Sen Kennedy would not receive care in the UK on grounds of his age. https://www.youtube.com/watch?v=QZK8ffUpL60

[100] http://www.foreignpolicy.com/articles/2009/08/18/the_most_outrageous_us_lies_about_global_healthcare?page=0,0

[101] "Bloggers debate British healthcare". *BBC News*. August 12, 2009. Retrieved May 23, 2010.

[102] http://www.spectator.co.uk/alexmassie/5255761/stephen-hawking-has-not-yet-been-murdered-by-the-nhs.thtml

[103] Points for pain: waiting list priority scoring systems by Rhiannon Tudor Edwards. *British Medical Journal*. 1999 February 13; 318 (7181): 412–414. Accessed September 1, 2009.

[104] Martin, S. (1999). "Rationing by waiting lists: an empirical investigation". *Journal of Public Economics*. **71**: 141–164. doi:10.1016/S0047-2727(98)00067-X.

[105] Ezra Klein (June 17, 2009). "A Rational Look At Rationing". *The Washington Post*. Retrieved September 7, 2009.

[106] Gratzer, David (June 9, 2009). "Canada's ObamaCare Precedent". *OpinionJournal.com*. *The Wall Street Journal*. Retrieved September 1, 2009.

[107] Doug Bandow. "Uwe Reinhardt on Health Care Rationing". CATO Institute. Retrieved September 7, 2009.

[108] http://www.healthcarecommission.org.uk/_db/ _documents/Full_2007_results_with_historical_ comparisons_-_tables.doc   Healthcare   Commission: 'Survey of adult inpatients in the NHS 2007'

[109] http://www.businessweek.com/magazine/content/07_28/ b4042072.htm *Business Week*: The doctor will see you in 3 months

[110] "There's rationing in health care now, and there still would be under reform bill". PolitiFact. Retrieved September 7, 2009.

[111] Cass Business School: Academics challenge A&E waiting times

[112] BBC News:Anger at 'patient stacking' claim

[113] copy of original Observer story from Guardian website

[114] http://www.londonambulance.nhs.uk/publications/areport/ London%20Ambulance%20Service%20AR%2006-07.pdf

[115] Triggle, Nick (June 28, 2005). "Minister blasted over A&E target". *BBC News*. Retrieved May 23, 2010.

[116] http://www.18weeks.nhs.uk/Content.aspx?path= /What-is-18-weeks/patient 18 week NHS target

2.13   Spanish National Health System

The **Spanish National Health System** (Spanish: *Sistema Nacional de Salud*, SNS) is the agglomeration of public health services that has existed in Spain since it was established through and structured by the *Ley General de Sanidad* (the "General Health Law") of 1986. Management of these services has been progressively transferred to the distinct autonomous communities of Spain, while some continue to be operated by the National Institute of Health Management (*Instituto Nacional de Gestión Sanitaria*, INGESA), part of the Ministry of Health and Social Policy (which superseded the Ministry of Health and Consumer Affairs— *Ministerio de Sanidad y Consumo*—in 2009). The activity of these services is harmonized by the Interterritorial Council of the Spanish National Health Service (*Consejo Interterritorial del Servicio Nacional de Salud de España*, CISNS)

in order to give cohesion to the system and to guarantee the rights of citizens throughout Spain.

Article 46 of the *Ley General de Sanidad* establishes the fundamental characteristics of the SNS:

- a. Extension of services to the entire population.

- b. Adequate organization to provide comprehensive health care, including promotion of health, prevention of disease, treatment and rehabilitation.

- c. Coordination and, as needed, integration of all public health resources into a single system.

- d. Financing of the obligations derived from this law will be met by resources of public administration, contributions and fees for the provision of certain services.

- e.   The provision of a comprehensive health care, seeking high standards, properly evaluated and controlled.[1]

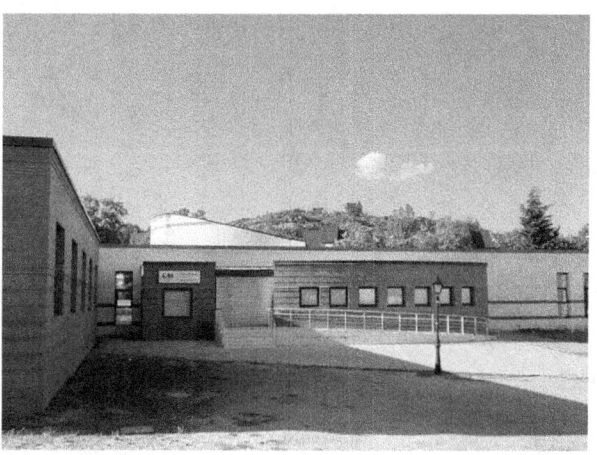

Health center in Torrelodones (Community of Madrid).

2.13.1   Antecedents to the SNS in Spain

Public intervention in collective health problems has always been of interest to governments and societies, especially in the control of epidemics through the establishment of naval quarantines, the closing of city walls and prohibitions on travel in times of plague, but also in terms of hygienic and palliative measures. Al-Andalus—Muslim-ruled medieval Spain—was distinguished by its level of medical knowledge relative to the rest of Europe, particularly among the physicians of the Golden age of Jewish culture in Spain. In the years after the *Reconquista*, the *Real Tribunal del Protomedicato* regulated the practice of medicine in Spain and in its colonies. However, the system of medical faculties at the various universities was very decentralized. Surgery and pharmacy were quite separate from medicine and were considerably less prestigious; the systems of Galen and Hippocrates dominated medical practice during most of the era of the *Antiguo Régimen*.

Medicine was one of the principal fields of activity for the *novatores* of the late 17th century, but their initiatives were individualized and localized. There is some continuity from their work to the broader work during the Age of Enlightenment, such as through the Colegio de Cirugía de San Carlos ("San Carlos College of Surgery") in Madrid. At the beginning of the 19th century, the Balmis Expedition (1803) to administer the smallpox vaccine throughout the Spanish colonies was a public health undertaking of unprecedented geographical scope.

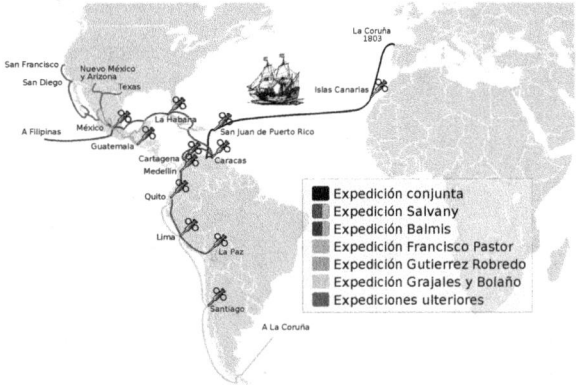

The Balmis Expedition of 1803 was a public health undertaking of unprecedented geographical scope.

The Cádiz Cortes debated a sanitary code (the *Código Sanitario de 1812*), but nothing was approved due to lack of scientific and technical consensus about the actions to be undertaken. During the bienio progresista, the Law of 28 November 1855 established the basis for a General Health Directorate (*Dirección General de Sanidad*), which was created a few years later and which would last into the 20th century. The Royal Decree of 12 January 1904 approved the General Health Instruction (*Instrucción General de Sanidad*), which altered little of the 1855 scheme besides the name; the name would later change to General Inspectorate of Health (*Inspección General de Sanidad*).

After the Spanish Civil War, the *Ley de Bases de 1944* perpetuated this . The Law of 14 December 1942 create a system of obligatory health insurance under the already extant National Insurance Institute (*Instituto Nacional de Previsión*, INP). The system was based on a percentage tax linked to employment. This was further modified by the General Law of Social Security (*Ley General de la Seguridad Social*) in 1974, toward the end of the Franco regime.[2] Social Security had taken on an increasing number of dis-

eases within its package of services, as well as covering a larger number of individuals and communities.

The General Health Law (*Ley General de Sanidad*) of 25 April 1986 and the creation of Health Councils (*Consejerías de Sanidad*) and a Ministry of Health, fulfilled the mandate of the Spanish Constitution of 1978, in particular Articles 43 and 49 which made protection of health a right of all citizens, and Title VIII, which foresaw that purview over matters of health would devolve to the autonomous communities.[3]

2.13.2 Laws regulating the Spanish National Health System

The General Health Law of 1986

The General Health Law of 1986 (*Ley 14/1986 General de Sanidad*) was formulated on two bases. First, it carries out a mandate of the Spanish Constitution, whose articles 43 and 49 establish the right of all citizens to protection of their health. The law recognizes a right to health services for all citizens and for foreigners resident in Spain.

Second, Title VIII of the Constitution confers upon the autonomous communities broad purview in matters of health and health care. The autonomous communities have first-order importance in this area, and the law permits devolution of these functions from the central government to the autonomous communities, in order to provide a health care system sufficient for the needs of their respective jurisdictions. Article 149.1.16 or the Constitution, a further basis for the present law, establishes substantive principles and criteria that allow general and common characteristics to be consistent throughout the new system, providing a common basis for health services throughout Spanish territory.

The administrative device set up by the law is the National Health System. The presumption underlying the adopted model is that in each autonomous community, authorities are adequately equipped with necessary territorial perspective, so that the benefits of autonomy do not conflict with the needs of management efficiency.

> The National Health System is thus conceived as the set of health services of the Autonomous Communities properly coordinated.[4]

Thus, the various health services fall under the responsibility of the respective autonomous communities, but also under basic direction and coordination by the central state. The respective health services of the autonomous communities would gradually realize a transfer of health resources from the central government to the autonomous communities.

Law of Cohesion and Quality (2003)

The General Health Law was complemented in 2003 by the Law of Cohesion and Quality of the National Health System (*Ley 16/2003 de cohesión y calidad del Sistema Nacional de Salud*), which maintained the basic lines of the General Health Law, but modified and broadened the articulation of that law to reflect existent social and political reality. By 2003, all of the autonomous communities had gradually assumed purview in matters of health and had established stable models to finance the assumed purview. Meanwhile, in the 17 years since the original law, Spanish society had undergone many cultural, technological and socioeconomic changes that affected people's ways of life and affected the country's patterns of disease and illness. These posed new challenges to the National Health System.

Therefore, the 2003 law establishes coordination and cooperation of public health authorities as a means to ensure citizens the right to health protection, with the common goal of ensuring equity, quality and social participation National Health System. The law defines a core set of functions common to all of the autonomous health services. Without interfering with the diversity of forms of organization, management and services inherent in a decentralized system, it attempts to establish certain basic, common safeguards throughout the country. This law attempts to establish collaboration of public health authorities with respect to benefits provided, pharmacy, health professionals, research, health information systems, and the overall quality of the health system.

Toward these ends, the law created or empowered several specialized organs and agencies, all of which are open to the participation of the autonomous communities. Among these are the Agency of Evaluation of Technologies (*Agencia de Evaluación de Tecnologías*, Spanish Agency of Medicines and Medical Products (*Agencia Española de Medicamentos y Productos Sanitarios*), the Human Resources Committee (*Comisión de Recursos Humanos*), the Committee to Assess Health Research (*Comisión Asesora de Investigación en Salud*), the Charles III Institute of Health (*Instituto de Salud Carlos III*), the Institute of Health Information (*Instituto de Información Sanitaria*), the Quality Agency of the National Health System (*Agencia de Calidad del Sistema Nacional de Salud*) and the Observatory of the National Health System (*Observatorio del Sistema Nacional de Salud*).

The basic organ of cohesion is the Interterritorial Council of the Spanish National Health Service (*Consejo Interterritorial del Servicio Nacional de Salud de España*), which has great flexibility in decision making, as well as mechanisms to build consensus and to bring together the parties taking such decisions. A system of inspection, the *Alta Inspección*, assures that accords are followed.[5]

Royal Decree-Law of Urgent Measures to Guarantee the Sustainability of the Sistema Nacional de Salud and Improve the Quality and Security of its Prestations (2012)

The Royal Decree-Law 16/2012[6] was introduced on April 20, 2012. It puts into law severe cuts in the Spanish National Health System, including the following:

- Refusal to give assistance to unregistered foreigners (in effect from September 1, 2012). This hasn't been applied by all the comunidades autónomas.

- Increase of the percentage of medicines paid by the user:[7]

    - Senior citizens didn't pay for medicines before the reform, but now they pay 10% (limited to €8/month if their income is ≤€18,000 a year, €18/month if their income is >€18,000 and ≤€100,000 a year, or €60/month if their income is >€100,000 a year).

    - Workers now pay 40% if their income is ≤€18,000 a year, 50% if their income is >€18,000 and ≤€100,000 a year, or 60% if their income is >€100,000 a year.

2.13.3　Governing agencies

Ministry of Health and Social Policy

The Ministry of Health and Social Policy develops the policies of the Government of Spain in matters of health, in planning and delivery of services, as well as exercising the purview of the General Administration of the State to assure citizens the right to protection of their health. The ministry has its headquarters on the Paseo del Prado in Madrid, across the street from the Museo del Prado.

The Royal Decree 1041/2009 of 29 June lays out the basic organic structure of the Spanish Ministry of Health and Social Policy. From the date of that decree, the new ministry assumed the functions of, and superseded the former Ministry of Health and Consumption (*Ministerio de Sanidad y Consumo*) and Secretary of State for Social Policy, Family, and Attention to Dependency and Disability (*Secretaría de Estado de Política Social, Familia y Atención a la Dependencia y a la Discapacidad*).

The objective of this reorganization is to reinforce the role of the single ministry as the instrument of cohesion for the National Health System (SNS), adding to the portfolio of the Secretary General of Health purview in matters of the quality of the SNS by adding to it the Agency of Quality

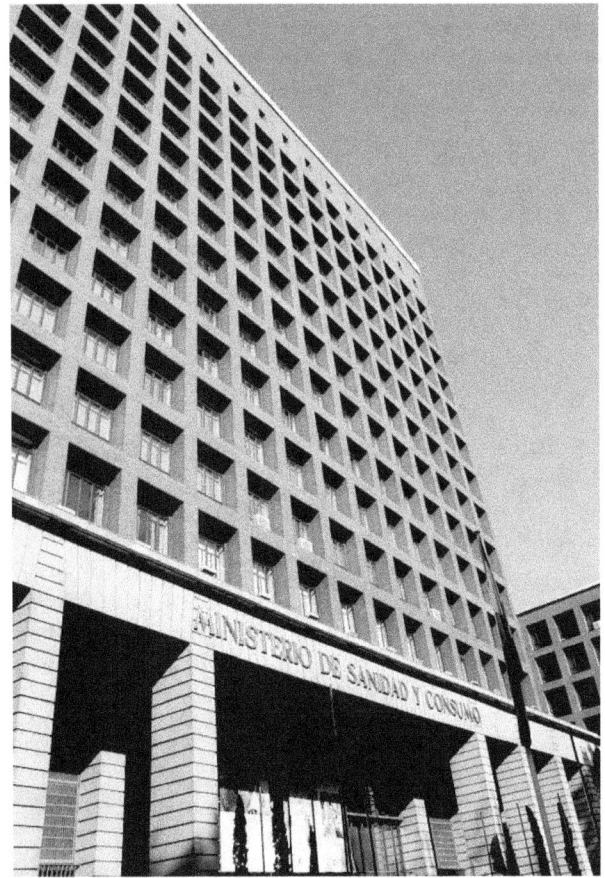

Seat of the Ministry of Health and Social Policy

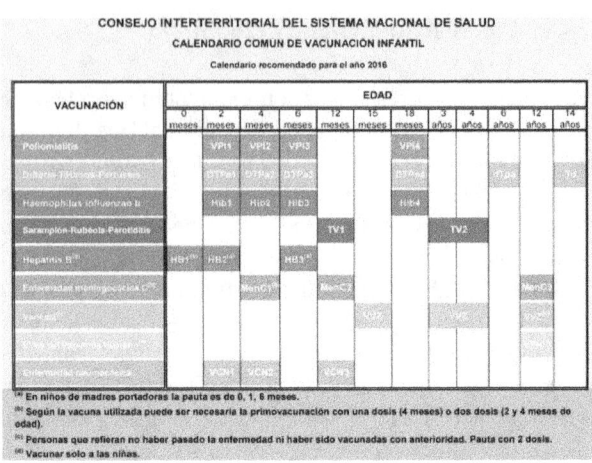

Childhood vaccination calendar, promoted by the CISNS.

of the National Health System (*Agencia de Calidad del Sistema Nacional de Salud*) and the General Directorate of Advanced Therapies and Transplants (*Dirección General de Terapias Avanzadas y Trasplantes*).[8]

Interterritorial Council of the Spanish National Health Service

The General Health Law of 1986 created the Interterritorial Council of the Spanish National Health Service (*Consejo Interterritorial del Servicio Nacional de Salud*, CISNS) as the organ of general coordination in matters related to health between the central State and the autonomous communities who were given authority in health matters under that law. It is jointly composed, and coordinates the basic lines of health policy in matters affecting contracts; acquisition of health and pharmaceutical products, as well as other related goods and services; as well as basic health personnel policies.

The 2003 Law of Cohesion and Quality of the SNS introduced significant changes in the composition, functioning, and purview of the CISNS. Under this law, the CISNS func-

tions variously as a plenary body, by delegated committees, through technical commissions, and through work groups. It meets as a plenary body at the initiative of its president or at the initiative of one-third of its members; plenary meetings occur at least four times a year. To some extent, this is a formality: resolutions from CISNS commissions are typically adopted by consensus. Cooperation agreements to conduct joint health actions are formalized in CISNS agreements.

Under the Law of Cohesion, CISNS functions mainly through the adoption of and compliance with joint accords, through the political use of the plenary sessions, with each member making an uncompromising defense of the interests of its region.

Presentations, committees, and working groups have been very important, some more than others. Important committees include:[9]

- Public Health Committee (*Comisión de Salud Pública*)

- Permanent pharmacy committee (*Comisión permanente de farmacia*)

- Scientific-technical committee of the National Health System (*Comisión científico-técnica del sistema Nacional de Salud*)

- Committee to monitor the health cohesion fund (*Comisión de seguimiento del fondo de cohesión sanitaria*)

- Permanent committee on insurance, funding, and benefits (*Comisión permanente de aseguramiento, financiación y prestaciones*)

- Committee against gender violence (*Comisión contra la violencia de género*)

- Transplant committee (*Comisión de trasplantes*)

Articles 69, 70 and 71 of the Law of Cohesion regulate the principal functions of the Interterritorial Council of the SNS. The principal aspects of the Interterritorial Council are:

The Interterritorial Council is constituted by the Minister of Health and Consumer Affairs [now of Health and Social Policy], who holds its presidency, and by the Councilors with purview over matters of health of the autonomous communities. The vicepresidency of the body will be fulfilled by one of the Councilors with purview over matters of health of the autonomous communities, elected by all of the Councilors who make up the body.[10]

The CISNS will come to know, debate among other things, and, as appropriate, make recommendations on the following matters:

- a) The development of the portfolio of services corresponding to the Catalog of Services of the National Health System, as well as its actualization.

- b) The establishment of health services complementary to the basic services of the National Health System on the part of the autonomous communities.

- c) Minimal guarantees of safety and quality for the authorization of the opening and placing into function of the health centers, services and establishments.

- d) The general and common criteria for the development of collaboration between pharmacy offices.

- e) The basic criteria and conditions of the convocations of professionals to assure their mobility throughout the State.

- f) Declaration of the necessity to realize coordinated actions in matters of public health to which this law refers.

- g) General criteria for the public financing of medicines, medical products and their variables.

- h) Establishment of criteria and mechanisms in order to guarantee at all times the financial sufficiency of the system.

The prior functions shall be exercised without prejudice to the legislative purview of the Cortes Generales and, as appropriate, the norms of the General Administration of the State; likewise the normal developmental, executive and organizational purview of the autonomous communities.[11]

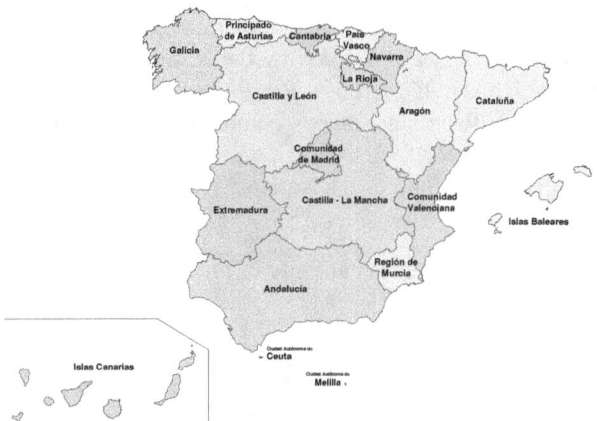

Map of the autonomous communities of Spain.

Purview of the autonomous communities in matters of health

Article 41 of the General Health Law establishes that:

- The autonomous communities exercise the purview assumed in their statutes [of autonomy] and those that the state transfers to them or, as appropriate, delegates to them.

- The public policies and actions foreseen in this Act which are not expressly reserved for the state will be deemed to have been delegated to the autonomous communities.[12]

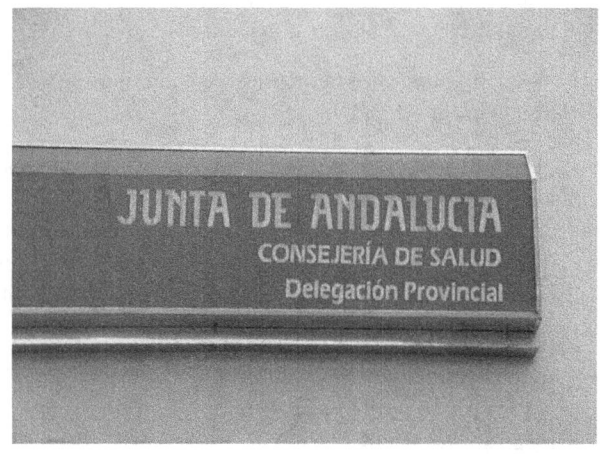

*Sign for the headquarters of a Health Office (*Delegación de Salud*) in Andalusia.*

The State finances, through general taxes, all health benefits and a percentage of pharmaceutical benefits. This tax is shared among the several autonomous communities according to various sharing criteria now that the communities are responsible for health in their respective territories.

Each year the CISNS, after deliberation, establishes the portfolio of services covered by the National Health System, which is published by a Royal Decree of the Ministry of Health. Each autonomous community then establishes its respective portfolio of services, which includes at least the service portfolio of the National Health System.

Purview of local governments in matters of health

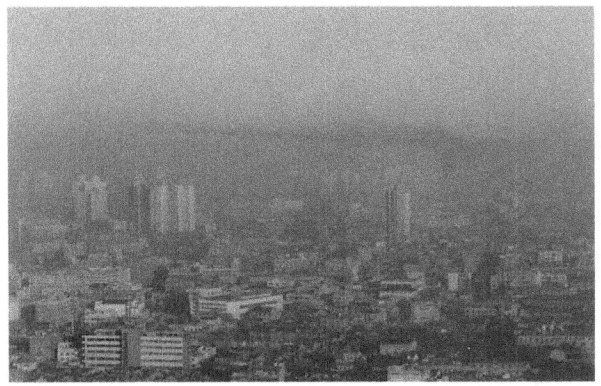

Air pollution; this photo is from Shanghai, China.

Article 42 of the General Health Law sets out that *ayuntamientos*—municipal governments—have the following responsibilities with respect to health, without prejudice to the purview of other public administrative bodies:

- a) Health control of the environment: air pollution, water supply [and water quality], wastewater treatment, urban and industrial residue.

- b) Health control of industries, activities and services, transport, noise and vibrations.

- c) Health control of buildings and places of human residence or gathering, especially of food centers, hairdressers, saunas and centers of personal hygiene, hotels and residential centers, schools, tourist campsites and areas of physical activity for sports and recreation.

- d) Health control of perishable food distribution and supply, beverages and other products directly or indirectly related to human use or consumption, such as means of transport.

- e) Health control of cemeteries and mortuary health policy.[13]

2.13.4   Territorial organization

As a consequence of the decentralization contemplated by the Spanish Constitution, each autonomous community has received adequate transfers to create a Health Service, the administrative structure that manages all of the centers, services and establishments of the community itself, as well as its deputations, municipal governments, and whatever other territorial administrations fall within that community. The Law of Cohesion establishes the Interterritorial Council (CISNS) as the organ of coordination and cooperation of the SNS.

In the autonomous cities of Ceuta and Melilla the corresponding health services are provided by the National Institute of Health Management, INGESA.

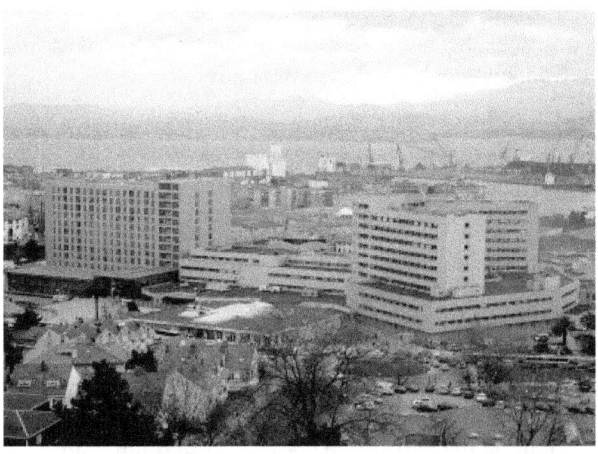

Marqués de Valdecilla University Hospital, part of the Cantabrian Health Service.

2.13.5   Health coverage in Spain

Under Chapter III of the 1978 Spanish Constitution, all Spanish citizens are beneficiaries of public health services. Concretely, it establishes that:

- Article 39: The public powers assure social, economic and juridical protection of the family.

- Article 43: The right to health protection is recognized. It is the responsibility of public authorities to organize and act as guardian over public health through preventive measures and the provision of necessary services. The Law will establish the rights and duties of all in this respect. The public powers will promote health education, physical education and sports.

- Article 49. The public powers will bring into existence a policy of prevention, treatment, rehabilitation and integration of those with physical, sensory or psychological disabilities.[16]

Further, the Organic Law 4/2000 (*Ley Orgánica 4/2000*) establishes the rights and liberties of foreigners resident in

Spain. Its effect on the healthcare provision can be seen in the following articles:

- Article 3. Foreigners will enjoy in Spain, in equal conditions with the Spanish, the rights and liberties recognized in Title I of the Constitution and in the laws that develop it, in terms established in this Organic Law.

- Article 10. Foreigners will have the right to engage in remunerated activity in self-employment or working for others, such as access to the Social Security System, in terms foreseen in this Organic Law and in the dispositions that develop it.

- Article 12. Foreigners who are registered in Spain in the municipality in which they are habitually resident have the right to health services on the same conditions as the Spanish. Foreigners who are in Spain have the right to urgent health services in the event of contracting severe illness or having an accident, whatever may be the cause, and the continuity of this care until the time of discharge. Foreign minors of less than 18 years who are in Spain have the right to health care on the same conditions as the Spanish. Pregnant foreigners who are in Spain have the right to health care during the pregnancy, while giving birth, and *post partum*.[17]

2.13.6   Financing of the health system

Article 10 of the Law of Cohesion establishes that the financing of the Spanish health system is the responsibility of the autonomous communities in conformity with the accords of transfer and the current system of autonomic financing, notwithstanding the existence of a third party liable to pay. Sufficient financing of services is determined by the resources assigned to the autonomous communities in conformity to what is established in the laws of autonomic financing.

Inclusion of a new service in the catalog of services of the National Health System is accompanied by an economic memo that contains the positive or negative financial impact it is expected to imply. This memo is brought up to the Council of Fiscal Policy and Finance for analysis and approval as to whether to proceed.

Fairness in financing

Prior to 1986, public financing of health care occurred mostly through highly regressive payroll taxes. In 1986, the law that established the Spanish National Health System also shifted financing toward progressive general taxes and away from payroll taxes.[18] In a 2000 report, the World

Health Organization ranked Spain 26th of 191 countries in its fairness in financing.[19]

In 1999, reform to income tax deductions allowed high income earners to deduct more for private insurance. Although this reform was intended to decrease overconsumption of health care services, it had the side effect of more regressive financing of public health services. Nevertheless, that same year payroll taxes were completely phased out while higher indirect taxes (on excise goods such as alcohol and tobacco) were earmarked for health care.[20]

2.13.7   Functional organization

Individual health card

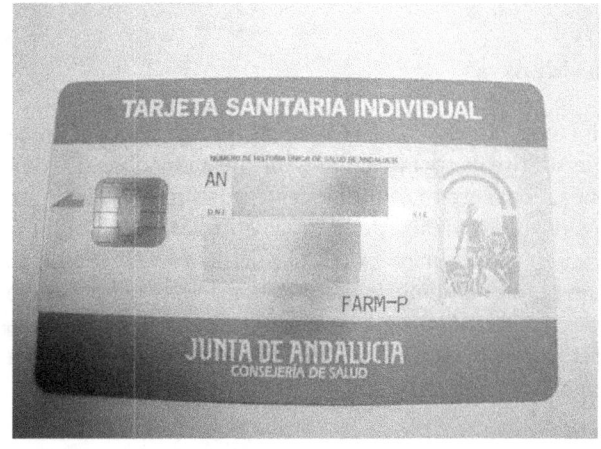

A health card (tarjeta sanitaria) *for the Andalusian Health Service (2010)*

Article 57 of the Law of Cohesion establishes that citizens' access to health services will be facilitated by use of an individual health card (*tarjeta sanitaria individual*), as the administrative document that accredits its holder and provides certain basic data.

In order to best facilitate collaboration, quality, and continuity of services, the each card includes a standardized form of basic identification data for the holder, and indicates in which autonomic health service the person is enrolled. In particular, the cards incorporate a digital form of this information; health facilities throughout Spain have appropriate equipment to read the digital information from the cards. A cardholder should thereby be able to access all the services of all relevant health professionals throughout the country.

Clinical history

A patient's clinical history is a medical-legal document that arises from the interactions between health professionals and their clients. From a medical and legal point of view, the clinical history is the only document valid to track this history of interactions. In primary care, where methods of health promotion are important, the clinical history document is sometimes known as a "health history" (*historia de salud*) or "life history" (*historia de vida*).

Clinical histories in the SNS   The Clinical History of the [Spanish] National Health System (*Historia Clínica Digital del Sistema Nacional de Salud*, HCDSNS) is intended to guarantee citizens and health professionals access to whatever clinical information is relevant for medical care of a particular patient. This history should be available at all authorized locations, but nowhere else: except as needed for treatment, the information is considered confidential and access is restricted.[21]

Health Areas

The term "Health Area" (**Área de Salud**) refers to an administrative district that brings together a functional and organizational group of health centers and primary care professionals. A Health Area may be exclusively focused on primary care or may include specialists as well. Some autonomous communities use different term, such as Direction of a sector (*Dirección de sector*), or of a comarca, district, department, or other territorial unit used in that autonomous community.[22]

Basic Health Zones

Although the autonomous communities differ among themselves in layering subdivisions of their health areas, all eventually come down to a Health Zone (*Zona de Salud*) or Basic Health Zone (*Zona Básica de Salud*) as the unit for a primary health care team. In Andalusia, for example, each existing Basic Health Zone takes care of a population between 5,000 and 20,000 inhabitants. The Basic Health Zone is served by a single general hospital and specialists' center.[23]

Primary Care

Article 12 of the Law of Cohesion establishes the concept of "primary care," the basic level of patient care that guarantees the comprehensiveness and continuity of care throughout the patient's life, acting as manager and coordinator of cases and regulator of issues. Primary care includes health promotion, health education, prevention of illness, health care, maintenance and recuperation of health, as well as physical rehabilitation and social work. Primary health care includes service provided either on-demand, scheduled, or urgently, both in the clinic as well as in the patient's home.

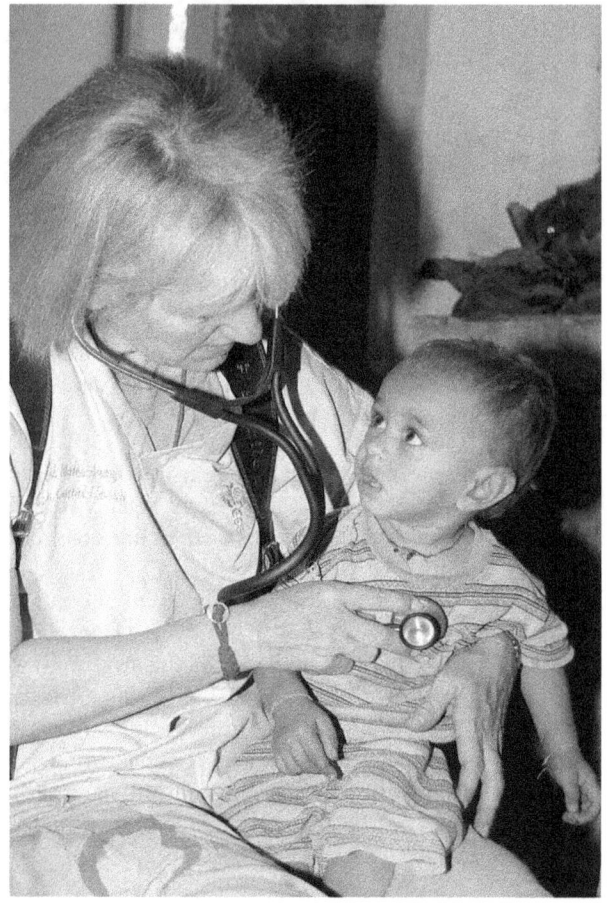

Cardiac auscultation, a protocol used in primary care for initial diagnosis of diseases and syndromes of the heart.

Specialized care

Article 13 of the Law of Cohesion regulates characteristics of health care offered in Spain by medical specialists, which is provided at the request of primary care physicians. This may be in-patient hospital care or out-patient consultation at specialist centers or day hospitals. It includes care, diagnosis, therapy, rehabilitation and certain preventive care, as well as health promotion, health education and prevention of illness whose nature makes it appropriate to handle at this level. Specialized care guarantees the continuity of integrated patient care once the capabilities of primary care have been exhausted and until matters can be returned to that level. Insofar as patient condition allows, specialized care is offered in out-patient consultation and in day hospitals. As of 2010, Spain recognizes fifty distinct medical specialties.[24]

Social-health care

Article 14 of the Law of Cohesion defines social-health care (*atención sociosanitaria*) as the combination of care for those patients, generally those with a chronic illness, whose would benefit from the simultaneous and synergistic provision of health services and social services to increase their personal autonomy, palliate their limitation or hardships, and facilitate their social reinsertion. This group includes:

- a) Longterm health care.

- b) Health care connected to convalescence.

- c) Rehabilitation after illness

2.13.8 Registered health professionals

2000 data from the INE (Spain's National Institute of Statistics) counts 616,232 individuals credentialed by a professional association as health care professionals. The largest number of these are nursing professionals; that is also the profession with the highest percentage of women. The following table is a breakdown of some of the INE statistics. No exact breakdown is available to indicate what number of these might be related to mental health and psychotherapy or clinical psychology.

2.13.9 Health establishments

Healthcare centers

Royal Decree 1277/2003, of 10 October, establishes the general bases for authorization of health centers, services and establishments. It defines "healthcare center" (*centro sanitario*) as the organized combination of technical means and installations in which trained professionals, identified by their official certification or professional qualification, undertake basic health care activities with the purpose of improving people's health. These may be integrated into one or more health services, which constitute its healthcare portfolio.[26]

Consultorios

Certain healthcare centers (*centros sanitarios*) are referred to as *consultorios*, a term roughly equivalent to British English "surgery" or American English "doctor's office."

These are offices that, while not full-fledged health centers (*centros de salud*), nonetheless provide care beyond primary care. Some terms used are *consultorios rurales, consultorios locales*, and *consultorios periféricos* (respectively, rural, local and "peripheral"; that last means a center located in a community other than the main settlement of a municipality), but other terms may exist, analogous to those that refer to various types of health centers.[27]

According to the 2008 National Catalog of Hospitals (*Catálogo Nacional de Hospitales 2008*), Spain in 2007 had a total of 10,178 *consultorios* that allowed health professionals to provide more local services than the health centers in their respective zones, with the purpose of bringing basic services closer to people who reside in nuclei dispersed through rural areas that tend to have an older than average population.[28]

Health centers

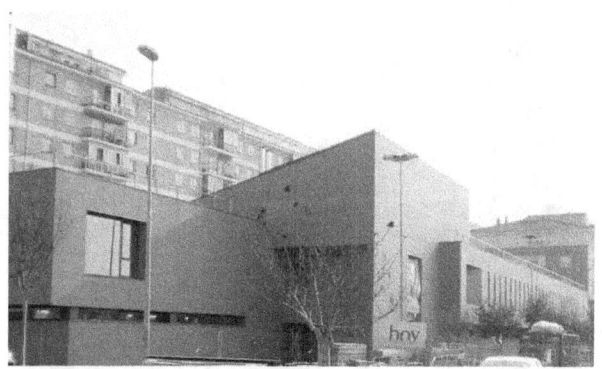

Health center in Ansoáin (Navarre)

A health center (*centro de salud*, distinct from the smaller "healthcare center" *centro sanitario*) in Spain's SNS is main physical and functional structure devoted to coordinated global, integral, permanent and continuing primary care, based in a team of health care professionals and other professionals who work there as a team.[29]

Health centers basically practice the general medicine or family medicine, providing a unity of care in which a specialist in community and family medicine is responsible to provide preventive care, health promotion, diagnosis and basic treatment on an outpatient basis. According to the 2008 National Catalog of Hospitals (*Catálogo Nacional de Hospitales*), in 2007 Spain had 2,913 health centers.[30]

Specialized centers

Specialized centers are healthcare centers where different health care professionals provide services to particular group identified by common pathologies, age, or other common characteristics. Among these are:

Dental clinics Focused on care of the teeth and mouth.

Centers for assisted human reproduction Biomedical teams focused on assisted reproductive technology.

Centers for voluntary interruption of pregnancy Provide abortion services in legally permitted cases.

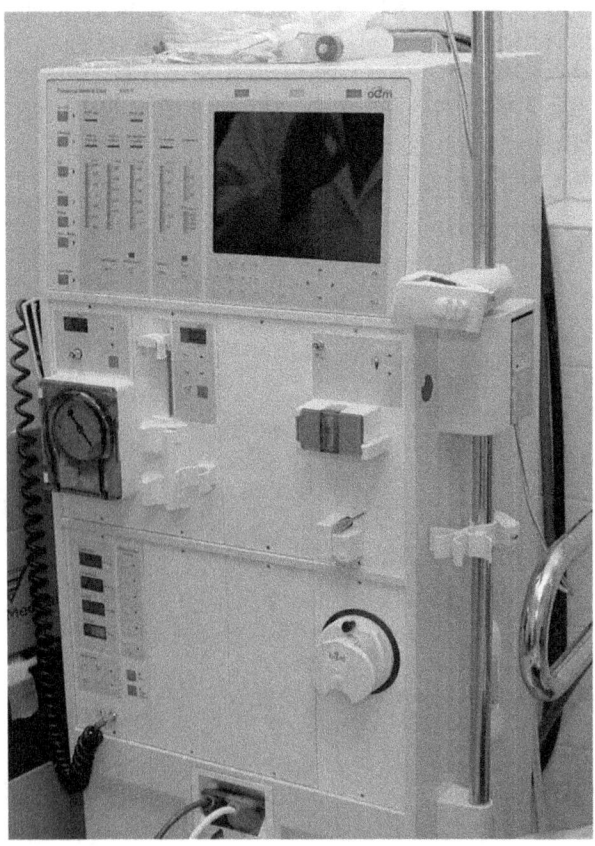

Hemodialysis machine.

Centers for major outpatient surgery Provide surgery and subsidiary services including general, local and regional anesthesia and sedation. For surgeries that require only brief post-operative care and therefore do not require overnight hospitalization.

Dialysis centers For patients with failed kidneys.

Diagnostic centers Dedicated to diagnostic, analytic and imaging services.

Mobile health care centers Carry human and technical means for the purpose of health care activities.

Transfusion centers Carry out all activities related to the extraction and verification of human blood and its components, and of treatment, storage, and distribution.

Tissue banks Conserve and guarantee the quality of tissues after they are obtained and until they are used as allografts or autografts.

Medical inspection centers (*Centros de reconocimiento médico*), where examinations and other tests of ability are carried out for applicants or holders of medical and other health care permits or licenses.

Mental health centers Diagnose and treat mental illness on an outpatient basis.

Specialized health care establishments

Specialized health care establishments are private centers that provide a suite of health care products, ranging from medicines to sophisticated prostheses. These establishments are grouped by specialty and, on that account, must have accredited or certified technical personnel. Among these establishments are:

Pharmacies Private establishments operated in the public interest, subject to health care planning established by the autonomous communities, which provide the public with basic services recognized in Article 1 of Law 16/1997, of 25 April, that regulates pharmacy services (*Ley 16/1997, de 25 de abril, de regulación de los servicios de las oficinas de farmacia*).

Botiquines (singular: *Botiquín*) are authorized to hold, conserve and dispense medicines and health care products in places where there would be special difficulties of accessibility of a pharmacy.

Optometric offices (Ópticas) Evaluate visual capacity using optometric techniques; crafting, sale, verification and control of adequate means for the prevention, detection, protection, and improvement of visual acuity.

Orthopedia centers Dispense orthopedic health care products such as prostheses and orthotics, technical devices to alleviate loss of autonomy, functionality, or physical capacity.

Audioprosthesis centers Dispense health care products, intended for the correction of auditory deficiencies, such as hearing aids, with adaptation individualized to each patient.

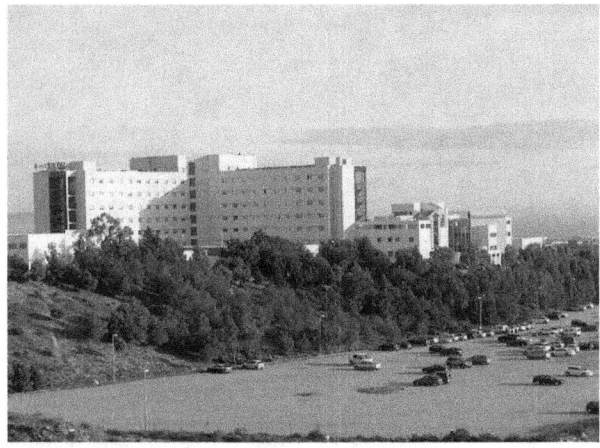

Hospital General Torrecárdenas, Almería.

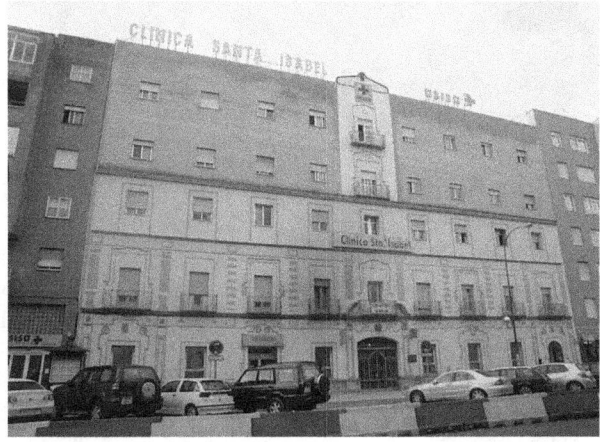

ASISA private clinic in Seville.

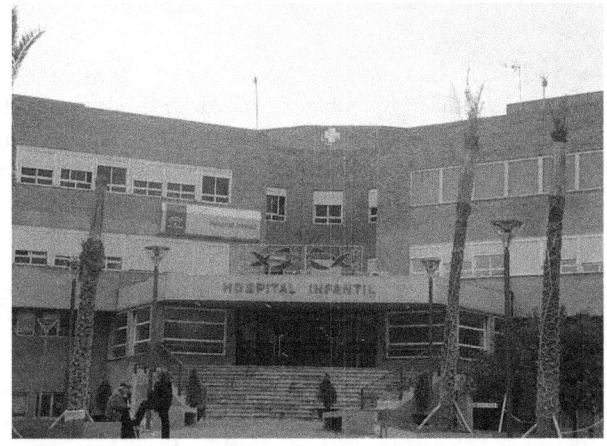

Children's hospital in Seville.

Hospitals

A hospital is a health care establishment that provides inpatient care and specialized (and other) care, providing such services as are needed in its geographical area. A hospital can be a single structure or a hospital complex, even including branch buildings off of its main campus; it can also integrate any number of specialized centers.[31]

A similar concept to a hospital is a *clinic*. In Spain, a clinic (*clínica*) is a health center, typically a private one, where patients can receive health coverage in a broad range of specialties. Some of these clinics include very up-to-date operating theaters capable of providing minimally invasive surgery, and "hospitalization zones" where patients can recuperate on an inpatient basis. In large Spanish cities, there are numerous clinics. These are the facilities that are normally used by health care professionals whose medical societies cover it: ASISA, Adeslas, etc.[32]

The General Health Law of 1986 establishes that the level of specialized care provided in hospitals and their dependent specialty centers will focus care on complex health problems. Hospital centers will develop, besides their functions strictly related to health care, functions of health promotion, prevention of illnesses and investigation and teaching, in accord with the programs of each of health, with the object of complementing their activities with those developed by the primary care network.[33]

As elsewhere in the world, the size of hospitals in Spain is often gauged by the number of "installed beds" (*camas instaladas*). This is the number of hospital beds with fixed locations; at any given time, some beds may be out of commission.

General and specialized hospitals General hospitals treat a broad range of pathologies and typically provide services including surgery, obstetrics and gynecology, and pediatrics. Other hospitals are more specialized. The following list includes most of the common types of specialized hospitals in Spain, but is not intended to be exhaustive.

Health care contracts Spanish government-run healthcare administrations sign health care contracts (*conciertos sanitarios*) with privately run entities that provide health care services. They are regulated by the provisions of the General Health Law and the current rules of government contracting. There are some special cases where the relation between the hospital and the managing entity is regulated by a special arrangement called a *Convenio de Vinculación* or *Convenio Singular* ("Linkage Convention" or "Singluar Convention").[34] In Catalonia there are also centers integrated into the Network of Hospitals for Public Use (Red de Hospitales de Utilización Pública, XHUP) as outlined in the supplement to Decree 124/2008 of the Department of Health of the Autonomous Government of Catalonia (*Anexo del Decreto 124/2008 del Departamento de Salud* *de la Generalitat de Catalunya).*

Patrimonial dependency The patrimonial dependency (*dependencia patrimonial*) of a hospital (or other health care facility) is the individual or other juridical entity that owns, at least, the building occupied by the facility. Hospitals that are under the dependency of Spanish Social Security belong primarily to the General Treasury of Social Security, although there is a special group within Social Security for the Mutuals of Accidents and Occupational Diseases (*Mutuas de Accidentes de Trabajo y Enfermedades Profesionales*, MATEP). There are also a few cases where patrimony is shared by two or more public entities on a consortium basis.

The 2009 National Catalog of Hospitals contains information about the patrimonial dependency of hospitals, summarized as follows; hospital complexes are each counted here as a single hospital:[35]

40 percent of stays in private hospitals are arranged and paid for by the public system.[35]

The 2008 National Catalog of Hospitals gives the following breakdown of types of hospitals.[36]

High technology resources

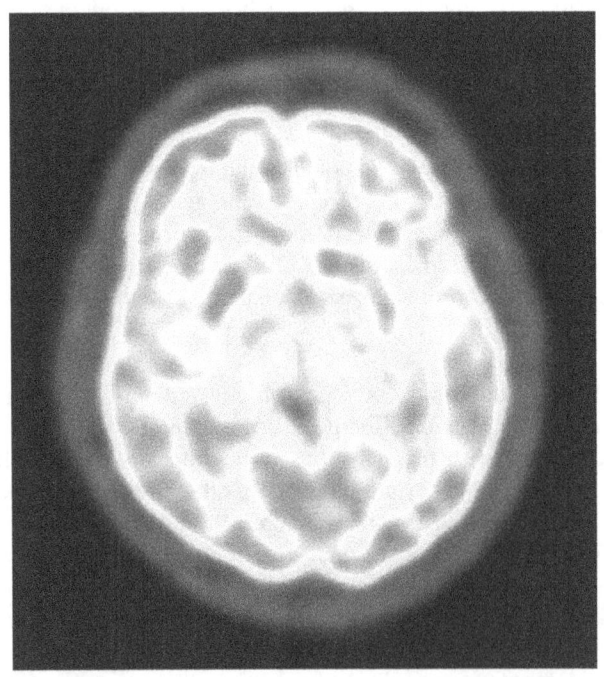

Positron emission tomography (PET) scan of a typical brain.

Health care centers, principally hospitals and specialty centers, have high technology capabilities used primarily to perform better patient diagnoses. The following breakdown

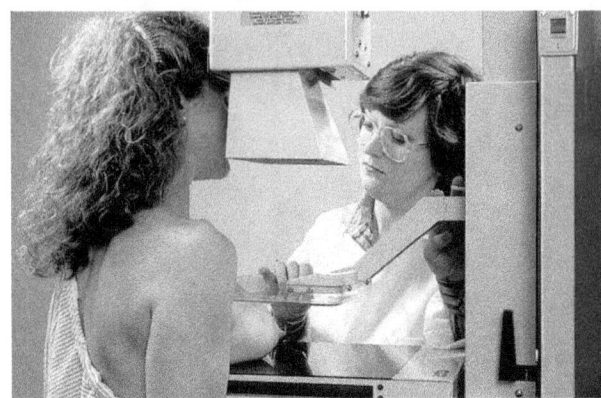

Performing a mammogram. The image is from the United States.

of such facilities is based on the 2008 National Catalog of Hospitals.

2.13.10 Services

Article 7 of the Law of Cohesion establishes the catalog of services of the National Health System, with the object of guaranteeing the basic and common conditions for an adequate level of integrated, continuous health care. Health care services include prevention, diagnosis, therapy and rehabilitation, as well as promotion and maintenance of citizens' health.

Article 11 of the law establishes the basic lines of public health services:

- 1. The public health service is the ensemble of initiatives organized by public administrations to preserve, protect and promote the health of the population. It is a combination of sciences, capabilities and attitudes directed to the maintenance and improvement of the health of all persons through collective and social acts.

- 2. The services in this ambit include the following activities: Epidemiological information and vigilance. Protection of health. Promotion of health. Vigilance and control of possible health risks derived from the importation, exportation and transit of merchandise and of international travel. Promotion and protection of environmental safety. Promotion and protection of health on the job.

- 3. Public health services are to be exercised with an integral character, from public health structures to administrations and the infrastructure of primary care of the National Health System.[38]

Primary care services

Primary care services constitute the majority of the services of the SNS; this is true of health promotion and education, prevention of illness, hands-on health care, health maintenance, recuperation, rehabilitation, and social work.

The following catalog demonstrates preventive activities, health promotion and education, family care and community care as performed in primary care centers.[39]

- Inculcate healthy life habits in adolescents with respect to the use of tobacco, alcohol and recreational drugs as well as harmful eating disorders and healthy conduct with respect to sexuality.

- Orientation of women during pregnancy and birth, early diagnosis of gynecological cancers and breast cancer, detection and care of problems related to menopause. Family planning.

- Pediatrics, including infant and child health care, nutrition, general counsel on child development, health education and childhood accidents. Vaccinations.

- Care for adults in risk groups or with chronic conditions. Counsel on healthy life styles and detection of health problems.

- Geriatrics: promotion of health and prevention of illness. Homecare for the housebound.

- Detection of violence against women and domestic abuse, as well as child abuse, elder abuse, and abuse of the disabled.

- Dentistry: Care, diagnosis and therapy, health promotion and education, and illness prevention related to the teeth and mouth.

- Care of terminal patient: integral, individual and continual care either in the home or at a health center.

- Mental health care: prevention and promotion to maintain mental health, in coordination with specialists.

Specialized care

At times, patients will require specialized health care services. These may be provided in external consultations, day hospitals, or on an inpatient basis.

Examples of specialized services are intensive and critical care, anesthesia, defibrillation, but also some forms of hemotherapy, rehabilitation, and even nutrition, diet, postpartum treatment, and family planning, especially assisted

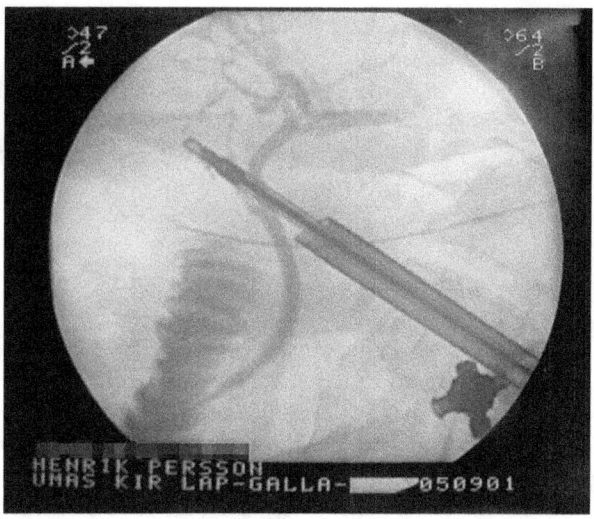

Laparoscopy is a specialized diagostic tool. Here, a laproscopic image from a cholecystectomy.

reproductive technology. Specialized treatment can also be involved in detecation, prescription and implementation of diagnostic and therapeutic procedures, especially those related to prenatal diagnosis in risk groups, diagnosis by imaging, interventionist radiology, hemodynamics, nuclear medicine, neurophysiology, endoscopy, lab tests, biopsies, radiotherapy, radiosurgery, renal lithotripsy, dialysis, techniques of respiratory therapy, organ transplants and other tissue and cell transplants.[40]

Urgent care

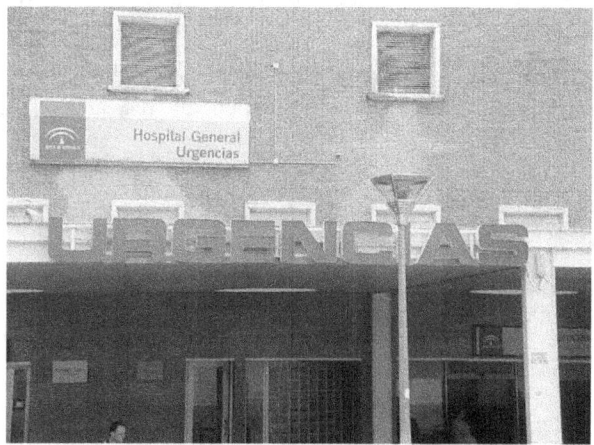

Emergency room of the Virgen del Rocío hospital, Seville.

Emergency medicine is health care provided in cases where emergency care is needed. Emergency medicine is practiced both in healthcare facilities and at the site of work accidents, traffic accidents, etc. or in the home of a patient whose condition prevents them from getting to a health-care facility. Emergency medicine is a 24-hour-a-day service provided, in particular, by physicians and other medical professionals in hospital emergency rooms, but also in ambulances, medical evacuation helicopters, etc. *en route* to such facilities.[41]

Pharmaceutical services

Medications in Spain are regulated under Law 29/2006 of 26 July, of guarantees and rational use of medications and health care products (*Ley 29/2006, de 26 de julio, de garantías y uso racional de los medicamentos y productos sanitarios*).[42] One of the SNS's priorities with respect to pharmaceuticals is to teach patients to make rational use of medications and to avoid, insofar as possible, unsupervised self-medication.

Pharmaceutical services include medications and health products are provided to patients according to their clinical needs, in precise doses and over an adequate period at the least cost possible. Medications are dispensed by pharmacies, each of which is headed by a licensed pharmacist.

All medications to be prescribed to patients must either be authorized and registered by the Spanish Agency of Medications and Health Care Products (*Agencia Española de Medicamentos y Productos Sanitarios*), or must be formulations prepared by licensed pharmacists. Exceptions to this requirement are cosmetics, dietetic products, dental products and other sanitary products, as well as drugs classified as advertising, homeopathic medicines, and articles and accessories advertised to the general public and where the purchaser pays the full price (that is, no money comes from SNS-related sources).

Spanish patients make a copayment when they acquire pharmaceuticals. The distribution of the cost is as follows:[43]

- Medications dispensed as part of hospitalization are free to the patient.

- Other prescriptions are financed as follows

    - Most pensioners and their beneficiaries receive their medicines for free. Pensioners who were public functionaries and are protected by MU-FACE (Mutualidad General de Funcionarios Civiles del Estado) pay 30 percent of prescription cost.

    - Non-pensioners pay 40 percent of the price of prescription drugs. Active functionaries protecte by MUFACE pay 30 percent.

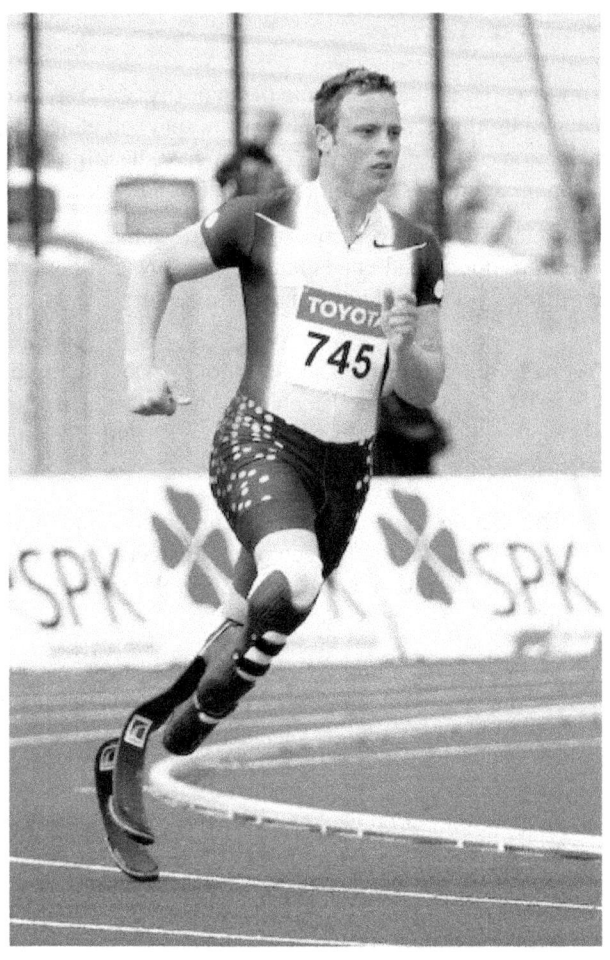

Runner Oscar Pistorius, with his orthopedic leg.

- Communities affected by toxic oil syndrome and patients with AIDS receive their prescriptions for free.

- Individuals with toxic treatments pay 10 percent, up to a maximum of 2.64 euros per prescription.

Orthoprosthetic and complementary services

Orthoprosthetic services can be permanent surgically implanted prostheses, external prostheses, special orthoses and prostheses including hearing aids and earmolds for children up to age 16 suffering from bilateral hearing impairments.[44][45]

"Complementary services" include complex dietary therapies, vehicles for invalids, and home oxygen therapy.[44][45]

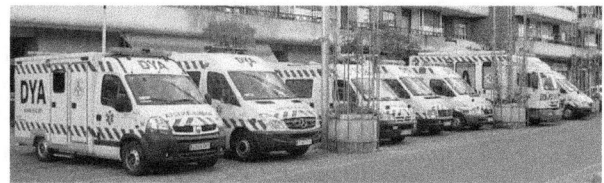

DYA ambulances in the Basque Country.

Health care transport

The health care transport infrastructure transports people who are ill, accident victims, or otherwise in need of medical attention. It includes ambulances, as well as air ambulances: helicopters and airplanes whose interiors are specially modified for the purpose. For most purposes, of course, ground transport is preferred, but sometimes distances or the difficulty of reaching particular locations make air transport more practical.

2.13.11   Demographics of Spain

According to data from the National Institute of Statistics (*Instituto Nacional de Estadística*, INE), as of January 1, 2009, Spain has a population of 46,754,807, of whom 23,116,988 (49,44%) are male and 23,628,919 (50.56%) female. In recent years, this population has been increasing slowly but progressively. In the last decade, the increase has been largely through immigration: 5,268,762 Spanish residents are foreigners.

These numbers count only citizens and legal immigrants. The health care system must also provide services for thousands of illegal immigrants and for the many tourists who visit Spain each year.

Population pyramid

Analysis of the population pyramid shows that

- 19 percent of the total population is under 20 years of age.

- 32 percent of the total population is 20 to 40 years of age.

- 28 percent of the total population is 40 to 60 years of age.

- 21 percent of the total population is at least 60 years old.

This structure is typical of a modern demographic regimen, with an evolution toward an aging population and a declin-

ing birth rate. This means that Spain has to expect an increase in use of the services that are targeted at older adults. This effect is further exacerbated by a steadily increasing life expectancy.

2.13.12   See also

- National Transplant Organization achieved the highest rate of donors in the world in 2006.

- Miguel de Cervantes Health Care Centre

- Social Security in Spain

2.13.13   Notes

[1]
- a. La extensión de sus servicios a toda la población.

- b. La organización adecuada para prestar una atención integral a la salud, comprensiva tanto de la promoción de la salud y prevención de la enfermedad como de la curación y rehabilitación.

- c. La coordinación y, en su caso, la integración de todos los recursos sanitarios públicos en un dispositivo único.

- d. La financiación de las obligaciones derivadas de esta Ley se realizará mediante recursos de las Administraciones públicas, cotizaciones y tasas por la prestación de determinados servicios.

- e. La prestación de una atención integral de la salud procurando altos niveles de calidad debidamente evaluados y controlados.

Ley 14/1986 General de Sanidad. Organización General de Sistema Sanitario Público, noticias.juridicas.com.

[2] Decreto 2065/1974, de 30 de mayo

[3] Ley 14/1986, de 25 de abril, General de Sanidad, *BOE* number 102 of 1986-04-29, pages 15207–15224. (Text of the law, in Spanish.)

[4] *El Sistema Nacional de Salud se concibe así como el conjunto de los servicios de salud de las Comunidades Autónomas convenientemente coordinados.* - Preamble to the General Health Law of 1986.

[5] "LEY 16/2003, de 28 de mayo, de cohesión y calidad del Sistema Nacional de Salud.". Jefatura del Estado (*BOE* número 128 de 29/5/2003). Retrieved 2010-01-08.

[6] Available online at http://boe.es/buscar/doc.php?id=BOE-A-2012-5403

[7] http://boe.es/buscar/doc.php?id=BOE-A-2012-5403. Article 2, section Trece. Checked on March 18, 2013.

[8] "Organización del Ministerio de Sanidad y Política Social (España)". msps.es. Retrieved 2010-01-09.

[9] Colectivo El Bosque (2008-10-15). "Qué es, como funciona el Consejo Interterritorial del Sistema Nacional de Salud (CISNS)". e-ras. Revista on.line de información sanitaria. Retrieved 2010-01-11.

[10] *El Consejo Interterritorial está constituido por el Ministro de Sanidad y Consumo, que ostentará su presidencia, y por los Consejeros competentes en materia de sanidad de las comunidades autónomas. La vicepresidencia de este órgano la desempeñará uno de los Consejeros competentes en materia de sanidad de las comunidades autónomas, elegido por todos los Consejeros que lo integran.* (from Article 70 of the Ley de cohesión y calidad de SNS.)

[11] *El CISNS conocerá, debatirá entre otros aspectos, y, en su caso, emitirá recomendaciones sobre las siguientes materias:*

- *a) El desarrollo de la cartera de servicios correspondiente al Catálogo de Prestaciones del Sistema Nacional de Salud, así como su actualización.*

- *b) El establecimiento de prestaciones sanitarias complementarias a las prestaciones básicas del Sistema Nacional de Salud por parte de las comunidades autónomas.*

- *c) Las garantías mínimas de seguridad y calidad para la autorización de la apertura y puesta en funcionamiento de los centros, servicios y establecimientos sanitarios.*

- *d) Los criterios generales y comunes para el desarrollo de la colaboración de las oficinas de farmacia.*

- *e) Los criterios básicos y condiciones de las convocatorias de profesionales que aseguren su movilidad en todo el territorio del Estado.*

- *f) La declaración de la necesidad de realizar las actuaciones coordinadas en materia de salud pública a las que se refiere esta ley.*

- *g) Los criterios generales sobre financiación pública de medicamentos y productos sanitarios y sus variables.*

- *h) El establecimiento de criterios y mecanismos en orden a garantizar en todo momento la suficiencia financiera del sistema.*

Las anteriores funciones se ejercerán sin menoscabo de las competencias legislativas de las Cortes Generales y, en su caso, normativas de la Administración General del Estado, así como de las competencias de desarrollo normativo, ejecutivas y organizativas de las comunidades autónomas. "Capítulo X. Ley de cohesión y calidad de SNS. Del Consejo Interterritorial". *BOE*. Retrieved 2010-01-12.

[12]
- *Las comunidades autónomas ejercerán las competencias asumidas en sus estatutos y las que el estado les transfiera o, en su caso, les delegue.*

- *Las decisiones y actuaciones publicas previstas en esta ley que no se hayan reservado expresamente al estado se entenderán atribuidas a las comunidades autónomas.*

[13]
- *a) Control sanitario del medio ambiente: Contaminación atmosférica, abastecimiento de aguas, saneamiento de aguas residuales, residuos urbanos e industriales.*

- b) *Control sanitario de industrias, actividades y servicios, transportes, ruidos y vibraciones.*

- c) *Control sanitario de edificios y lugares de vivienda y convivencia humana, especialmente de los centros de alimentación, peluquerías, saunas y centros de higiene personal, hoteles y centros residenciales, escuelas, campamentos turísticos y áreas de actividad físico deportivas y de recreo.*

- d) *Control sanitario de la distribución y suministro de alimentos perecederos, bebidas y demás productos, directa o indirectamente relacionados con el uso o consumo humanos, así como los medios de su transporte.*

- e) *Control sanitario de los cementerios y policía sanitaria mortuoria.*

[14] "Transferencias del Insalud" (PDF). Madrid: Ministerio de Sanidad y Política Social (Ministry of Health and Social Policy). Retrieved 2010-01-06.

[15] "Cifras de población referidas al 01/01/2009. Resumen por Comunidades Autónomas.". Instituto Nacional de Estadística (Spain). Retrieved 2010-01-06.

[16]
- *Artículo 39: Los poderes públicos aseguran la protección social, económica y jurídica de la familia.*

- *Artículo 43: Se reconoce el derecho a la protección de la salud. Compete a los poderes públicos organizar y tutelar la salud pública a través de medidas preventivas y de las prestaciones y servicios necesarios. La Ley establecerá los derechos y deberes de todos a ete respecto. Los poderes públicos fomentarán la educación sanitaria, la educación física y el deporte.*

- *Artículo 49. Los poderes públicos realizarán una política de previsión, tratamiento, rehabilitación e integración de los disminuidos físicos, sensoriales y psíquicos.*

"Constitución Española. Capítulo III". noticias.jurídicas.com. Retrieved 2010-01-12.

[17]
- *Artículo 3. Los extranjeros gozarán en España, en igualdad de condiciones que los españoles, de los derechos y libertades reconocidos en el Título I de la Constitución y en sus leyes de desarrollo, en los términos establecidos en esta Ley Orgánica.*

- *Artículo 10. Los extranjeros tendrán derecho a ejercer una actividad remunerada por cuenta propia o ajena, así como al acceso al Sistema de la Seguridad Social, en los términos previstos en esta Ley Orgánica y en las disposiciones que la desarrollen.*

- *Artículo 12. Los extranjeros que se encuentren en España inscritos en el padrón del municipio en el que residan habitualmente, tienen derecho a la asistencia sanitaria en las mismas condiciones que los españoles. Los extranjeros que se encuentren en España tienen derecho a la asistencia sanitaria pública de urgencia ante la contracción de enfermedades graves o accidentes, cualquiera que sea su causa, y a la continuidad de dicha atención hasta la situación de alta médica. Los extranjeros menores de dieciocho años que se encuentren en España tienen derecho a la asistencia sanitaria en las mismas condiciones que los españoles. Las extranjeras embarazadas que se encuentren en España tendrán derecho a la asistencia sanitaria durante el embarazo, parto y postparto.*

"Ley Orgánica 4/2000, de 11 de enero, sobre derechos y libertades de los extranjeros en España y su integración social." (pdf). Boletín Oficial del Estado. Retrieved 2010-01-12.

[18] Costa-Font, Joan; Gil, Joan (December 2009). "Exploring the pathways of inequality in health, health care access and financing in decentralized Spain". *Journal of European Social Policy.* **19** (5): 446–458.

[19] World Health Organisation, World Health Staff, (2000), Haden, Angela; Campanini, Barbara, eds., The world health report 2000 - Health systems: improving performance (PDF), Geneva, Switzerland: World Health Organisation, ISBN 92-4-156198-X

[20] Puig-junoy, Jaume; Rovira, Joan (June 2004). "Issues raised by the impact of tax reforms and regional devolution on health-care financing in Spain, 1996 - 2002". *Environment and Planning C: Government and Policy.* **22** (3): 453–464.

[21] msc.es (ed.). "Historia Clínica Digital del Sistema Nacional de Salud (España)". Retrieved 2010-01-12.

[22] "Catálogo de Centros de Atención Primaria del Sistema Nacional de Salud 2009". msc.es. Retrieved 2010-01-12.

[23] "Organización del Sistema Nacional de Salud (España)" (pdf). msps.es. Retrieved 2009-12-28.

[24] "Especialidades médicas en España". ortopedia.rediris.es. Retrieved 2010-01-11.

[25] "Profesionales sanitarios colegiados por tipo de profesional, años y sexo.". INE. Retrieved 2010-01-13.

[26] "Real Decreto 1277/2003, de 10 de octubre, por el que se establecen las bases generales sobre autorización de centros, servicios y establecimientos sanitarios.". *BOE* nº254 23 de octubre de 2003. Retrieved 2010-01-14.

[27] "Centros de Sanitarios del SNS". msc.es. Retrieved 2010-01-12.

[28] "Recursos y actividades del SNS" (pdf). msps.es. Retrieved 2010-01-12.

[29] "Real Decreto 1277/2003, de 10 de octubre. ANEXO II Definiciones de centros, unidades asistenciales y establecimientos sanitarios. Centro de salud.". *BOE* nº254 23 de octubre de 2003. Retrieved 2010-01-14.

[30] "Actividades y recursos del SNS" (pdf). msps.es. Retrieved 2010-01-12.

[31] "Definición de hospital". definicionabc.com. Retrieved 2010-01-07.

[32] "Un nuevo concepto de clínica". clinicastarte.com. Retrieved 2010-01-15.

[33] "Funciones de los hospitales". noticias.juridicas.com. Retrieved 2010-01-07.

[34] "Ley 2/2002, de 17 de abril, de Salud. Colaboración con la iniciativa privada.". noticias.juridicas.com. Retrieved 2010-01-07.

[35] "Recursos y actividades del SNS. Hospitales." (pdf). msps.es Ministerio de Sanidad. Retrieved 2010-01-12.

[36] "Recursos y actividades del SNS. Hospitales" (pdf). msps.es Ministerio de Sanidad. Retrieved 2010-01-12.

[37] "Recursos sanitarios de alta tecnología" (PDF). msps.es. Retrieved 2010-01-17.

[38]   • 1. La prestación de salud pública es el conjunto de iniciativas organizadas por las Administraciones públicas para preservar, proteger y promover la salud de la población. Es una combinación de ciencias, habilidades y actitudes dirigidas al mantenimiento y mejora de la salud de todas las personas a través de acciones colectivas o sociales.

        • 2. Las prestaciones en este ámbito comprenderán las siguientes actuaciones: Información y vigilancia epidemiológica. Protección de la salud. Promoción de la salud. Vigilancia y control de los posibles riesgos para la salud derivados de la importación, exportación o tránsito de mercancías y del tráfico internacional de viajeros. Promoción y protección de la sanidad ambiental. Promoción y protección de la salud laboral.

        • 3. Las prestaciones de salud pública se ejercerán con un carácter de integralidad, a partir de las estructuras de salud pública de las Administraciones y de la infraestructura de atención primaria del Sistema Nacional de Salud.

[39] "Prestaciones sanitarias del Sistema Nacional de Sald. Atención primaria" (PDF). msps.es. Retrieved 2010-01-16.

[40] "Prestaciones de la Atención Esppecializada" (PDF). msps.es.

[41] "Urgencia médica". tuotromedico.com.

[42] "Ley 29/2006, de 26 de julio, de garantías y uso racional de los medicamentos y productos sanitarios" (PDF). *boe.es. BOE.* Retrieved 2010-01-18.

[43] "Prestaciones famaceúticas del Sistema Nacional de Salud". seg-social.es. Retrieved 2010-01-18.

[44] "Prestaciones complementarias". seg-social.es. Retrieved 2010-01-18.

[45] "Prestaciones complementarias". Servei Català de la Salut.
      Retrieved 2010-08-13.

[46] "Revisión del Padrón municipal 2008. Datos por municip-
      ios. Población por sexo, municipios y edad (grupos quinque-
      nales). España". Instituto Nacional de Estadística, España.
      Retrieved 2010-01-15.

[47] ". Serie histórica de población. España". Instituto Nacional
      de Estadística (INE) España. Retrieved 2010-01-15.

Chapter 3

Universal Healthcare Topics (in Alphabetical Order)

3.1 Canada Health Act

The **Canada Health Act** (**CHA**) (French: *Loi canadienne sur la santé*) is a piece of Canadian federal legislation, adopted in 1984, which specifies the conditions and criteria with which the provincial and territorial health insurance programs must conform in order to receive federal transfer payments under the Canada Health Transfer. These criteria require universal coverage of all insured services (for all "insured persons")[1] "Insured health services" means hospital services, physician services and surgical-dental services provided to insured persons, if they are not otherwise covered, for example by Workers Safety Insurance.[2]

The CHA deals only with how the system is financed. Because of the constitutional division of powers among levels of government, adherence to CHA conditions is voluntary. However, the fiscal levers have helped to ensure a relatively consistent level of coverage across the country. Although there are disputes as to the details, the CHA remains highly popular.

In popular discussion, the CHA is often conflated with the health care system in general. However, the CHA is silent about how care should be organized and delivered, as long as its criteria are met. The Act states that "the primary objective of Canadian health care policy is to protect, promote and restore the physical and mental well-being of residents of Canada and to facilitate reasonable access to health services without financial or other barriers."[3]

Another cause for debate is the scope of what should be included as "insured services". For historical reasons, the CHA's definition of insured services is largely restricted to care delivered in hospitals or by physicians. As care has moved from hospitals to home and community, it increasingly has been moving beyond the terms of the CHA. International data shows that approximately 70% of Canadian health expenditures are paid from public sources,[4] placing Canada below the OECD average.[5] However, health insurance covers surgery and services, including psychotherapy, in clinics and doctors' offices as well as dental surgery at dental offices and laboratory tests.

3.1.1 History: Federalism

Main article: Canadian federalism

Canada is a federal country in which power is distributed between the national government and the ten provinces. The division of power was spelled out in the British North America Act 1867 (renamed the *Constitution Act, 1867* in 1982). Section 92(7) lists as one of the "exclusive powers of provincial legislatures" "The Establishment, Maintenance, and Management of Hospitals, Asylums, Charities, and Eleemosynary Institutions in and for the Province, other than Marine Hospitals." [6] Although this language does not specifically give authority over 'health care,' subsequent court cases and interpretations have generally established the provinces have paramount authority in this area.

Over time, the mismatch between fiscal resources and fiscal capacity became increasingly problematic. If Canadians were to have similar levels of service, it would be necessary for the national government to somehow equalize the ability to pay for it. Yet attempts by the national government to implement programs directly encountered resistance from the provinces. This resulted in several legal battles. In a few cases, where there was agreement that the federal government should take the lead, adverse court decisions were handled by amending the constitution (e.g., in 1940, in response to a court decision that federal unemployment insurance was unconstitutional, the Constitution Act, 1867 was amended to give the national Parliament jurisdiction over unemployment insurance).[7] More commonly, however, other approaches have been used. Canadian health policy has accordingly been strongly related to Fiscal federalism and questions as to how best to address Fiscal imbalance. In consequence, Canada does not have - and arguably cannot have - a national health care system.

The Constitution Act does give potential powers over elements of health care to the federal government through various clauses (e.g., quarantine), but the role of the federal government has been highly debated. As summarized by a Senate Committee led by Michael Kirby,[8] the federal government has a number of roles to play, including assisting the provinces in paying for health services. Although this has not been tested in court, the federal government has assumed that it is entitled to use its spending powers to set national standards. However, the extent to which 'strings' can be (and are) attached to federal transfers has remained contentious, and most federal governments have been unwilling to antagonize the provinces.

Health insurance before the CHA

The development of Canadian health insurance has been well described by Malcolm Taylor, who participated in many of the negotiations in addition to studying it as an academic.[9] Unlike the UK, Canada never implemented a National Health Service; health care was and largely remains privately delivered. For many decades, it was also privately financed through a variety of programs. In consequence, as Taylor wrote, most Canadians "daily faced the potentially catastrophic physical and financial consequence of unpredictable illness, accident, and disability," and providers, unwilling to deny needed care, had growing bad debts. A number of efforts to establish social insurance systems in Canada had been unable to overcome provincial opposition to federal 'incursion' into their jurisdiction. These included the 1937 Rowell-Sirois Commission on Dominion-Provincial Relations, and the 1945 Green Book proposals of Prime Minister Mackenzie King as part of the post-World War II reconstruction. At the same time, Canada resembled other developed economies in its receptivity to a more expansive government role in improving social welfare, particularly given the widespread sacrifices during World War II and the still active memories of the Great Depression.

Accordingly, following the collapse of the conference proposals in 1946, in 1947, the social democratic premier of Saskatchewan, Tommy Douglas of the Co-operative Commonwealth Federation (CCF), decided to go it alone, and established Canada's first publicly funded hospital insurance plan. Other provinces - including British Columbia, Alberta, and Ontario, introduced their own insurance plans, with varying degrees of coverage, and varying degrees of success. When Newfoundland joined Canada, it brought along its system of cottage hospitals. These policy initiatives increased pressure on the federal government to get

involved, both to assist those provinces which had introduced programs, and to deal with the perceived inequity in those provinces whose citizens did not yet have coverage for hospital care.

The federal government had also acted by using its spending power; in 1948, it introduced a series of National Health Grants to directly provide funds to the provinces/territories for such purposes as hospital construction, professional training, and public health. This increased the number of hospital beds, but did not address the issue of how their operating costs would be covered. The result was that the Progressive Conservative government of John Diefenbaker, who also happened to represent Saskatchewan, introduced and passed (with all-party approval) the *Hospital Insurance and Diagnostic Services Act of 1957*. This shared the costs of covering hospital services. By the start date (July 1, 1958) five provinces—Newfoundland, Manitoba, Saskatchewan, Alberta, and British Columbia—had programs in place which could receive the federal funds. By January 1, 1961, when Quebec finally joined, all provinces had universal coverage for hospital care.

Saskatchewan decided to take the money released by the federal contributions to pioneer again, and following lengthy consultations with the provincial medical association, introduced a plan to insure physician costs (The Saskatchewan Medical Care Insurance Plan). By this time, Douglas had moved to national politics, as leader of the federal New Democratic Party (NDP), The provincial plan precipitated a strike by the province's physicians (1962). It was eventually settled, but the CCF lost the 1964 election to Liberal Ross Thatcher. The plan, however, remained popular, and encouraged other provinces to examine similar programs. A policy debate ensued, with some arguing for universal coverage, and others (particularly the Canadian Medical Association) arguing for an emphasis on voluntary coverage, with the government assisting only those who could not afford the premiums. Three provinces - BC, Alberta, and Ontario - introduced such programs.

The federal reaction was to appoint a Royal Commission on Health Services. First announced by Prime Minister Diefenbaker in December 1960, it was activated in the following June. Its chair was Justice Emmett Hall, the chief justice of Saskatchewan, and a lifelong friend of Mr. Diefenbaker. Three years later, following extensive hearings and deliberations, it released an influential report, which recommended that Canada establish agreements with all provinces to assist them in setting up comprehensive, universal programs for insuring medical services, on the Saskatchewan model, but also recommended adding coverage for prescription drugs, prosthetic services, home care services, as well as optical and dental services for children and those on public assistance. (None of these have yet been added to the formal national conditions, although most provinces do have some sort of coverage for these services.)

By this time, the Liberals, under Lester B. Pearson were in power. Following intense debate, the Pearson government introduced the *Medical Care Act* which was passed in 1966 by a vote of 177 to two. These two Acts established a formula whereby the federal government paid approximately 50% of approved expenditures for hospital and physician services. (The actual formula was a complex one, based on a combination of average national expenditures and spending by each province. In practice, this meant that higher-spending provinces received more federal money, but that it represented a lower proportion of their expenditures, and vice versa for lower-spending provinces.) By 1972, all provinces and territories had complying plans. However, the fiscal arrangements were seen as both cumbersome and inflexible. By 1977, a new fiscal regimen was in place.

Change in fiscal arrangements: the 1977 act

In 1977, HIDS, the Medical Care Act, and federal funds for post-secondary education (also under provincial jurisdiction) were combined into a new *Federal-Provincial Fiscal Arrangements and Established Programs Financing Act of 1977* (known as EPF). This legislation de-coupled the legislation governing the amount of the federal transfer from the legislation establishing the terms and conditions to be met to receive it.

Under this new arrangement, cost sharing was no more. Provinces/territories now had more flexibility, as long as the federal terms and conditions continued to be met. The federal government had more predictability. Rather than an open-ended commitment, EPF established a per capita entitlement (not adjusted for age-sex or other demographic factors) which would be indexed to inflation. This money would go into provincial general revenues. To simplify a complex formula, the EPF entitlement could be seen as consisting of two components. Part of the funds were in the form of "tax transfers" whereby "the federal government agreed with provincial and territorial governments to reduce its personal and corporate income tax rates, thus allowing them to raise their tax rates by the same amount. As a result, revenue that would have flowed to the federal government began to flow directly to provincial and territorial governments."[10] This transfer could not be reversed by subsequent governments, meaning that the federal government had no fiscal leverage over this component of the transfer. (Indeed, there has been an ongoing controversy as to whether this component should even be considered part of the federal contribution.[11]) The remainder of the entitlement was in the form of cash grants. Although the per capita amount was intended to be escalated to inflation, sub-

sequently, the federal government tried to deal with its fiscal position by unilaterally first reducing and then freezing the inflation escalator. As the cash portion threatened to disappear, in 1996, the federal government combined the EPF transfers with another cost-shared program, the Canada Assistance Plan (CAP), to form the Canada Health and Social Transfer (CHST). This enabled the federal government to both cut the total transfers (by approximately the amount in the CAP) while retaining a 'cash floor' on the total amount. In 2004, these transfers were split into the Canada Health Transfer (CHT) and the Canada Social Transfer. The federal Department of Finance publishes brief guides to these programs.[12] Nonetheless, many argue that there has been no explicit federal transfer for health care since 1977, since these programs are no longer tied to specific spending.

The second component of the federal plan, specification of the terms and conditions which provincial/territorial insurance plans must meet, continued to be those established in HIDS and the Medical Care Act. (Note that there were almost no conditions attached to the CAP or post-secondary education components of the transfers.) The genesis of the CHA was recognition of the extent to which the federal ability to control provincial behaviour had been reduced. One particular problem was the absence of any provision for graduated withholding of the federal contribution. Because there was little desire to withhold the full contribution for minor violations of terms and conditions, provinces increasingly were permitting extra billing for insured services. In response to the resulting political uproar, the federal government again turned to Justice Emmett Hall and asked him to report on the future of medicare. His 1979 report, 'Canada's National-Provincial Health Program for the 1980s' noted some of the areas recommended in his earlier report which had not yet been acted on, and warned that accessibility to health care was being threatened through rising user fees. The federal response was to pass the 1984 *Canada Health Act* which replaced both HIDS and the Medical Care Act and clarified the federal conditions.

3.1.2 The 1984 act

On December 12, 1983, the Canada Health Act was introduced by the Liberal government, under Trudeau, spearheaded by then Minister of Health Monique Bégin. As she noted, the government decided not to expand coverage (e.g., to mental health and public health), but instead to incorporate much of the language from the HIDS and Medical Care Acts.[13] The Canada Health Act was passed unanimously by Parliament in 1984, and received Royal Assent on 1 April. Following election of a Conservative government under Brian Mulroney in September 1984, in June 1985, after consultation with the provinces, new federal Health Minister Jake Epp wrote a letter to his provincial counterparts that clarified and interpreted the criteria points and other parts of the new act.

Key features of the CHA

The preamble of the act states that the objective of Canadian Health Care policy is "that continued access to quality health care without financial or other barriers will be critical to maintaining and improving the health and well-being of Canadians. The primary objective of the Act is "to protect, promote and restore the physical and mental well-being of residents of Canada and to facilitate reasonable access to health services without financial or other barriers." (Section 3).

To do so, the act lists a set of criteria and conditions that the provinces must follow in order to receive their federal transfer payments: Public administration, Comprehensiveness, Universality, Portability, and Accessibility. There is also a requirement that the provinces ensure recognition of the federal payments and provide information to the federal government.[14] An overview published by the federal government clarifies the conditions as follows:

Public administration   The health insurance plans must be "administered and operated on a non-profit basis by a public authority, responsible to the provincial/territorial governments and subject to audits of their accounts and financial transactions." (Section 8). This condition is the most frequently misunderstood; it does not deal with delivery, but with insurance. However, it does reduce the scope for private insurers to cover insured services (although they are still able to cover non-insured services, and/or non-insured persons).

Comprehensiveness   The health care insurance plans must cover "all insured health services provided by hospitals, medical practitioners or dentists" (Section 9). The Act lists, in the Definitions (Section 2), what is meant by insured services - in general, this retains the restriction to hospital and physician services arising from the earlier legislation. The provinces are allowed, but not required, to insure additional services. Note that the CHA refers to "surgical dental services" but only if these must be provided within a hospital. In practice, this almost never occurs, and the annual health expenditure data published by the Canadian Institute for Health Information (CIHI) confirm that Canadian dental services are almost entirely financed privately. Lobbying by other providers, including nurses, led the act to speak of 'practitioners' rather than physicians; physician services had to be covered, but provinces were allowed, but not required, to define other health professions as qualifying under the

Act. To date, this provision has been used only occasionally; for example, some provinces have added Midwifery, which means that their services are also fully publicly paid for.

Universality   All insured persons must be covered for insured health services "provided for by the plan on uniform terms and conditions" (Section 10). This definition of insured persons excludes those who may be covered by other federal or provincial legislation, such as serving members of the Canadian Forces or Royal Canadian Mounted Police, inmates of federal penitentiaries, persons covered by provincial workers' compensation, and some Aboriginal people. Some categories of resident, such as landed immigrants and Canadians returning to live in Canada from other countries, may be subject to a waiting period by a province or territory, not to exceed three months, before they are classified as insured persons; this waiting period arises from the portability provisions.[15]

Portability   Because plans are organized on a provincial basis, provisions are required for covering individuals who are in another province. The conditions attempt to separate temporary from more permanent absences by using three months as the maximum cut-off. As the above-mentioned summary clarifies, "Residents moving from one province or territory to another must continue to be covered for insured health care services by the "home" province during any minimum waiting period, not to exceed three months, imposed by the new province of residence. After the waiting period, the new province or territory of residence assumes health care coverage." The portability provisions are subject to inter-provincial agreements; there is variation in what is considered emergency (since the portability requirement does not extend to elective services), in how out-of-country care is covered (since there is no 'receiving' province), in how longer absences are dealt with (e.g., students studying in another province), whether the care will be paid for at home province or host province rates, and so on.

Accessibility   Finally, the insurance plan must provide for "reasonable access" to insured services by insured persons, "on uniform terms and conditions, unprecluded, unimpeded, either directly or indirectly, by charges (user charges or extra-billing) or other means (age, health status or financial circumstances);" (Section 12.a). This section also provides for "reasonable compensation for...services rendered by medical practitioners or dentists" and payments to hospitals that cover the cost of the health services provided. Note that neither reasonable access nor reasonable compensation are defined by the CHA, although there is a presupposition that certain processes (e.g., negotiations between the provincial governments and organizations representing the providers) satisfy the condition. The CHA allows for dollar-for-dollar withholding of contributions from any provinces allowing user charges or extra-billing to insured persons for insured services. As noted below, this provision was effective in 'solving' the extra-billing issue.

Additional conditions   Section 13 lists two additional conditions which must be met by the province in order to receive its full share of the federal transfers. The first condition is that the federal Minister of Health is entitled to specific information relating to a province's insured & extended health care services. This information is used in drafting annual reports, presented to parliament, on how the province administered its health care services over the previous year. Again, there was - and continues to be - controversy as to how detailed this information should be.

The second condition is that the province must "give recognition" to the federal government "in any public documents, or in any advertising or promotional material, relating to insured health services and extended health care services in the province" (Section 13.b). Again, this is controversial.

Violations and penalties

In order to document compliance with the act, the federal Minister of Health annually reports to the Canadian Parliament on how the act has been administered by each province over the course of the previous fiscal year.

For non-compliance with any of the five criteria listed above, the federal government may withhold all or a part of the transfer payment with "regard to the gravity of the default" (Section 15). Thus far all non-compliance issues have been settled through discussion or negotiation. Some argue that the federal government has not actively attempted to enforce these conditions, with particular issues around handling of portability (e.g., the reduction of coverage for residents while traveling abroad) and comprehensiveness (e.g., de-insuring of some medical procedures).

In accordance with section 20, if a province were to violate the prohibition on extra-billing or user charges, the corresponding amount of that collected would be deducted from the transfer payment. Details about these amounts are available from the Canadian government websites.

One aspect of the CHA was provision for reimbursement of funds withheld for extra-billing and user charges if these were eliminated within three years. Although often contentious (e.g., Ontario's physicians went on strike), all provinces complied with the provisions of the Act. Although the amounts withheld were relatively modest—financial penalties totaling $246,732,000 were withheld

from the provinces in the first two years—provinces found it difficult to resist the pressure. (They found that many interest groups seeking additional funds would argue that it could be afforded if the province/territory eliminated their extra billing/user fees. Faced with multiple claims on the same pot, most provinces decided that the easiest path was to eliminate these charges.)

In 1993, British Columbia allowed approximately 40 medical practitioners to use extra-billing in their practices. In response, the federal government reduced B.C.'s EPF payments by a total of $2,025,000 over the course of four years.

In 1996, Alberta had their EPF payment reduced by a total of $3,585,000 over the course of a few years due to the use of private clinics that charged user fees. Newfoundland suffered the loss of $323,000 until 1998 and Manitoba lost a total of $2,056,000 until 1999 from user fees being charged at private clinics. Nova Scotia has also forgone EPF payment for their use of user fees in private clinics.

As required by section 23 of the Canada Health Act, the federal government publishes a yearly report describing the extent to which each province and territory has complied with the Act.

- Reports: *Canada Health Act* Annual Reports

3.1.3 Weaknesses of the CHA

Pro-choice advocates have pointed out that the Canada Health Act fails to meet its criteria in providing access to abortion. Abortion, as a medical service, does not meet the basic principles of the Canada Health Act: public administration, comprehensiveness, universality, portability, and accessibility. Joyce Arthur concludes that "Abortion services fail at least 4 out 5 of these tests." The delivery of abortion services fails comprehensiveness because clinics are not equally funded, universality because of lack of equal access across the country and especially in rural areas, portability because abortion is excluded from the standard reciprocal billing between provinces, accessibility because of lack of clinics in some provinces, and possibly public administration because private clinics are forced to administer its costs.[16]

3.1.4 See also

- Canada Health Transfer

- Canada Health and Social Transfer

- Indian Health Transfer Policy (Canada)

- Health care in Canada

- Canada's Health Care providers, 2007

- Canadian Institute for Health Information

- Canadian and American health care systems compared

- Royal Commission on the Future of Health Care in Canada

- Medicare (Canada)

- Medical Services Plan of British Columbia

- Ontario Health Insurance Plan

3.1.5 References

[1] "Canada Health Act, Section 9". Government of Canada. 1984-04-01. Retrieved 2012-12-14.

[2] "Canada Health Act, Section 2". Government of Canada. 1984-04-01. Retrieved 2012-12-14.

[3] "Canada Health Act, Section 3". Government of Canada. 1984-04-01. Retrieved 2012-12-14.

[4] Canadian Institute for Health Information (September 27, 2005), *CIHI exploring the 70-30 split*, ISBN 1-55392-655-2, retrieved 2010-12-15.

[5] Organisation for Economic Co-operation and Development (2010), *OECD Health Data 2010: How Does Canada Compare* (pdf), retrieved 2010-12-15.

[6] Canada, "Archived copy". Archived from the original on 2011-06-05. Retrieved 2010-11-07. Retrieved on 2010-12-15.

[7] Reference Archived November 21, 2007, at the Wayback Machine. re Employment Insurance Act (Can.), ss. 22 and 23, 2005 SCC 56, [2005] 2 Supreme Court of Canada 669.

[8] Standing Senate Committee on Social Affairs, Science and Technology (March 2001), *The Health of Canadians – The Federal Role, Interim Report, Volume One – The Story So Far* (pdf), Canada, retrieved 2007-12-26.

[9] Malcolm G. Taylor. *The Seven Decisions That Created the Canadian Health Insurance System and Their Outcomes.* Second edition. McGill-Queen's University Press, 1987. ISBN 978-0-7735-0629-9

[10] Health Canada (2002), *The Canada Health and Social Transfer*, Canada, archived from the original (– Scholar search) on December 18, 2007, retrieved 2007-12-26 .

[11] Raisa Deber (July 11, 2000), "Who Wants To Pay For Health Care", *Canadian Medical Association Journal*, **163** (1): 43, retrieved 2007-12-26.

[12] Department of Finance. "A Brief History of the Health and Social Transfers". *Federal provincial cost sharing programs.* Canada. Archived from the original on 2007-12-17. Retrieved 2007-12-27.

[13] Monique Begin. Medicare: Canada's Right to Health. 1988 ISBN 978-0-88890-219-1.

[14] Health Canada (November 25, 2002). "Canada Health Act Overview, 2002". *About Health Canada.* Canada. Archived from the original on December 17, 2007. Retrieved 2007-12-26.

[15] "Canada Health Act, Section 10". Government of Canada. 1984-04-01. Retrieved 2012-12-14.

[16] Arthur, Joyce (November 2001). "Canada Health Act Violates Abortion Services: Five Basic Principles Not Met". Pro Choice Action Network. Retrieved 2012-12-14.

General references

- Canada Health Act

- Epp Letter, 1985

- Marleau Letter, 1994

- Overview of the Act by Health Canada

- Madore's Overview And Options, 2003

- Madore, Private Health Care Funding and Delivery under the Canada Health Act, 2005

- Maple Leaf Web: The Canada Health Act

- Health Canada page linking to key Federal reports and commissions and their background material, including Romanow Report and Kirby Commission

3.2 EMBRACE Healthcare Reform Plan

The **E**xpanding **M**edical and **B**ehavioral **R**esources with **A**ccess to **C**are for **E**veryone (EMBRACE) plan is a healthcare system reform proposal introduced by a group called Healthcare Professionals for Healthcare Reform (HPfHR). The plan incorporates elements of private health insurance, Single-payer and fee-for-service models in one comprehensive system. It has been referred to as a "Single System" healthcare system.[1] First published in the Annals of Internal Medicine in April 2009,[2] the plan got some early discussion in the healthcare community, but appeared to have come out too late to have had any impact in the development of the Patient Protection and Affordable Care Act (PPACA), the 111th Congress' landmark health insurance reform legislation.[3][4][5] A book outlining the EMBRACE plan in more detail was authored in 2016 by Dr. Gilead Lancaster, a cofounder of HPfHR.[6]

3.2.1   The origins of EMBRACE

In 2007 HPfHR was established in an effort to advise politicians on healthcare issues from the point of view of healthcare professionals. They felt that the only effective way to fix the American healthcare system was with a complete overhaul based on science-based guidelines, also known as evidence-based medicine.

The group identified five important parts of the American healthcare system that they felt needed to be addressed in their new system. These included inefficiencies in medical offices and hospitals due to a cumbersome insurance and reimbursement system; coverage of the entire United States population for basic healthcare services while preserving the quality and feel of the current delivery system of healthcare; promotion and integration of scientifically validated diagnostic and therapeutic modalities into the system so it becomes the driving force of the healthcare system; and depoliticizing healthcare and allowing for a more manageable way to finance it. In addition, the group felt that it was important that the plan was completely portable throughout the country and did not depend on income, age or employment status.

3.2.2   The scope of reform under EM-BRACE

The EMBRACE system would require a comprehensive reorganization of the entire United States healthcare system, but would attempt to preserve important elements of the current infrastructure. Current Procedural Terminology (CPT) and International Statistical Classification of Diseases and Related Health Problems (ICD) codes that are currently being used to report services and determine reimbursement to doctors, hospitals and other care providers would be maintained. There would also be an attempt to allow doctors and other healthcare providers to keep private offices and clinics as independent businesses.[2]

The new system would change 4 fundamental things: It would classify diseases and their therapies into 3 distinct tiers, separate private insurance from public insurance but keep them in the same system, create a politically quasi-independent 'healthcare board' funded by Congress to supervise the U. S. healthcare system, and develop a simpli-...eb-based electronic billing and reimbursement sys-...fundamental reforms would change many other ...ent healthcare system. For example,

healthcare coverage would be completely portable from job to job and from state to state and would not be tied to employment.

3.2.3   The Tier system

EMBRACE would establish 3 tiers of diagnoses and treatments founded on evidence-based medicine (EBM), and its funding will be tier-specific and separate:

The base level (**Tier 1**) would cover all medical, surgical and psychiatric therapies shown to be life saving, life sustaining and/or preventative and would cover the entire population "from cradle to grave" without registration, deductibles or fee payments. It would also be completely portable and independent of employment status, economic status, race, gender or pre-existing conditions.

Funding of Tier 1 services would be overseen by a healthcare board (see below) that is in turn funded by Congress. The method of raising this revenue could be similar to the present funding of Medicare (e.g. Federal Insurance Contributions Act tax) and Medicaid. Since there will be no requirement for employer-based insurance under EMBRACE, payroll taxes (indexed to salary), a tax on businesses based on the number of employees (and their wages) or a combination of these could also be considered.

Tier 2 would cover all conditions affecting quality of life and their therapies. In addition, this tier will include all services of Tier 1 conditions and treatments that do not have sufficient evidence for a Tier 1 indication.

Private insurance carriers would be invited to cover Tier 2 services through a menu of plans developed by the Board that is similar to the Medigap Plans A to N[7] now offered through the Centers for Medicare & Medicaid Services. Although each insurance carrier does not have to offer all the plans listed on the menu, the plans that are offered by the insurance carrier must cover all the services stipulated by the Board. This assures that consumers (whether state governments, unions, employers or individuals) can compare the price of the plans and can be confident of the scope of their coverage. In addition, if an insurance provider offers a specific plan in one state, it will be required to offer it in all other states; assuring portability of all tier 2 coverage. Except for these two stipulations, the private insurance provider will be free to set their fee (on an individual basis), set deductibles and co-pays and even deny coverage. The Tier 2 plans can be broad (covering most Tier 2 services) or can be customized for specific groups: a geriatric plan that covers extended care facilities but not fertility care, a heavy laborer plan that includes chiropractic therapy, or a Workman's Compensation plan purchased by employers, employees or unions.

Tier 3 would apply to all medical and surgical issues considered luxury or cosmetic (examples are Lasik surgery or Botox treatments). Funding for Tier 3 would not be covered under this system (as is true in the current system) and all bills would go to the patient. However, billing would still be made through the web-based universal billing form discussed below.

Pharmaceuticals will have similar Tier assignments as medical coverage: Tier 1 would be formulations and therapies that have good evidence-based data for treatment or prevention of Tier 1 illnesses and would mostly be paid by public funds or be heavily subsidized. Tier 2 would apply to those drugs and therapies that enhance quality of life or have not yet had adequate evidence for effectiveness for a particular condition. These Tier 2 pharmaceuticals would be covered by private insurance or out of pocket. Tier 3 would be for "luxury" items and would likely be 'out of pocket'.

3.2.4 Oversight

The entire health system would be overseen by a healthcare panel known as "The Board". Although the details of the exact composition of the Board has not been discussed in detail by HPfHR, it would be composed of physicians and other healthcare professionals, public health experts, economists specializing in health care, business representatives, insurance representatives, representatives from the pharmaceutical industry and representatives of patients. This Board's mission would be to promote the health of Americans in a socially responsible and economically sound way. Similar to the "Federal Health Board" proposed by Tom Daschle,[8] it would be a quasi-independent organization resembling the Federal Reserve, which it is hoped would make it less beholden to political pressures. It would be headed by a chairperson who would be appointed to a 10-year term by the president and require Senate confirmation. The Board would have oversight of a significantly revised Center for Medicare & Medicaid Services, and input into the Food and Drug Administration and the National Institutes of Health. It would use the already established Diagnosis-related group (DRG), Ambulatory Payment Classification (APC) and International Classification of Diseases (ICD) codes. The Board would decide which diagnoses and services are covered by Tier 1, 2 or 3 based on the medical importance (using evidence-based data such as practice guidelines developed by expert medical panels, Cochrane Library database reviews and other sources), public health considerations and economic impact. This would be updated periodically as more evidence and research becomes available. When evidence is not available, the Board would have the option to commission the National Institutes of Health and the Food and Drug Administration to direct research focused specifically to use

in the Tier assignments. Among the prerequisites to the implementation of this system would be delineation of the specific relationships between the Board and existing agencies within the Department of Health and Human Services, in particular the Food and Drug Administration and the National Institutes of Health. Some reorganization of these government agencies might be warranted to optimize interagency interactions. To address local variations in health and social concerns, the health Board would establish several local health-boards (possibly in each state). These local branches would not only handle local health issues, but may be used to establish peer review boards to hear ethical and malpractice issues.

3.2.5 Hospital and office billing

To simplify claim submissions by healthcare providers (physicians, and hospitals), a "Universal Reimbursement Form" would be created by the Board and would be implemented electronically using a web-based tool available to hospitals and physician offices. This Universal Reimbursement Form (URF) will be the only form of billing for all providers, will be internet-based and will be simple to use. It will transmit data to a "Central Billing System", which will decide if the condition/service is Tier 1, Tier 2 or Tier 3. Tier 1 services will be reimbursed directly to the provider. Tier 2 services will trigger a search (by the computer) for insurance coverage; if insurance is found the insurance carrier would be billed, if not the patient would be billed. Bills for Tier 3 would be sent directly to the patient. To help in cases where there is some question about which tier a particular service will be charged, there will be a "Billing Inquiry" feature on the Central Billing System available to providers and consumers that allows inquiries of tier assignment in advance. Although the CBS will be secured with encryption and other anti-hacking devices, the internet platform that the URF is based on will be open-sourced and available for entrepreneurial development. Similar to the open sourced platform of the iPhone, the URF platform would allow for the development of "Health Information Technology" on a single fully interactive web-based platform.

3.2.6 Financing the EMBRACE healthcare system

The budget for the EMBRACE system will be determined by the United States Congress, with one comprehensive bill a year that will fund the entire public healthcare system in the United States. Because the Healthcare Board will have to justify the budget, Congress will continue to have full control on expenditures for the healthcare system.

3.2.7   References

[1] "EMBRACE single system healthcare reform". *The Hill.* March 7, 2017.

[2] Lancaster GI, O'Connell R, Katz DL, et al. (April 7, 2009). "The Expanding Medical and Behavioral Resources with Access to Care for Everyone Health Plan". *Annals of Internal Medicine.* **150** (7): 490. doi:10.7326/0003-4819-150-7-200904070-00113.

[3] The Editors (April 7, 2009). "Perspectives on Health Care Reform". *Annals of Internal Medicine.* **150** (7): 498. doi:10.7326/0003-4819-150-7-200904070-00116.

[4] http://www.annals.org/content/150/7/490.full#responses

[5] Gilead I. Lancaster; Ryan O'Connell; David L. Katz (November 3, 2009). "Comments and Critiques on the EMBRACE Health Care Reform Plan". *Annals of Internal Medicine.* **151** (9): 672. doi:10.7326/0003-4819-151-9-200911030-00020.

[6] Lancaster, Gilead (2016). *EMBRACE: A Revolutionary New Healthcare System for the Twenty-First Century.* North Charleston, SC: CreateSpace. ISBN 978-1532803963.

[7] Centers for Medicare & Medicaid Services. "2011- Choosing a Medigap Policy: A Guide to Health Insurance for People with Medicare" (PDF). Centers for Medicare & Medicaid Services (CMS) and the National Association of Insurance Commissioners (NAIC). Retrieved 2011-05-19.

[8] Tom Daschle, Scott S. Greenberger, and Jeanne M. Lambrew, Critical: What We Can Do About the Health-Care Crisis, Thomas Dunne, 2008. ISBN 978-0-312-38301-5

3.2.8   External links

- Healthcare Professionals for Healthcare Reform (HPfHR) website

- EMBRACE plan in the Annals of Internal Medicine

- Website for the book about EMBRACE called **EMBRACE: A Revolutionary New Healthcare System for the Twenty-First Century**

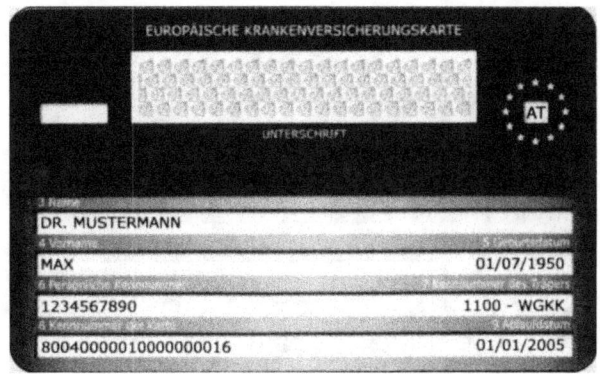

Sample European Health Insurance Card from Austria (reverse).

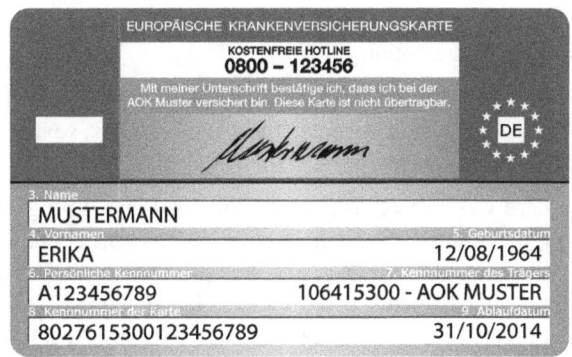

German card

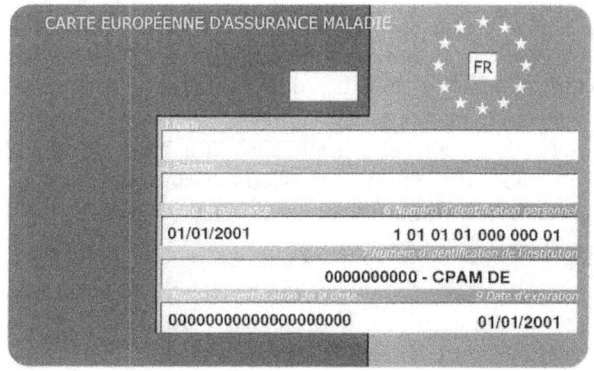

Sample French EHIC

3.3   European Health Insurance Card

The **European Health Insurance Card** (or **EHIC**) is issued free of charge and allows anyone who is insured by or covered by a statutory social security scheme of the EEA countries and Switzerland to receive medical treatment in another member state free or at a reduced cost, if that treatment becomes necessary during their visit (for example, due to illness or an accident), or if they have a chronic pre-existing condition which requires care such as kidney dialysis. The term of validity of the card varies according to the issuing country.

The intention of the scheme is to allow people to continue their stay in a country without having to return home for medical care; as such, it does not cover people who have visited a country for the purpose of obtaining medical care, nor does it cover care, such as many types of dental treatment, which can be delayed until the individual returns to

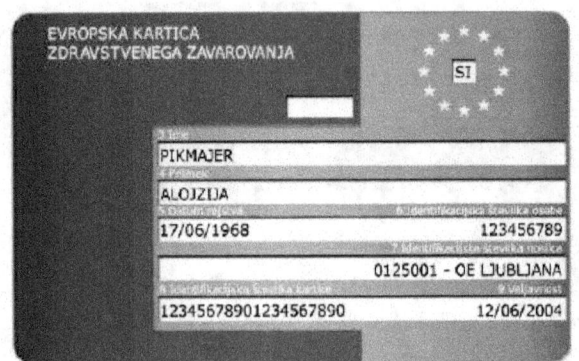

Slovenian card

his or her home country.

It only covers healthcare which is normally covered by a statutory health care system in the visited country, so it does not render travel insurance obsolete.

The card was phased in from 1 June 2004 and throughout 2005, becoming the sole healthcare entitlement document on 1 January 2006. The card is applicable in all French overseas departments (Martinique, Guadeloupe, Réunion and French Guiana) as they are part of the EEA, but not non-EEA dependent territories such as Jersey, the Isle of Man, Aruba or French Polynesia.[1] However, there are agreements for the use of the EHIC in the Faroe Islands and Greenland,[2] even though they are not in the EEA.

The reason for the existence of this card, is that the right to health care in Europe is based on the country of legal residence, not the country of citizenship. Therefore, a passport is not enough to receive health care. It is however possible that a photo ID document is asked for, since the European Health Insurance Card does not contain a photo.

In some cases, even if a person is covered by the health insurance of an EU country, one is not eligible for a European Health Insurance Card. For instance, in Romania, a person who is currently insured has to have been insured for the previous five years to be eligible.[3]

It replaced the following medical forms:

- E110 - For international road hauliers

- E111 - For tourists

- E119 - For unemployed people/job seekers

- E128 - For students and workers in another member state

3.3.1 Third party application processors

European Health Insurance cards are provided free to all legal residents of participating countries. There are however various businesses who act as non-official agents on behalf of individuals, arranging supply of the cards in return for payment, often offering additional services such as the checking of applications for errors and general advice or assistance.[4] This has proved extremely controversial. In 2010 the British government moved against companies that invited people to pay for the free EHIC, falsely implying that through payment the applicant could speed up the process.[5][6] Despite this, the practice continues.[7][8]

3.3.2 Participating member states

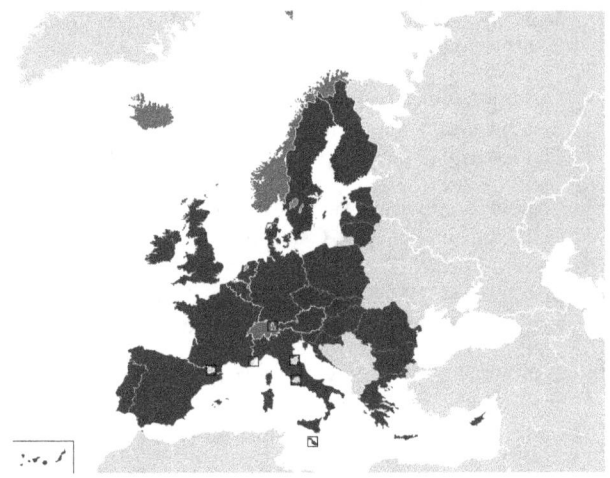

32 participating member states, coinciding with 28 EU (blue) and 4 EFTA (green).

As of 2013, 32 countries in Europe participate: the 31 member states of the European Economic Area (EEA) plus Switzerland. This coincides with the 28 member states of the European Union (EU) and 4 member states of the European Free Trade Association (EFTA).

The Channel Islands and Isle of Man do not supply coverage under the EHIC, and their residents are not eligible for EHICs.

3.3.3 Controversy

In August 2015 the *Daily Mail* ran a story about abuse of the EHIC system in which a card was issued to its undercover Hungarian reporter who "obtained the card after visiting the UK for less than one day" after another journalist posed as her landlord and presented a GP with the tenancy agreement of a property that neither occupied in order to get an NHS number. It claimed that "foreigners were charging the NHS for care in their own country." As *The Guardian* pointed out, the NHS issued a card to an individual that wasn't eligible to receive the card because a GP was duped into issuing an NHS number, and it was unclear what benefit would accrue as a result.[9]

With no active investigation branch, the likelihood of NHS authorities discovering fraud is extremely low. The *Huffington Post* reported that only nine instances of low-level fraud involving the EHIC in the UK had been discovered in five years with a combined cost of £712.56.[10]

3.3.4 See also

- Healthcare in the European Union
- Italian health insurance card
- Carte Vitale
- European driving licence

3.3.5 References

[1] "UK FCO Travel Advice: French Polynesia". Fco.gov.uk. 2012-09-12. Retrieved 2012-10-12.

[2] "UK FCO Travel Advice: Denmark". Fco.gov.uk. Retrieved 2012-10-12.

[3] "Cardul european de asigurări de sănătate, eliberat gratuit". Libertatea.ro. 2009-08-01. Retrieved 2012-10-12.

[4] "Third Party Application Processors". 2016-09-02. Retrieved 2016-06-03.

[5] "BBC News - European health card scam stopped by OFT". Bbc.co.uk. 2010-08-10. Retrieved 2012-10-12.

[6] "Consumers warned to be search engine savvy – Consumer Focus Wales". Consumerfocus.org.uk. 2011-06-22. Retrieved 2012-10-12.

[7] Ray Massey (2011-07-01). "Millions duped into paying for free EU health cards | Mail Online". Dailymail.co.uk. Retrieved 2012-10-12.

[8] James Coney (2012-06-20). "EHIC scam warning - don't pay for a card". This is Money. Retrieved 2012-10-12.

[9] "Are foreigners really gaming the NHS to pay for their medical treatment abroad?". Guardian. 11 August 2015. Retrieved 22 August 2015.

[10] "Exclusive: Migrant NHS Fraud Costs Only £700 Despite Fury Over Health Card Abuse. Government Accused Of 'Stoking Up Mistrust'". Huffington Post. 11 September 2015. Retrieved 18 September 2015.

3.3.6 External links

- Third Party EHIC Processor
- EHIC Renewal Third Party Processor
- Third Party UK EHIC Processor
- UK EHIC application
- General UK EHIC information
- EU site about the EHIC
- Irish EHIC site - includes details of coverage in various countries
- Dutch EHIC website
- Accessing healthcare in Switzerland

3.4 Health insurance cooperative

A **health insurance cooperative** is a cooperative entity that has the goal of providing health insurance and is also owned by the people that the organization insures. It is a form of mutual insurance.

3.4.1 United States

In the debate over healthcare reform, healthcare cooperatives are posited as an alternative to both publicly funded healthcare and single-payer healthcare.

It has been proposed as part of the healthcare reform debate in the United States by the Barack Obama administration as a possible compromise with Blue Dog Democrats (as well as with Republicans) in the search for universal healthcare in the United States.[1][2][3] As it is being proposed by President Obama and others, a future health insurance cooperative would not be government owned or run, but would instead receive an initial government investment and would then be operated as a non-profit organization.[4]

While a health insurance co-op is not strictly run by the government, hence not making it a public entity, it has been described by Senator Max Baucus of Montana, who is also the chairman of the United States Senate Committee on Finance as "tough enough to keep insurance companies' feet to the fire."[5] He has proposed a bill that includes a health insurance cooperative instead of the public option.[6]

There once were numerous rural health cooperatives established by the Farm Security Administration (FSA). Most of them closed or merged over the years, generally because they lacked a sufficient economy of scale (i.e., they were too small to function efficiently). Thus, co-operatives currently have so little market share as to be "invisible".[7]

The bill proposed by Max Baucus, the America's Healthy Future Act, which uses health insurance cooperatives, was estimated by the Congressional Budget Office to cost $829 billion over ten years, and because of the increase in taxes of $210 billion over 10 years[8] on premium insurance plans with high benefits, would lead to a reduction in the deficit of $81 billion.[9] It would expand coverage to 94 percent of all eligible Americans.[10]

Support

During a September 2009 report by John King of CNN, he stated that "supporters know, here in Minnesota and other farm states think co-ops could solve at least a big chunk of the healthcare access and affordability problem." He interviewed Bill Oemichen, President of the Cooperative Network, who remarked that "where co-ops are, they tend to be very, very high quality because it is the consumer who owns them, that is making sure that their health care provider is a quality health care provider." Oemichen also stated that 65% of those who switched from typical health insurance reported better coverage and service.[11]

In June 2009, Republican Senator Chuck Grassley told reporters, "if it's all done entirely within the private sector, you know, it doesn't seem to me it's got the faults that you have... by having the government institute something."[12] Steven Hill, a program director at the New America Foundation, has written for Salon.com that "co-ops may hold the key to a substantive compromise", comparing the U.S. reform proposals with health care in Germany. He argued that they can produce quality care for less money given that they would lack the profit motive, they would negotiate fees for service, and that they would end current market monopolies that insurance companies have in several states.[13]

Criticism

Howard Dean and other Democrats have criticized abandoning the idea of a federally run, statewide, public option in favor of co-ops, questioning whether the co-ops would have enough negotiating power to compete with private health insurers.[12] The activist groups SEIU and MoveOn.org have also stated their opposition.[12] Prominent economists such as 2008 Nobel Economics Laureate Paul Krugman and Robert Reich have also questioned co-ops' ability to become large enough to reduce health care costs significantly. Thus, they both support the public option instead, which they state has strong opposition from the insurance industry.[14][15]

3.4.2 Examples

- Everspring Health

- Kentucky Health Cooperative

- Evergreen Health Cooperative

- Consumers Mutual Health Insurance of Michigan

- Health Republic Insurance - New York, New Jersey, Oregon

- Nevada Health CO-OP - Nevada

3.4.3 See also

- Housing cooperative

3.4.4 References

[1] "White House appears ready to drop 'public option'" Retrieved on August 17, 2009

[2] "White House Appears Open to Insurance Co-ops" New York Times Retrieved on August 17, 2009

[3] "Chances Dim for a Public Plan" The Wall Street Journal Retrieved on August 18, 2009

[4] "President Obama Considering Insurance Co-Op" KKTV.com Retrieved on August 17, 2009

[5] "Co-op Health Plan Emerging as a Senate Option" New York Times Retrieved on August 17, 2009

[6] "Zen Health Reform" - Slate.com Retrieved September 18, 2009

[7] Michael R. Grey. New Deal Medicine: The Rural Health Programs of the Farm Security Administration. Baltimore: Johns Hopkins University Press. 1999.

[8] The Atlantic, "New CBO Score Of Baucus Bill" 07 Oct 2009

[9] "The Baucus Bill Cuts The Deficit" - theAtlantic.com Retrieved October 7, 2009

[10] "Health bill would cost $829B, help cover 94 pct" - Seattle Times Retrieved August 7, 2014

[11] John King (September 6, 2009). "Interview With Senators Klobuchar, Nelson; Interview With Governor Pawlenty". State of the Union with John King. Retrieved September 21, 2009.

[12] Wangsness, Lisa (June 21, 2009). "Health debate shifting to public vs. private". *Boston Globe*. Retrieved September 21, 2009.

[13] http://www.salon.com/opinion/feature/2009/10/12/ cooperatives/index.html

[14] Robert Reich's recent references to health insurance cooperatives

[15] Paul Krugman (September 17, 2009). "Baucus and the Threshold". *The New York Times*. Retrieved September 21, 2009.

3.4.5 External links

- Looking At Health Care Co-ops at Planet Money.

- *Health Democracy: How to Liberate Americans from Medical Insurers* (book).

3.5 Healthcare reform debate in the United States

See also: Health care reform in the United States, Health care in the United States, and Health insurance coverage in the United States

The **healthcare reform debate in the United States** has been a political issue for many years, focusing upon increasing coverage, decreasing the cost and social burden of healthcare, insurance reform, and the philosophy of its provision, funding, and government involvement.

3.5.1 Quality of care

According to a 2015 report from The Commonwealth Fund, the United States pays almost twice as much towards healthcare per capita than other wealthy countries with universal healthcare, although under ObamaCare the cost of healthcare ceased to rise. Despite the amount spent on healthcare, patient outcomes are poorer, life expectancy is lower, and the infant mortality rate is the highest and in some cases twice as high when compared with other Organisation for Economic Co-operation and Development (OECD) countries. Also highlighted in their report is data that shows that although Americans have one of the lowest percentages of daily smokers, they have the highest mortality rate for heart disease, a significantly higher obesity rate and more amputations due to diabetes. Other health related issues highlighted were that Americans over the age of 65 have a higher percentage of the population with two or more chronic conditions and the lowest percentage of that age group living (Squires and Anderson).

Some medical researchers say that patient satisfaction surveys are a poor way to evaluate medical care. Researchers at the RAND Corporation and the Department of Veterans Affairs asked 236 elderly patients in two different managed care plans to rate their care, then examined care in medical records, as reported in Annals of Internal Medicine. There was no correlation. "Patient ratings of health care are easy to obtain and report, but do not accurately measure the technical quality of medical care," said John T. Chang, UCLA, lead author.[1][2][3]

3.5.2 Cost and efficiency

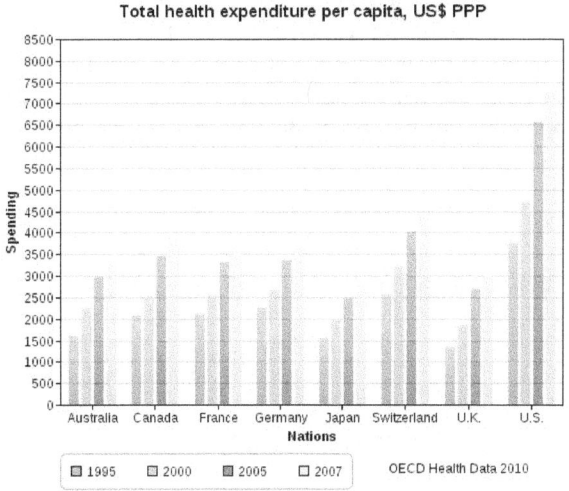

Health spending per capita, in US$ PPP-adjusted, compared amongst various first world nations.

The United States spends a higher proportion of its GDP on healthcare.

Proponents of healthcare reforms involving expansion of government involvement to achieve universal healthcare argue that the need to provide profits to investors in a predominantly free market health system, and the additional administrative spending, tends to drive up costs, leading to more expensive provision.[4]

According to economist and former US Secretary of Labor, Robert Reich, only a "big, national, public option" can force insurance companies to cooperate, share information, and reduce costs. Scattered, localized, "insurance cooperatives" are too small to do that and are "designed to fail" by the moneyed forces opposing Democratic health care reform.[5][6]

Impact on U.S. economic productivity

The adverse economic effects of the ACA on US economic productivity was a major factor in the election of Donald

Trump who has stated "Since March of 2010, the American people have had to suffer under the incredible economic burden of the Affordable Care Act—Obamacare. This legislation, passed by totally partisan votes in the House and Senate and signed into law by the most divisive and partisan President in American history, has tragically but predictably resulted in runaway costs, websites that don't work, greater rationing of care, higher premiums, less competition and fewer choices."[7]

On March 1, 2010, billionaire Warren Buffett said that the high costs paid by U.S. companies for their employees' healthcare under ObamaCare put them at a competitive disadvantage. He compared the roughly 17% of GDP spent by the U.S. on healthcare with the 9% of GDP spent by much of the rest of the world, noted that the U.S. has fewer doctors and nurses per person, and said, "that kind of a cost, compared with the rest of the world, is like a tapeworm eating at our economic body."[8]

Allegations of waste

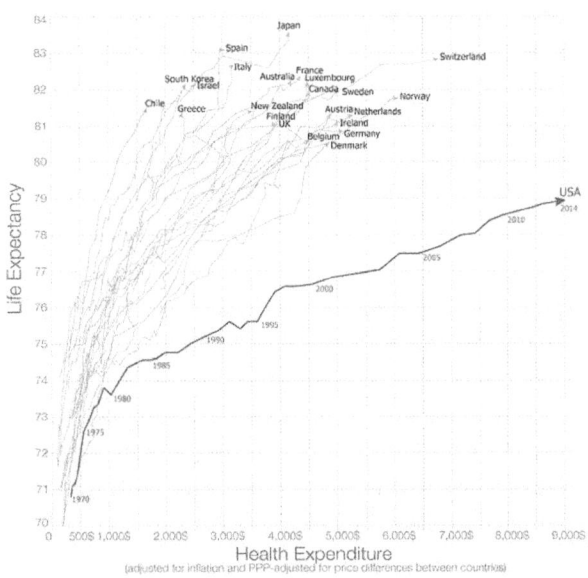

Life expectancy compared to healthcare spending from 1970 to 2008, in the US and the next 19 most wealthy countries by total GDP.[9]

In December 2011 following the ObamaCare reform the outgoing Administrator of the Centers for Medicare & Medicaid Services, Dr. Donald Berwick, asserted that 20% to 30% of healthcare spending is waste. He listed five causes for the waste: (1) overtreatment of patients, (2) the failure to coordinate care, (3) the administrative complexity of the system, (4) burdensome rules and (5) fraud.[10]

3.5.3 Proposed strategies for reform

Main article: Health care reforms proposed during the Obama administration

During a June 2009 speech, President Barack Obama outlined his strategy for reform. He mentioned electronic record-keeping, preventing expensive conditions, reducing obesity, refocusing doctor incentives from quantity of care to quality, bundling payments for treatment of conditions rather than specific services, better identifying and communicating the most cost-effective treatments, and reducing defensive medicine.[11]

President Obama further described his plan in a September 2009 speech to a joint session of Congress. His plan mentions: deficit neutrality; not allowing insurance companies to discriminate based on pre-existing conditions; capping out of pocket expenses; creation of an insurance exchange for individuals and small businesses; tax credits for individuals and small companies; independent commissions to identify fraud, waste and abuse; and malpractice reform projects, among other topics.[12][13]

OMB Director Peter Orszag described aspects of the Obama administration's strategy during an interview in November 2009: "In order to help contain [Medicare and Medicaid] cost growth over the long term, we need a new healthcare system that has digitized information... in which that information is used to assess what's working and what's not more intelligently, and in which we're paying for quality rather than quantity while also encouraging prevention and wellness." He also argued for bundling payments and accountable care organizations, which reward doctors for teamwork and patient outcomes.[14]

Mayo Clinic President and CEO Denis Cortese has advocated an overall strategy to guide reform efforts. He argued that the U.S. has an opportunity to redesign its healthcare system and that there is a wide consensus that reform is necessary. He articulated four "pillars" of such a strategy:[15]

- Focus on value, which he defined as the ratio of quality of service provided relative to cost;

- Pay for and align incentives with value;

- Cover everyone;

- Establish mechanisms for improving the healthcare service delivery system over the long-term, which is the primary means through which value would be improved.

Writing in *The New Yorker*, surgeon Atul Gawande further distinguished between the delivery system, which refers to how medical services are provided to patients, and the payment system, which refers to how payments for services are processed. He argued that reform of the delivery system is critical to getting costs under control, but that payment system reform (e.g., whether the government or private insurers process payments) is considerably less important yet gathers a disproportionate share of attention. Gawande argued that dramatic improvements and savings in the delivery system will take "at least a decade." He recommended changes that address the overutilization of healthcare; the refocusing of incentives on value rather than profits; and comparative analysis of the cost of treatment across various healthcare providers to identify best practices. He argued this would be an iterative, empirical process and should be administered by a "national institute for healthcare delivery" to analyze and communicate improvement opportunities.[16]

Use of comparative effectiveness research

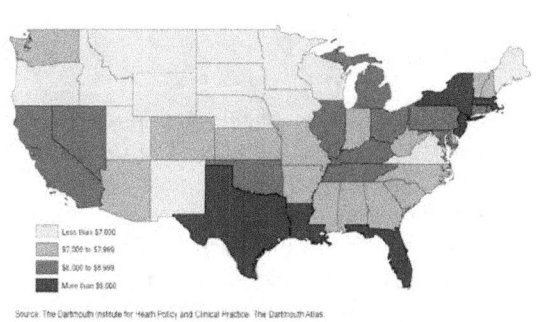

U.S. Medicare Spending Per Capita - 2006

Less than $7,000
$7,000 to $7,999
$8,000 to $8,999
More than $9,000

Source: The Dartmouth Institute for Health Policy and Clinical Practice. The Dartmouth Atlas.

Medicare spending per person varied significantly across states in 2006

Several treatment alternatives may be available for a given medical condition, with significantly different costs yet no statistical difference in outcome. Such scenarios offer the opportunity to maintain or improve the quality of care, while significantly reducing costs, through comparative effectiveness research. Writing in the New York Times, David Leonhardt described how the cost of treating the most common form of early-stage, slow-growing prostate cancer ranges from an average of $2,400 (watchful waiting to see if the condition deteriorates) to as high as $100,000 (radiation beam therapy):[17]

> Some doctors swear by one treatment, others by another. But no one really knows which is best. Rigorous research has been scant. Above

all, no serious study has found that the high-technology treatments do better at keeping men healthy and alive. Most die of something else before prostate cancer becomes a problem.

According to economist Peter A. Diamond and research cited by the Congressional Budget Office (CBO), the cost of healthcare per person in the U.S. also varies significantly by geography and medical center, with little or no statistical difference in outcome.[18]

> Although the Mayo Clinic scores above the other two in terms of quality of outcome, its cost per beneficiary for Medicare clients in the last six months of life ($26,330) is nearly half that at the UCLA Medical Center ($50,522) and significantly lower than the cost at Massachusetts General Hospital ($40,181)... The American taxpayer is financing these large differences in costs, but we have little evidence of what benefit we receive in exchange.

Comparative effectiveness research has shown that significant cost reductions are possible. OMB Director Peter Orszag stated: "Nearly thirty percent of Medicare's costs could be saved without negatively affecting health outcomes if spending in high- and medium-cost areas could be reduced to the level of low-cost areas."[19]

Reform of doctor's incentives

ObamaCare reformed doctor's compensation in 2010.

Insurance reforms

The issue of concentration of power by the insurance industry has also been a focus of debate as in many states very few large insurers dominate the market.

Tax reform

The Congressional Budget Office has also described how the tax treatment of insurance premiums may affect behavior:[20]

> One factor perpetuating inefficiencies in health care is a lack of clarity regarding the cost of health insurance and who bears that cost, especially employment-based health insurance. Employers' payments for employment-based health insurance and nearly all payments by employees

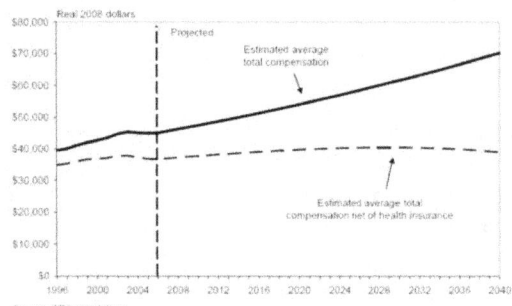

Compensation – Gross and Net of Health Insurance Premiums

Health insurance premiums paid on behalf of workers are increasingly offsetting compensation

for that insurance are excluded from individual income and payroll taxes. Although both theory and evidence suggest that workers ultimately finance their employment-based insurance through lower take-home pay, the cost is not evident to many workers.... If transparency increases and workers see how much their income is being reduced for employers' contributions and what those contributions are paying for, there might be a broader change in cost-consciousness that shifts demand.

In November 2009, *The Economist* estimated that taxing employer-provided health insurance (which is presently exempt from tax) would add $215 billion per year to federal tax revenue during the 2013–2014 periods.[21] Peter Singer wrote in the *New York Times* that the current exclusion of insurance premiums from compensation represents a $200 billion subsidy for the private insurance industry and that it would likely not exist without it.[22] In other words, taxpayers might be more inclined to change behavior or the system itself if they were paying $200 billion more in taxes each year related to health insurance. To put this amount in perspective, the federal government collected $1,146 billion in income taxes in 2008,[23] so $200 billion represents a 17.5% increase in the effective tax rate.

Independent advisory panels

President Obama has proposed an "Independent Medicare Advisory Panel" (IMAC) to make recommendations on Medicare reimbursement policy and other reforms. Comparative effectiveness research would be one of many tools used by the IMAC. The IMAC concept was endorsed in a letter from several prominent healthcare policy experts, as

summarized by OMB Director Peter Orszag:[24]

> Their support of the IMAC proposal underscores what most serious health analysts have recognized for some time: that moving toward a health system emphasizing quality rather than quantity will require continual effort, and that a key objective of legislation should be to put in place structures (like the IMAC) that facilitate such change over time. And ultimately, without a structure in place to help contain costs over the long term as the health market evolves, nothing else we do in fiscal policy will matter much, because eventually rising health care costs will overwhelm the federal budget.

Both Mayo Clinic CEO Dr. Denis Cortese and Surgeon/Author Atul Gawande have argued that such panel(s) will be critical to reform of the delivery system and improving value. Washington Post columnist David Ignatius has also recommended that President Obama engage someone like Cortese to have a more active role in driving reform efforts.[25]

Lowering obesity

Preventing obesity and overweight conditions presents a significant opportunity to reduce costs. The Centers for Disease Control reported that approximately 9% of healthcare costs in 1998 were attributable to overweight and obesity, or as much as $92.6 billion in 2002 dollars. Nearly half of these costs were paid for by the government via Medicare or Medicaid.[26] However, by 2008 the CDC estimated these costs had nearly doubled to $147 billion.[27] The CDC identified a series of expensive conditions more likely to occur due to obesity.[28] The CDC released a series of strategies to prevent obesity and overweight, including: making healthy foods and beverages more available; supporting healthy food choices; encouraging kids to be more active; and creating safe communities to support physical activity.[29][30] An estimated 25.6% of U.S. adults in 2007 were obese, versus 23.9% in 2005. State obesity rates ranged from 18.7% to 30%. Obesity rates were roughly equal among men and women.[31] Some have proposed a so-called "fat tax" to provide incentives for healthier behavior, either by levying the tax on products (such as soft drinks) that are thought to contribute to obesity,[32] or to individuals based on body measures, as is done in Japan.[33]

Rationing of care

Healthcare rationing may refer to the restriction of medical care service delivery based on any number of objective or subjective criteria. Republican Newt Gingrich argued that the reform plans supported by President Obama expand the control of government over healthcare decisions, which he referred to as a type of healthcare rationing.[34] President Obama has argued that U.S. healthcare is already rationed, based on income, type of employment, and medical pre-existing conditions, with nearly 46 million uninsured. He argued that millions of Americans are denied coverage or face higher premiums as a result of medical pre-existing conditions.[35]

Peter Singer wrote in the *New York Times* in July 2009 that healthcare is rationed in the United States and argued for improved rationing processes:[36]

> Health care is a scarce resource, and all scarce resources are rationed in one way or another. In the United States, most healthcare is privately financed, and so most rationing is by price: you get what you, or your employer, can afford to insure you for...Rationing healthcare means getting value for the billions we are spending by setting limits on which treatments should be paid for from the public purse. If we ration we won't be writing blank checks to pharmaceutical companies for their patented drugs, nor paying for whatever procedures doctors choose to recommend. When public funds subsidize healthcare or provide it directly, it is crazy not to try to get value for money. The debate over healthcare reform in the United States should start from the premise that some form of healthcare rationing is both inescapable and desirable. Then we can ask, What is the best way to do it?"

According to PolitiFact, private health insurance companies already ration healthcare by income, by denying health insurance to those with pre-existing conditions and by caps on health insurance payments. Rationing exists now, and will continue to exist with or without healthcare reform.[37] David Leonhardt also wrote in the *New York Times* in June 2009 that rationing is a part of economic reality: "The choice isn't between rationing and not rationing. It's between rationing well and rationing badly. Given that the United States devotes far more of its economy to healthcare than other rich countries, and gets worse results by many measures, it's hard to argue that we are now rationing very rationally."[38]

Palin's death panel remarks were based on the ideas of Betsy McCaughey.[39][40] During 2009, former Alaska Governor Sarah Palin wrote against alleged rationing, referring to what by her interpretation was a "downright evil" "death panel" in current reform legislation known as H.R. 3200 Section 1233.[40] However, Palin supported similar

end of life discussion and advance directives for patients in 2008.[41] Defenders of the plan indicated that the proposed legislation H.R. 3200 would allow Medicare for the first time to cover patient-doctor consultations about end-of-life planning, including discussions about drawing up a living will or planning hospice treatment. Patients could seek out such advice on their own, but would not be required to. The provision would limit Medicare coverage to one consultation every five years.[42] Rep. Earl Blumenauer, D-Ore., who sponsored the H.R. 3200 end of life counseling provision, said the measure would block funds for counseling that presents suicide or assisted suicide as an option, and called references to death panels or euthanasia "mind-numbing".[43] Republican Senator Johnny Isakson, who co-sponsored a 2007 end-of-life counseling provision, called the euthanasia claim "nuts".[44] Analysts who examined the end-of-life provision Palin cited agree that Palin's claim is incorrect.[45][46][47][48][49] According to TIME and ABC, Palin and Betsy McCaughey made false euthanasia claims.[40][50][51]

The federal requirement that hospitals help patients with things like living wills began when Republican George H. W. Bush was President. Section 1233 merely allows doctors to be paid for their time.[45] However, an NBC poll indicates that as of August, 2009, 45% of Americans believed in the death panel story.[52]

Slate columnist Christopher Beam used the term "deathers" to refer to those who believed rationing and euthanasia would become likely for senior citizens. *The Rachel Maddow Show* aired a program called "Obama and the Deathers" in which Maddow discussed conspiracy theories that included "a secret plot to kill old people." Daily Kos and other web sites had used the term for about a week before Hari Sevugan, national spokesman for the Democratic National Committee, sent out an email with the subject line "Murkowski: Deathers 'Lying' 'Inciting Fear.'" The message included an article about a town hall statement by Senator Lisa Murkowski, a Republican from Alaska, that no version of healthcare reform included "death panels".

Sevugan explained the term "deathers" to Patricia Murphy, who writes a *Politics Daily* column called "The Capitolist":

> By "deather," I mean an opponent of change who is knowingly spreading false information regarding the existence of an alleged "death panel" in health insurance reform plans despite the fact the claim has been repeatedly and unequivocally debunked by independent fact-checking organizations. Like "birthers", "deathers" are shamefully lying and trafficking in scurrilous rumors to incite fear and achieve their stated political objective of derailing the president of the United States.[53]

Others, such as former Republican Secretary of Commerce Peter G. Peterson, have indicated that some form of rationing is inevitable and desirable considering the state of U.S. finances and the trillions of dollars of unfunded Medicare liabilities. He estimated that 25–33% of healthcare services are provided to those in the last months or year of life and advocated restrictions in cases where quality of life cannot be improved. He also recommended that a budget be established for government healthcare expenses, through establishing spending caps and pay-as-you-go rules that require tax increases for any incremental spending. He has indicated that a combination of tax increases and spending cuts will be required. All of these issues would be addressed under the aegis of a fiscal reform commission.[54]

Medical malpractice costs and limits on redress (tort)

Critics have argued that medical malpractice costs are significant and should be addressed via tort reform.[55] At the same time, a Hearst Newspapers investigation concluded that up to 200,000 people per year die from medical errors and infections in the United States.[56] None of the three major bills under consideration lower recoverable damages in tort suits. Medical malpractice, such as doctor errors resulting in harm to patients, has several direct and indirect costs:

- jury awards to injured;

- workers' compensation;

- reduced worker productivity as a result of injury;

- pain and suffering of the injured;

How much these costs are is a matter of debate. Some have argued that malpractice lawsuits are a major driver of medical costs.[57] However, the direct cost of malpractice suits amounts to only about 0.5% of all healthcare spending, and a 2006 Harvard study showed that over 90% of the malpractice suits examined contained evidence of injury to the patient and that frivolous suits were generally readily dismissed by the courts.[58] A 2005 study estimated the cost around 0.2%, and in 2009 insurer WellPoint Inc. said "liability wasn't driving premiums."[59] Counting both direct and indirect costs, other studies estimate the total cost of malpractice "is linked to" between 5% and 10% of total U.S. medical costs.[59] A 2004 report by the Congressional Budget Office put medical malpractice costs at 2% of U.S. health spending and "even significant reductions" would do little to reduce the growth of health care expenses.[59]

Conservative columnist Charles Krauthammer argued that between $60–200 billion per year could be saved through tort reform. Physician and former Democratic National Committee Chairman Howard Dean explained why tort reform is not part of the bills under consideration: "When you go to pass a really enormous bill like that, the more stuff you put it in it, the more enemies you make, right?...And the reason tort reform is not on the bill is because the people who wrote it did not want to take on the trial lawyers in addition to everybody else they were taking on. That is the plain and simple truth."[60]

However, even successful tort reform might not lead to lower aggregate liability: for example, medical commentators have argued that the current contingent fee system skews litigation towards high-value cases while ignoring meritorious small cases; aligning litigation more closely with merit might thus increase the number of small awards, offsetting any reduction in large awards.[61] A New York study found that only 1.5% of hospital negligence led to claims; moreover, the CBO observed that "health care providers are generally not exposed to the financial cost of their own malpractice risk because they carry liability insurance, and the premiums for that insurance do not reflect the records or practice styles of individual providers but more-general factors such as location and medical specialty."[62] Given that total liability is small relative to the amount doctors pay in malpractice insurance premiums, alternative mechanisms have been proposed to reform malpractice insurance.[63]

Addressing Medicare fraud

The Office of Management and Budget reported that $54 billion in "improper payments" were made to Medicare ($24B), Medicaid ($18B) and Medicaid Advantage ($12B) during FY 2009. This was 9.4% of the $573 billion spent in these categories.[64] The Government Accountability Office lists Medicare as a "high-risk" government program due to its vulnerability to improper payments.[65][66][67] Fewer than 5% of Medicare claims are audited.[68] Medicare fraud accounts for an estimated $60 billion in Medicare payments each year, and "has become one of, if not the most profitable, crimes in America."[69] Criminals set up phony companies, then invoice Medicare for fraudulent services provided to valid Medicare patients who never receive the services. These costs appear on the Medicare statements provided to Medicare card holders. The program pays out over $430 billion per year via over 1 billion claims, making enforcement challenging.[69] Its enforcement budget is "extremely limited" according to one Medicare official. U.S. Attorney General Eric Holder said in an interview: "Clearly more auditing needs to be done and it needs to be done in real time."[69] The Obama administration is providing Medicare with an additional $200 million to fight fraud as part of its stimulus package, and billions of dollars to computerize medical records and upgrade networks, which should assist Medicare in identifying fraudulent claims.[69]

Single-payer payment system

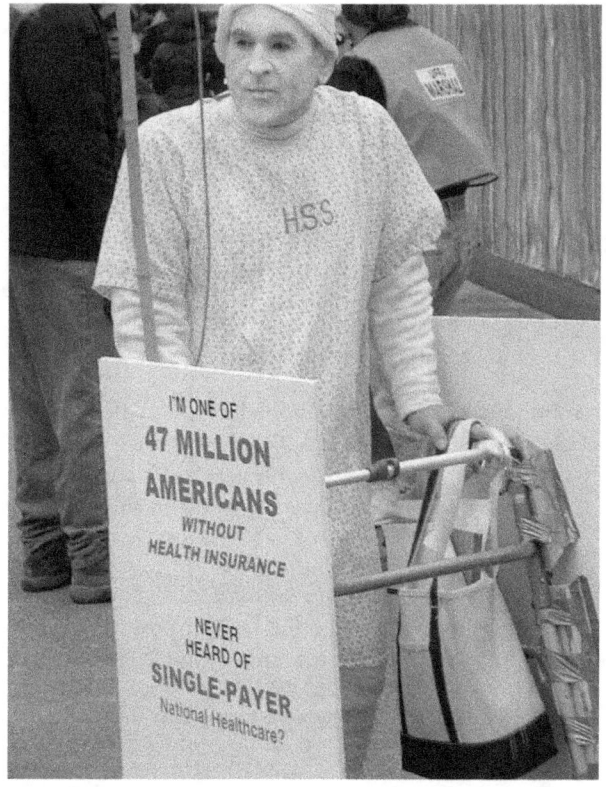

Costumed supporter of single-payer at an April 2009 protest in New York City.

See also: Single-payer_health_care § United_States, and United States National Health Care Act

In a single payer system the government or a government regulated non-profit agency channels health care payments to collect premiums and settle the bills of medical providers, instead of for-profit insurance companies. Many countries use single-payer systems to cover all their citizens.

The over 1,300 U.S. health insurance companies have different forms and processes for billing and reimbursement, requiring high costs on the part of service providers (mainly doctors and hospitals) to process payments. For example, the Cleveland Clinic, considered a low-cost, best-practices hospital system, has 1,400 billing clerks to support 2,000 doctors.[70] Further, the insurance companies have their own overhead functions and profit margins, much of which could be eliminated with a single payer system. Economist Paul Krugman estimated in 2005 that converting from the current private insurance system to a single-payer system would save $200 billion per year, primarily

via insurance company overhead.[71] One advocacy group estimated savings as high as $400 billion annually for 2009 and beyond.[72]

The U.S. system is often compared with that of its northern neighbor, Canada (see Canadian and American health care systems compared). Canada's system is largely publicly funded. In 2006, Americans spent an estimated US$6,714 per capita on health care, while Canadians spent US$3,678.[73] This amounted to 15% percent of U.S. GDP in that year, while Canada spent 10%. A study by Harvard Medical School and the Canadian Institute for Health Information determined that some 31% of U.S. health care dollars (more than $1,000 per person per year) went to health care administrative costs.[74]

Advocates argue that shifting the U.S. to a single-payer health care system would provide universal coverage, give patients free choice of providers and hospitals, and guarantee comprehensive coverage and equal access for all medically necessary procedures, without increasing overall spending. Shifting to a single-payer system would also eliminate oversight by managed care reviewers, removing a potential impediment to the doctor-patient relationship.[75]

Although studies indicate Democrats tend to be more supportive of a single-payer system than Republicans, none of the reform bills debated in the U.S. Congress when the Democrats had a majority from 2007–10, included proposals to implement a single payer health care system. Advocates argue that the largest obstacle to single-payer, universal system in the U.S. is a lack of political will.[76]

Privatize Medicare with a voucher system

Main article: The Path to Prosperity

Rep. Paul Ryan (R) has proposed the *Roadmap for America's Future*, which is a series of budgetary reforms. His January 2010 version of the plan includes the transition of Medicare to a voucher system, meaning individuals would receive a voucher which could be used to purchase health insurance in the private market. This would not affect those near retirement or currently enrolled.[77] A series of graphs and charts summarizing the impact of the plan are included.[78] Economists have both praised and criticized particular features of the plan.[79][80] The CBO also partially scored the bill.[81]

3.5.4 Congressional Proposals for Health Care Reform

On November 7, 2009, the House passed their version of a health insurance reform bill, the Affordable Health Care for America Act, 220–215, but this did not become law.

On December 24, 2009, the Senate passed the Patient Protection and Affordable Care Act.[82][83] President Obama signed this into law in March 2010.

Republicans continue to claim that they had a workable bill to extend coverage to all Americans and not cost the taxpayer anything, though nothing has been publicly presented to back the claim.[84] The Empowering Patients First Act which was proposed as a replacing amendment to the Senate Bill during the bill mark-up. However, this alternative bill was rejected by the Senate Finance Committee. The Congressional Budget Office said that it would not reduce the percentage of working age people who do not have insurance over the next 10 years, and that it estimated it would encourage health insurers to reduce rather than increase insurance coverage as it would remove mandated coverage rules that currently apply in some states. This bill would have given the insurance industry greater access to government funds through new insurance subsidies.[85] It did not have any taxation provisions and though it would reduce the deficit over 10 years by $18 billion, this was a considerably smaller deficit reduction than either the House or the Senate bills.

Similarities between the House and Senate Bills

The two bills are similar in a number of ways. In particular, both bills:[93][94]

- Mandate minimum health insurance benefits for most Americans

- Remove insurer set annual and lifetime caps on coverage and limit co-pay amounts

- Remove co-pays on certain services such as health screenings and some vaccinations

- Impose a new excise tax on medical devices and drugs, including vaccines[95][96] (the federal government began taxing vaccines in 1987[97]).

- Establish health insurance exchanges making easier price and coverage comparisons and purchasing for people and small businesses buying health care coverage

- Prevent insurers selling in the exchange insurance policies that do not meet minimum coverage standards

- Prevent insurers from denying coverage to people with pre-existing health conditions

- Prevent sex discrimination by insurers (especially the current discrimination against women) in setting premiums

- Limit age discrimination by insurers when setting policy premiums

- Restrict the ability of insurers to rescind policies they have been collecting premiums on

- Require insurers to cover adult children up to their mid twenties as part of family coverage

- Expand Medicaid eligibility up the income ladder (to 133% of the poverty line in the Senate bill and 150% in the House bill)

- Offer tax credits to certain small businesses (under 25 workers) who provide employees with health insurance

- Impose a penalty on employers who do not offer health insurance to their workers

- Impose a penalty on individuals who do not have health insurance (except American Indians (currently covered by the Indian Health Service), people with religious objections and people who can show financial hardship)

- Provide health insurance assistance subsidies for those earning up to 400% of the federal poverty level that must buy insurance for themselves

- Offer a new voluntary long-term care insurance program

- Pay for new spending, in part, through cutting over-generous funding (under existing law) given to private insurers that sell privatised health care plans to seniors (so called Medicare Advantage plans), slowing the growth of Medicare provider payments , reducing Medicare and Medicaid drug prices , cutting other Medicare and Medicaid spending through better reward structures, and raising taxes on very generous health care packages (typically offered to senior executives) and penalties on larger firms not providing their employees with health care coverage and certain persons who do not buy health insurance.

- Impose a $2,500 limit on contributions to a flexible spending account (FSAs), pre-tax health benefits, to pay for health care reform costs.

Differences in the House and Senate Bills

The biggest difference between the bills, currently, is in how they are financed. In addition to the items listed in the above bullet point, the House relies mainly on a surtax on income above $500,000 ($1 million for families). The Senate, meanwhile, relies largely on an "excise tax" for high cost 'Cadillac' insurance plans, as well as an increase in the Medicare payroll tax for high earners.[94][98]

Most economists believe the excise tax to be best of the three revenue raisers above, since (due to health care cost growth) it would grow fast enough to more than keep up with new coverage costs, and it would help to put downward pressure on overall health care cost growth.[99][100] In contrast, the House bill's insurance mandate has been described as "an economic assault on the young" by, for example, Robert J. Samuelson for The Washington Post.[101]

Unlike the House bill, the Senate bill would also include a Medicare Commission which could modify Medicare payments in order to keep down cost growth.

Services marketed as preventive care are a subject of continuing debate. Years of study have shown that most common services provide no benefit to patients.[102][103] The House and Senate bills would mandate the purchase of policies that pay 100% of the cost of certain services, with no co-pay; when the Senate bill was amended to mandate paying for tests that a federal panel and U.S. News & World Report said "do more harm than good,"[104] The New York Times wrote, "This sorry episode does not bode well for reform efforts to rein in spending on other procedures based on sound scientific evidence of their potential benefits and risks for patients."[105]

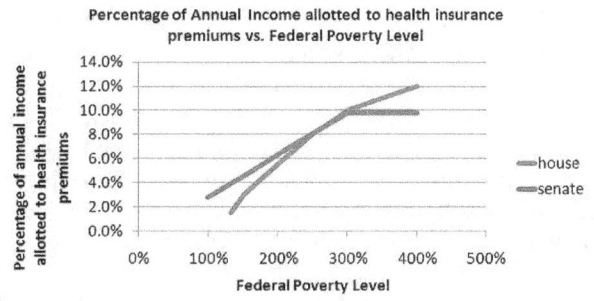

The relationship between a family's poverty level and the percentage of their income that is allotted to pay for health insurance. Note that the Senate Bill provides for Medicaid coverage up to 133% of the federal poverty level while the House Bill provides for Medicaid coverage up to 150% of the federal poverty level. Adapted from the texts of the House Bill and Senate Bill.

Differences in how each chamber determines subsidies
How each bill determines subsidies also differs. Each bill subsidizes the cost of the premium and the out-of-pocket costs but are more or less generous based on the relationship of the family's income to the federal poverty level.

The amount of the subsidy given to a family to cover the cost of a premium is calculated using a formula that includes the family's income relative to the federal poverty level. The

federal poverty level is related to a determined percentage that defines how much of that family's income can be put towards a health insurance premium. For instance, under the House Bill, a family at 200% of the federal poverty level will spend no more than 5.5% of its annual income on health insurance premiums. Under the Senate Bill, the same family would spend no more than 6.3% of its annual income on health insurance premiums. The difference between the family's maximum contribution to health insurance premiums and the cost of the health insurance premium is paid for by the federal government. To understand how each bill can affect different poverty levels and incomes, see the Kaiser Family Foundation's subsidy calculator

Subsidies Under House Bill The House plan subsidizes the cost of the plan and out-of-pocket expenses. The cost of the plan is subsidized according to the family's poverty level, decreasing the subsidy as the poverty level approaches 400%. The out-of-pocket expenses are also subsidized according to the poverty level at the following rates. The out-of-pocket expenses are subsidized initially and are not allowed to exceed a particular amount that will rise with the premiums for basic insurance.

Subsidies Under Senate Bill The Senate plan subsidizes the cost of the plan and out-of-pocket expenses. The cost of the plan is subsidized according to the family's poverty level, decreasing the subsidy as the poverty level approaches 400%. The out-of-pocket expenses are also subsidized according to the poverty level at the following rates. The out-of-pocket expenses are subsidized initially and are not allowed to exceed a particular amount that will rise with the premiums for basic insurance.

The Senate Bill also seeks to reduce out-of-pocket costs by setting guidelines for how much of the health costs can be shifted to a family within 200% of the poverty line. A family within 150% of the FPL cannot have more than 10% of their health costs incurred as out-of-pocket expenses. A family between 150% and 200% of the FPL cannot have more than 20% of their health costs incurred as out-of-pocket expenses.

The House and Senate bill would differ, somewhat, in their overall impact. The Senate bill would cover an additional 31 million people, at a federal budget cost of nearly $850 billion (not counting unfunded mandates) over ten years, reduce the ten-year deficit by $130 billion, and reduce the deficit in the second decade by around 0.25% of GDP. The House bill, meanwhile, would cover an additional 36 million people, cost roughly $1050 billion in coverage provisions, reduce the ten-year deficit by $138 billion, and slightly reduce the deficit in the second decade.[94]

Commentary on the cost analysis

It is worth noting that both bills rely on a number of "gimmicks" to get their favorable deficit reduction numbers. For example, both institute a public long-term care insurance known as the CLASS Act – because this insurance has a 5-year vesting period, it will appear to raise revenue in the first decade, even though all the money will need to be paid back. If the CLASS Act is subtracted from the bills, the Senate bill would reduce the deficit by $57 billion over ten years, and the House by $37 billion. In addition to the CLASS Act, neither bill accounts for the costs of updating Medicare physician payments, even though the House did so on a deficit-financed basis shortly after passing their health care bill.[106]

The Senate bill also begins most provisions a year later than the House bill in order to make costs seem smaller:

- 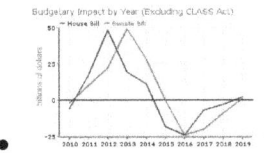 Budgetary Impact of House and Senate Bills

- 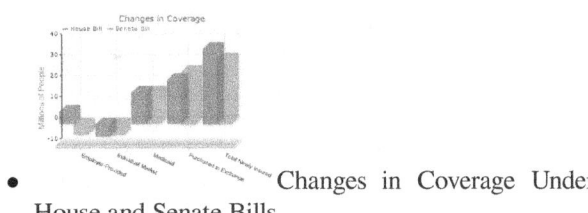 Changes in Coverage Under House and Senate Bills

- 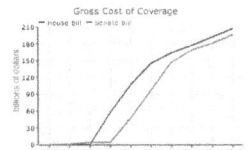 Gross Cost of Coverage Provisions in House and Senate Bills

Surgeon Atul Gawande wrote in *The New Yorker* that the Senate and House bills passed contain a variety of pilot programs that may have a significant impact on cost and quality over the long-run, although these have not been factored into CBO cost estimates. He stated these pilot programs cover nearly every idea healthcare experts advocate, except malpractice/tort reform. He argued that a trial and error strategy, combined with industry and government partnership, is how the U.S. overcame a similar challenge in the agriculture industry in the early 20th century.[107]

3.5.5 Lobbying

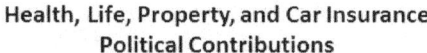
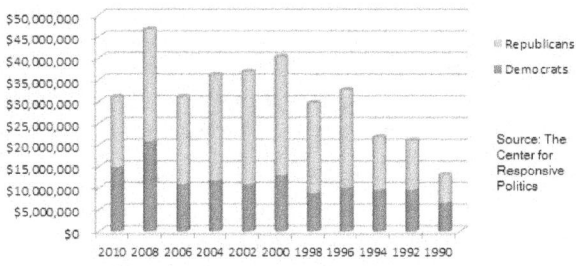

U.S. insurance health, life, property, and car insurance industry related political contributions from 1990 to 2010

The health and insurance sectors gave nearly $170 million to House and Senate members in 2007 and 2008, with 54% going to Democrats, according to data compiled by the Center for Responsive Politics. The shift in parties was even more pronounced during the first three months of 2009, when Democrats collected 60% of the $5.4 million donated by health care companies and their employees, the data show. Lawmakers that chair key committees have been leading recipients, some of whom received over $1.0 million in contributions.[108]

Matt Taibbi wrote in *Rolling Stone* that President Obama and key senators who have advocated single-payer systems in the past are unwilling to face the insurance companies and their powerful lobbying efforts. Key politicians on the Senate Finance Committee involved in crafting legislation have received over $2 million in campaign contributions from the healthcare industry. Several of the firms invited to testify at the hearings sent lobbyists that had formerly worked for Senator Max Baucus, the chair of the committee. Mr. Baucus stated in February 2009 that: "There may come a time when we can push for single-payer. At this time, it's not going to get to first base in Congress."[109]

George McGovern wrote that significant campaign funds were given to the chairman and ranking minority member of the Senate Finance Committee, which has jurisdiction over health care legislation: "Chairman Max Baucus of Montana, a Democrat, and his political action committee have received nearly $4 million from the health-care lobby since 2003. The ranking Republican, Charles Grassley of Iowa, has received more than $2 million. It's a mistake for one politician to judge the personal motives of another. But Sens. Baucus and Grassley are firm opponents of the single-payer system, as are other highly placed members of Congress who have been generously rewarded by the insurance lobby."[110]

3.5.6   Debate about political organizing methods

Much of the coverage of the debate has involved how the different sides are competing to express their views, rather than the specific reform proposals. The health care reform debate in the United States has been influenced by the Tea Party protest phenomenon, with reporters and politicians spending time reacting to it.[111][112][113] Supporters of a greater government role in healthcare, such as former insurance PR executive Wendell Potter of the Center for Media and Democracy- whose funding comes from groups such as the Tides Foundation-[114] argue that the hyperbole generated by this phenomenon is a form of corporate astroturfing, which he says that he used to write for CIGNA.[115] Opponents of more government involvement, such as Phil Kerpen of Americans for Prosperity- whose funding comes mainly from the Koch Industries corporation-[116] counterargue that those corporations oppose a public-plan, but some try to push for government actions that will unfairly benefit them, such as forcing private companies to buy health insurance for their employees.[117] Journalist Ben Smith has referred to mid-2009 as "The Summer of Astroturf" given the organizing and co-ordinating efforts made by various groups on both pro- and anti-reform sides.[113]

3.5.7   Arguments concerning health care reform

Liberal arguments

Some have argued that health care is a fundamental human right. Article 25 of the Universal Declaration of Human Rights states: "Everyone has the right to a standard of living adequate for the health and well-being of himself and of his family, including food, clothing, housing and medical care and necessary social services."[118] Similarly, Franklin D. Roosevelt advocated a right to medical care in his 1944 proposal for a Second Bill of Rights.[119]

Liberals were the primary advocates of both Social Security and Medicare, which are often targeted as significant expansions of government that has overwhelming satisfaction among beneficiaries.[120] President Obama argued during a September 2009 joint session of Congress that the government has a moral responsibility to ensure quality healthcare is available to all citizens. He also referred to a letter from the late Senator Ted Kennedy.[121]

Economist and New York Times columnist Paul Krugman has argued that Republican and conservative strategies in opposing healthcare are based on spite: "At this point, the guiding principle of one of our nation's two great political parties is spite pure and simple. If Republicans think

something might be good for the president, they're against it – whether or not it's good for America." He argued that Republican opposition to Medicare savings proposed by the President is "utterly at odds both with the party's traditions and with what conservatives claim to believe. Think about just how bizarre it is for Republicans to position themselves as the defenders of unrestricted Medicare spending. First of all, the modern G.O.P. considers itself the party of Ronald Reagan – and Reagan was a fierce opponent of Medicare's creation, warning that it would destroy American freedom. (Honest.) In the 1990s, Newt Gingrich tried to force drastic cuts in Medicare financing. And in recent years, Republicans have repeatedly decried the growth in entitlement spending – growth that is largely driven by rising health care costs."[122] More recently he urged the House of representatives to pass the Senate's bill, which he called "centrist."[123]

Conservative and libertarian arguments

Conservatives and libertarians have historically argued for a lesser role of government in healthcare.

For example, Conservative GOP columnist Bill Kristol advocated several free-market reforms instead of the Clinton plan during the 1993–1994 period.[124] Investigative reporter and columnist John Stossel has remarked that "Insurance invites waste. That's a reason health care costs so much, and is often so consumer-unfriendly. In the few areas where there are free markets in health care – such as cosmetic medicine and Lasik eye surgery – customer service is great, and prices continue to drop."[125] Republican Senator and medical doctor Tom Coburn has stated that the healthcare system in Switzerland should serve as a model for U.S. reform. He wrote for *New York Sun* that reform should involve a market-based method transferring health care tax benefits to individuals rather than employers as well as giving individuals extra tax credits to afford more coverage.[126]

Some critics of the bills passed in 2009 call them a "government take over of health care."[127] FactCheck called the phrase an unjustified "mantra."[128] (Factcheck has also criticized a number of other assertions made during 2009 by advocates on both sides of the debate).[129] CBS News described it as a myth "mixed in with some real causes for concern."[130] President Obama disputes the notion of a government takeover and says he no more wants government bureaucrats meddling than he wants insurance company bureaucrats doing so.[131] However, other sources contend the bills do amount to either a government takeover or a corporate takeover, or both.[132][133][134][135][136] This debate occurs in the context of a "revolution...transforming how medical care is delivered:" from 2002 to 2008, the percentage of medical practices owned by doctors fell from more than 70% to below 50%; in contrast to the traditional practice in which most doctors cared for patients in small, privately owned clinics, by 2008 most doctors had become employees of hospitals, nearly all of which are owned by corporations or government.[137]

Republicans also argue the proposed excise tax on medical devices and drugs would increase the tax burden on vaccine makers.[96][138]

Some conservatives argue that forcing people to buy private insurance is unconstitutional;[139] legislators in 38 states have introduced bills opposing the new law,[140] and 18 states have filed suit in federal court challenging the unfunded mandates on individuals and states.[141][142][143][144]

Senator Judd Gregg (R) said in an interview regarding the passage of healthcare reform: "Well, in my judgment we're moving down a path towards... Europeanization of our nation. And our great uniqueness, what surrounds American exceptionalism, what really drives it is that entrepreneurial individualistic spirit which goes out and takes a risk when nobody else is willing to do it or comes up with an idea that nobody else comes up with and that all gets dampened down the larger and more intrusive government becomes, especially if you follow a European model."[145]

3.5.8 See also

- Health care compared – tabular comparisons of the US, Canada, and other countries.

- Health policy

- Health economics

- Health insurance cooperative

- History of health care reform in the United States

- List of healthcare reform advocacy groups in the United States

- Public opinion on health care reform in the United States

3.5.9 References

[1] Wessel, David (September 7, 2006). "Capital: In health care, consumer theory falls flat". Wall Street Journal. Retrieved 2013-10-10.

[2] "Rand study finds patients' ratings of their medical care do not reflect the technical quality of their care" (Press release). RAND Corporation. May 1, 2006. Retrieved August 27, 2007.

[3] Chang JT, Hays RD, Shekelle PG, et al. (May 2006). "Patients' global ratings of their health care are not associated with the technical quality of their care". Ann. Intern. Med. 144 (9): 665–72. doi:10.7326/0003-4819-144-9-200605020-00010. PMID 16670136.

[4] For-Profit Hospitals Cost More and Have Higher Death Rates, Physicians for a National Health Program

[5] "Robert Reich Public Option Video".

[6] "How Pharma and Insurance Intend to Kill the Public Option, And What Obama and the Rest of Us Must Do".

[7] "Healthcare Reform to Make America Great Again". Trump-Pence. Retrieved 4 December 2016.

[8] Funk, Josh (Mar 1, 2010). "Buffett says economy recovering but at slow rate". San Francisco Chronicle (SFGate.com). Archived from the original on March 6, 2010. Retrieved April 3, 2010.

[9] Kenworthy, Lane (July 10, 2011). "America's inefficient health-care system: another look". Consider the Evidence (blog). Retrieved September 11, 2012.

[10] Pear, Robert (Dec 3, 2011). "Health Official Takes Parting Shot at 'Waste'". New York Times. Retrieved Dec 20, 2011.

[11] "Remarks by the President to the AMA-June 15, 2009". Whitehouse.gov. Retrieved January 12, 2012.

[12] "Summary of Obama Plan" (PDF). Retrieved January 12, 2012.

[13] "Remarks by the President to a Joint Session of Congress-September 2009". Whitehouse.gov. Retrieved January 12, 2012.

[14] "Charlie Rose-Peter Orszag Interview Transcript". November 3, 2009. Retrieved January 12, 2012.

[15] "Denis Cortese Interview on Charlie Rose Show-July 2009".

[16] "The New Yorker-The Cost Conundrum-June 2009".

[17] "NYT-Leonhardt-In Health Reform, A Cancer Offers and Acid Test". The New York Times. July 8, 2009. Retrieved May 4, 2010.

[18] "Peter Diamond-Healthcare and Behavioral Economics-May 2008" (PDF).

[19] "The New Yorker-Gawande-The Cost Conundrum-June 2009".

[20] "CBO-Testimony to Senate Finance Committee-June 2008" (PDF).

[21] "The Economist-Stemming the Tide-November 2009". The Economist. November 19, 2009. Retrieved January 12, 2012.

[22] "NYT-Singer-Why We Must Ration Healthcare-July 15, 2009". *The New York Times*. July 19, 2009. Retrieved May 4, 2010.

[23] "CBO Historical Tables" (PDF).

[24] "OMB Director Orszag-IMAC".

[25] Ignatius, David (August 20, 2009). "Washington Post-Paging Dr. Reform-August 2009". *The Washington Post*. Retrieved May 4, 2010.

[26] "CDC Home Page-Economic Consequences of Overweight and Obesity-Retrieved October 6, 2009". Cdc.gov. March 28, 2011. Retrieved January 12, 2012.

[27] Mckay, Betsy (July 28, 2009). "WSJ-Cost of Treating Obesity Soars-July 28, 2009". *The Wall Street Journal*. Retrieved January 12, 2012.

[28] "CDC Home Page-Health Consequences of Obesity and Overweight-Retrieved October 6, 2009". Cdc.gov. March 3, 2011. Retrieved January 12, 2012.

[29] "WebMD-Retrieved October 6, 2009-Obesity Costs U.S. $147 billion per year". Webmd.com. Retrieved January 12, 2012.

[30] "CDC-Recommended Community Strategies and Measurements to Prevent Obesity in the U.S.- July 24, 2009". Cdc.gov. Retrieved January 12, 2012.

[31] Reinberg, Steven (July 17, 2008). "Washington Post-U.S. Obesity Epidemic Continues to Grow-July 17, 2008". *The Washington Post*. Retrieved January 12, 2012.

[32] Leonhardt, David (August 12, 2009). "NYT-Leonhardt-The Way We Live-Fat Tax-Aug 9". *The New York Times*. Retrieved January 12, 2012.

[33] Wang, Shirley S. (June 13, 2008). "WSJ-Another Thing Big in Japan-Measuring Waistlines-June 2008". *The Wall Street Journal*. Retrieved January 12, 2012.

[34] "LA Times-Gingrich-Healthcare Rationing-Real Scary". *Los Angeles Times*. August 16, 2009. Retrieved May 4, 2010.

[35] "NYT-President Obama-Why We Need Healthcare Reform-August 15, 2009". *The New York Times*. August 16, 2009. Retrieved May 4, 2010.

[36] "NYT-Singer-Why We Must Ration Healthcare-July 2009". *The New York Times*. July 19, 2009. Retrieved May 4, 2010.

[37] PolitiFact, There's rationing in health care now, and there still would be under reform bill

[38] "NYT-Leonhardt-Healthcare Rationing Rhetoric Overlooks Reality-June 2009". *The New York Times*. June 17, 2009. Retrieved May 4, 2010.

[39] Jim Dwyer, August 25, 2009, Distortions on Health Bill, Homegrown, The New York Times, Distortions on Health Bill, Homegrown

[40] Angie Drobnic Holan, PolitiFact, PolitiFact's Lie of the Year. Accessed August 5, 2010.

[41] "Office of the Governor of Alaska-Healthcare Decisions Day". Archived from the original on 2010-01-05.

[42] Farber, Dan (August 8, 2009). "CBS News-Palin Weighs In On Healthcare Reform-August 2009".

[43] Matthew Daly, August 14, 2009, The Chicago Tribune, AP story, Palin stands by 'death panel claim

[44] Ezra Klein, August 10, 2009, The Washington Post, Is the Government Going to Euthanize your Grandmother? An Interview With Sen. Johnny Isakson.

[45] Alonso-Zaldivar, Ricardo (August 15, 2009). "Palin is wrong: There's no 'death panel' in health care bill". *Alaska Journal of Commerce*. Archived from the original on 2010-11-29.

[46] Connolly, Ceci (August 1, 2009). "Talk Radio Campaign Frightening Seniors". *The Washington Post*.

[47] Farber, Daniel (August 8, 2009). "Palin Weighs In on Health Care Reform". CBS News. Retrieved August 11, 2009.

[48] Holan, Angie Drobnic (August 10, 2009). "Palin 'death panel' claim sets Truth-O-Meter ablaze". PolitiFact.com. Retrieved August 27, 2009.

[49] PolitiFact, August 7, 2009, Sarah Palin falsely claims Barack Obama runs a 'death panel'

[50] TIME, August 12, 2009, Ezekiel Emanuel, Obama's 'Deadly Doctor,' Strikes Back

[51] ABC News, Jake Tapper, August 7, 2009, Palin Paints Picture of 'Obama Death Panel' Giving Thumbs Down to Trig

[52] Mark Murray, August 18, 2009, NBC, Americans still skeptical about Obama's plans

[53] Murphy, Patricia (August 13, 2009). "Democrats Shift Criticism From 'Birthers' to 'Deathers'". *Politics Daily*. Retrieved October 1, 2009.

[54] "Peter G. Peterson on Charlie Rose-July 3, 2009-About 17 min in".

[55] "RCP-Roth-The High Cost of Medical Malpractice-August 2009".

[56] "Health care bills sidestep medical errors issue". *Chron.com*. Archived from the original on 2011-07-11.

[57] Philip K. Howard (July 31, 2009). "Health Reform's Taboo Topic". *The Washington Post*.

[58] "The Medical Malpractice Myth".

[59] "Bloomberg-Malpractice Lawsuits are Red Herring in Obama Plan". June 16, 2009.

[60] "RCP-Roundtable on Health Reform Costs-August 2009".

[61] "The Medical Malpractice Insurance Crisis, Again". Medscape.com. Retrieved 2013-10-10.

[62] "CBO – Limiting Tort Liability for Medical Malpractice".

[63] "Alternative malpractice insurance mechanisms". Archived from the original on 2011-09-28.

[64] ""White House Reports Billions of Improper Payments in 2009" CNN, November 2009" (URL). November 18, 2009. Retrieved November 18, 2009.

[65] ""High-Risk Series: An Update" U.S. Government Accountability Office, January 2009 (PDF)" (PDF). Retrieved November 13, 2009.

[66] U.S. Government Accountability Office, Medicare: More Effective Screening and Stronger Enrollment Standards Needed for Medical Equipment Suppliers, GAO-05-656 September 22, 2005

[67] Medicare Fraud and Abuse: DOJ Continues to Promote Compliance with False Claims Act Guidance, GAO Report to Congressional Committees, April 2002

[68] Carrie Johnson, "Medical Fraud a Growing Problem: Medicare Pays Most Claims Without Review," The Washington Post, June 13, 2008

[69] Ira Rosen and Joel Bach, producers, CBS-60 Minutes-Medicare Fraud-A $60 Trillion Business, CBS News, October 25, 2009

[70] "Newsweek-The Hospital That Could Cure Healthcare-December 7, 2009". *Newsweek*. November 26, 2009. Archived from the original on 2010-04-19. Retrieved January 12, 2012.

[71] Krugman, Paul (June 13, 2005). "Krugman-One Nation, Uninsured-June 2005". *The New York Times*. Retrieved January 12, 2012.

[72] "PNHP-Single Payer". Pnhp.org. Retrieved January 12, 2012.

[73] "OECD Health Data 2008: How Does Canada Compare" (PDF). Archived from the original (PDF) on 2012-06-16.

[74] Costs of Health Administration in the U.S. and Canada. Woolhandler, et al., NEJM 349(8) Sept. 21, 2003

[75] Physicians for a National Health Program. "What is Single Payer?"

[76] Timid ideas will not fix health mess. By Marie Cocco, Sacramento Bee, February 10, 2007

[77] "Republican Website-Roadmap for America's Future". Roadmap.republicans.budget.house.gov. January 26, 2011. Retrieved January 12, 2012.

[78] "Roadmap for America's Future-Charts & Graphs-February 2010". Roadmap.republicans.budget.house.gov. Retrieved January 12, 2012.

[79] "Washington Post-Robert Samuelson-Paul Ryan's Lonely Challenge-February 2010". *The Washington Post*. February 12, 2010. Retrieved January 12, 2012.

[80] "Forbes-Bartlett-Paul Ryan's Budgetary Holy Grail-February 2010". *Forbes*. February 12, 2010. Retrieved January 12, 2012.

[81] "CBO-Ryan Roadmap Letter-January 2010" (PDF). Retrieved January 12, 2012.

[82] "Patient Protection and Affordable Care Act" (PDF). Retrieved January 12, 2012.

[83] "CNN-Senate Passes Healthcare Bill-December 24, 2009". CNN. December 24, 2009. Retrieved January 12, 2012.

[84] Herszenhorn, David M. (January 29, 2010). "Searching for Some Light Amid the Heat". *The New York Times*. Retrieved May 4, 2010.

[85] "CBO.gov" (PDF). Retrieved January 12, 2012.

[86] Rau, Jordan (2009-12-24). "A Consumer's Guide To Health Reform". NPR. Retrieved 2013-10-10.

[87] Whitelaw, Kevin. "Next Step: Getting A Health Bill To Obama's Desk". NPR. Retrieved 2013-10-10.

[88] "Compare the Senate and House Health Reform Bills". PBS. 2009-12-21. Retrieved 2013-10-10.

[89] Section 1322 of H.R. 3590

[90] "Accessed 24 December 2009". Pbs.org. December 21, 2009. Retrieved January 12, 2012.

[91] "CBO Letter to John Dingle-November 20, 2009" (PDF). Retrieved January 12, 2012.

[92] "CBO Letter to Harry Reid-Corrected-December 19, 2009" (PDF). Retrieved January 12, 2012.

[93] Hossain, Farhana (February 23, 2009). "NYtimes.com". *The New York Times*. Retrieved January 12, 2012.

[94] "Updated Health Care Charts". Committee for a Responsible Federal Budget - Crfb.org. Retrieved 2013-10-10.

[95] Mundy, Alicia (October 30, 2009). "Drug Makers Face Tougher Measures". *The Wall Street Journal*.

[96] Frates, Chris (November 21, 2009). "Politico.com". Politico.com. Retrieved January 12, 2012.

[97] Klott, Gary (December 19, 1987). "Conferees Complete Bill For $23 Billion Tax Rise". *The New York Times*. Retrieved May 4, 2010.

[98] "Wallstreet Journal online". *The Wall Street Journal*. March 22, 2010. Retrieved January 12, 2012.

[99] "Understanding the Health Insurance Excise Tax | Committee for a Responsible Federal Budget". Crfb.org. Retrieved 2013-10-10.

[100] "Taxing Health Care Decisions | Committee for a Responsible Federal Budget". Crfb.org. Retrieved 2013-10-10.

[101] "Robert J. Samuelson on the health bill's burdens for the young". *The Washington Post*. November 23, 2009. Retrieved May 4, 2010.

[102] "Linkinghub.elsevier.com". Linkinghub.elsevier.com. Retrieved January 12, 2012.

[103] Kolata, Gina (August 12, 2003). "Annual Physical Checkup May Be an Empty Ritual". *The New York Times*. Retrieved May 4, 2010.

[104] "Health.usnews.com". Health.usnews.com. November 16, 2009. Retrieved January 12, 2012.

[105] "Senate Health Care Follies". *The New York Times*. December 6, 2009. Retrieved May 4, 2010.

[106] "The True Costs of Health Reform | Committee for a Responsible Federal Budget". Crfb.org. 2009-11-20. Retrieved 2013-10-10.

[107] Gawande, Atul (August 1, 2011). "Gawande-Testing, Testing-New Yorker-December 2009". Newyorker.com. Retrieved January 12, 2012.

[108] "Washington Post-Dan Eggen-Industry Cash Flowed to Drafters of Reform-July 2009". *The Washington Post*. July 21, 2009. Retrieved May 4, 2010.

[109] "Taibbi-Rolling Stone-Sick and Wrong-September 2009".

[110] McGovern, George S. (September 13, 2009). "McGovern Op Ed-Washington Post-September 2009". *The Washington Post*. Retrieved May 4, 2010.

[111] Bowser, Andre (August 22, 2009). "TEA Party protests health care reform plan". *East Valley Tribune*. Archived from the original on 2010-01-13. Retrieved August 26, 2009.

[112] Copeland, Mike (August 15, 2009). "Local Tea Party members protest Obama health care plan at Chet Edwards' Waco office". *Waco Tribune*. Retrieved August 26, 2009.

[113] Ben Smith (August 21, 2009). "The Summer of Astroturf". Politico. Retrieved August 28, 2009.

[114] "Financial Supporters". Center for Media and Democracy. Retrieved June 3, 2008.

[115] Wendell Potter (August 17, 2009). "Commentary: How insurance firms drive debate". CNN. Retrieved August 26, 2009.

[116] Evans, Will (October 6, 2008). "Secret Money Project". National Public Radio. Archived from the original on 2009-07-22. Retrieved September 1, 2009.

[117] "The Grass Is AstroTurf-er on the Other Side". Fox News. August 12, 2009. Archived from the original on 2011-08-05. Retrieved August 26, 2009.

[118] Asher, Judith (April 25, 2005). "Chapter 2 What is meant by the right to health?" (PDF). *The Right to Health: A Resource Manual for NGOs*. AAAS Science and Human Rights Program, 1200 New York Ave. NW, Washington, DC 20005. Archived from the original (PDF) on 2013-05-16.

[119] Franklin D. Roosevelt (January 11, 1944). "The Economic Bill of Rights". Archived from the original on 2009-02-25.

[120] Adler GS. "Medicare beneficiaries rate their medical care: new data from the MCBS (Medicare Current Beneficiary Survey)". *Health Care Financ Rev*. **16** (4): 175–87. PMC 4193523. PMID 10172473.

[121] Lee, Jesse (September 9, 2009). "President Obama Healthcare Speech of September 9, 2009".

[122] "NYT-Krugman-The Politics of Spite-October 2009". *The New York Times*. October 5, 2009. Retrieved May 4, 2010.

[123] Krugman, Paul (January 21, 2010). "Krugman-NYT-Do The Right Thing-January 21, 2010". *The New York Times*. Retrieved January 12, 2012.

[124] "WSJ-William Kristol-How to Oppose the Health Plan and Why-January 1994".

[125] John Stossel (October 16, 2006). "Health Insurance Isn't All It's Cracked Up to Be". ABC News.

[126] Tom Coburn (March 10, 2008). "Competition Solves Health Care". *New York Sun*.

[127] "Detailed Analysis: House Democrats' Government Takeover of Health Care Destroys Small Business Jobs". *Republicanleader.house.gov*. Archived from the original on 2010-06-13.

[128] "Factcheck.org". Factcheck.org. November 6, 2009. Retrieved January 12, 2012.

[129] "Factcheck.org". Factcheck.org. December 24, 2009. Retrieved January 12, 2012.

[130] "Fighting Myths of Health Care "Takeover"". *CBS News*. August 27, 2009.

[131] Jackson, David (August 11, 2009). "Obama: No government bureaucrats – or insurance bureaucrats". *USA Today*. Retrieved May 4, 2010.

[132] Douthat, Ross (December 17, 2009). "Obamanomics and Health Care". *The New York Times*. Retrieved May 4, 2010.

[133] "Washingtonexaminer.com". Washingtonexaminer.com. December 17, 2009. Retrieved January 12, 2012.

[134] "Cato.org". Cato.org. September 23, 2009. Retrieved January 12, 2012.

[135] "Heritage.org blog". Blog.heritage.org. November 4, 2009. Retrieved January 12, 2012.

[136] David Gratzer. *Why Obama's Government Takeover of Health Care Will Be a Disaster.* Encounter Broadsides. ISBN 9781594034602. Retrieved 2013-10-10.

[137] Harris, Gardiner (March 25, 2010). "More Doctors Giving Up Private Practices". *The New York Times.* Retrieved May 4, 2010.

[138] Fabian, Jordan (2009-11-21). "GOP: Health bill would tax H1N1 vaccine makers - The Hill's Blog Briefing Room". Thehill.com. Retrieved 2013-10-10.

[139] Seelye, Katharine Q. (September 26, 2009). "A Constitutional Debate Over a Health Care Mandate". *The New York Times.* Retrieved May 4, 2010.

[140] "PBS.org". PBS.org. April 1, 2010. Retrieved January 12, 2012.

[141] Fletcher, Pascal (April 7, 2010). "UPDATE 3-Florida says challenge to healthcare reform widens". *Reuters.*

[142] "Businessweek.com". *Bloomberg BusinessWeek.* Retrieved January 12, 2012.

[143] "14 states sue to block health care law". *CNN.* March 23, 2010. Retrieved May 4, 2010.

[144] Pierog, Karen (March 22, 2010). "UPDATE 3-U.S. states plan lawsuits against health reforms". *Reuters.*

[145] "Charlie Rose-Senator Judd Gregg Interview-March 2010". Retrieved January 12, 2012.

3.5.10 External links

- PBS Special Report:Healthcare Reform NOW on PBS

- Health Care Reform in the United States at DMOZ

- Malhotra, Umang, *Solving the American Healthcare Crisis*, iUniverse, 2010. ISBN 978-1-4401-8018-7

3.6 Hospital Insurance and Diagnostic Services Act

The **Hospital Insurance and Diagnostic Services Act** (HIDS) is a statute passed by the Parliament of Canada in 1957 that reimbursed one-half of provincial and territorial costs for hospital and diagnostic services administered under provincial and territorial health insurance programs.[1][2] Originally implemented on July 1, 1958, with five participating provinces, by January 1, 1961, all 10 provinces were enlisted.[2] The federal funding was coupled with terms and conditions borrowed from the Saskatchewan

Hospital Services Plan, introduced in 1947 as the first universal hospital insurance program in North America. In order to receive funding, services had to be universal, comprehensive, accessible and portable. This stipulation was dropped in 1977 with the Established Programs Financing Act and then reinstated in 1984 in the Canada Health Act. Widely acknowledged as the foundation for future developments in the Canadian health care system, the HIDS Act was a landmark example of federal-provincial cooperation in post-war Canada.[3]

3.6.1 Background

Prior to World War II, health care in Canada was privately funded and delivered, with the exception of services provided to the sick poor that were financed by local governments. The experience of the 1930s left many Canadians in challenging financial situations. As personal financial situations deteriorated, the municipal governments were overwhelmed. Though the provinces provided relief payments for food, clothing, and shelter, additional medical costs were beyond the capacity of most of the provincial budgets. Many Canadians were not receiving adequate medical care, and those that did, were overwhelmed with the associated costs. As such, preventable diseases and deaths were still common occurrences.[3]

Ten years of depression, followed by six years of war, formed the social context of the ambitious federal Green Book Proposals. In a bid for unprecedented cooperation between the federal and provincial governments, these initiatives formed the foundations of a national program for social security, including provisions for health insurance. However, the failure to come to a consensus on the required allocation of tax resources at the Dominion-Provincial Conference in August 1945 precluded adoption and delayed subsequent action.[3] Although the Green Book Proposals were not adopted, they effectively created an appetite for government-funded health services.[4]

Despite a lack of commitment for federal funding, Saskatchewan proceeded with a plan for provincial hospital insurance. From the collective efforts of the "wheat economy" came a cooperative movement towards efficient agencies to deliver services to Saskatchewan's sparse population. Strong local engagement contributed to creation of the union hospital system and municipal hospital care plans. However, a solution to the problem of providing medical and hospital services to a population reeling from the devastating effects of the depression required greater provincial contribution. The Co-operative Commonwealth Federation won their first majority government in 1944. Continuing the Liberal health insurance platform that introduced "A Bill Respecting Health Insurance," Tommy Douglas, as the

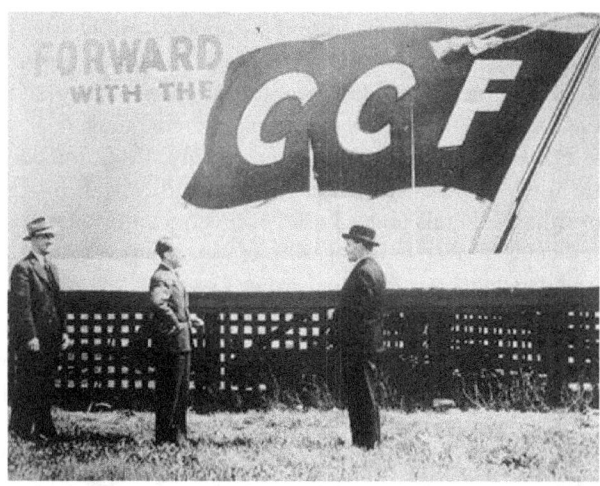

Cooperative Commonwealth Federation Party banner

new premier, signaled his commitment to the provision of health services by assuming the role of Health Minister as well. By 1947, Saskatchewan introduced the first universal hospital insurance program in North America.[3]

Saskatchewan's decision to launch the Saskatchewan Hospital Services Plan accelerated and influenced the development of other provincial insurance plans. The British Columbia Hospital Insurance Service was passed in early 1948, and followed soon after by the Alberta insurance system. The success of these provincial plans combined with the volume of illness and associated costs, in addition to provincial disparities in health coverage, fuelled debate on the topic of a federally funded health service. There was much disagreement as to the appropriate scope, funding allocation, and administration of such a plan.[3]

After several years of debate between the stakeholders, including Canadian medical professional associations and the provincial governments, the federal government made an offer to fund approximately one half of the national cost of diagnostic services and in-patient hospital care for provinces that implemented insurance plans. Five provinces, namely British Columbia, Alberta, Saskatchewan, Ontario, and Newfoundland, accepted the proposal, laying the groundwork for a Canadian health insurance plan.[3]

3.6.2   Overview

On May 1, 1957, the HIDS Act was formally legislated in Canada in response to the increasing pressures for national comprehensive health insurance.[3] Under the Act, the federal government agreed to fund approximately 50% of the costs of provincial or territorial insurance plans for hospital and diagnostic services.[5] Formally, federal funding comprised 25% of the per capita costs for hospital services in Canada plus 25% of the per capita costs for hospital services in the province or territory multiplied by the number of insured persons in that jurisdiction.[3] Funding was made available to any province or territory that agreed to make insured hospital services available to the region under uniform provisions.[6]

Provisions

Participating provinces and territories were obligated to satisfy four funding conditions as follows:[6]

- Comprehensiveness: All-encompassing in-patient and out-patient hospital services as well as diagnostic services were to be made available under the insurance plan.

- Universality: Services were to be made available to all residents of the province or territory.

- Accessibility: Services were to be made reasonably accessible to insured persons in a manner that did not preclude or impede access either directly or indirectly.

- Portability: Provincial plans were to provide coverage for out-of-province Canadian residents who were insured by home provincial or territorial plans.

Provinces and Territories were also obligated to limit co-payments and other "deterrent" fees to ensure that patients were not placed under financial burden at the point of care.[3] Though there was no other explicit provision preventing provinces and territories from demanding financial contribution for services from patients, such charges would have reduced the federal contribution since, under the cost-sharing arrangement, federal funding was proportional to provincial and territorial contributions.[7] Therefore, the Act intrinsically deterred provinces and territories from charging patients for services.

Coverage

Provincial and territorial insurance plans were to cover acute, convalescent, and chronic care of patients, including diagnostic services and in-patient drug administration in hospital facilities.[6] However, coverage was not provided for hospitals for tuberculosis, mental hospitals, nursing homes, capital expenditures, or administrative costs.[5]

Funding

Each province and territory was to be responsible for administering its own plan; therefore, each had the right to decide how to raise its proportion of funding for the insurance program, either through insurance premiums or taxation.[5]

Delivery

Under the Act, insured services could only be delivered by hospitals, most of which were private entities. Hospital employees including physicians, laboratory technicians, and radiologists were to be paid via a fee-for-service model negotiated with the provincial or territorial administrative body.[3]

The passage of the HIDS Act was the first milestone in the evolution of national health insurance in Canada and provided the foundation for all future Canadian Health legislation.[6]

3.6.3 Outcomes

By 1961, almost all Canadians were entitled to comprehensive hospital care benefits, protecting them from large hospital bills. The HIDS act enabled hospital operations that were not previously feasible and facilitated access to care for who could not otherwise afford it.[2]

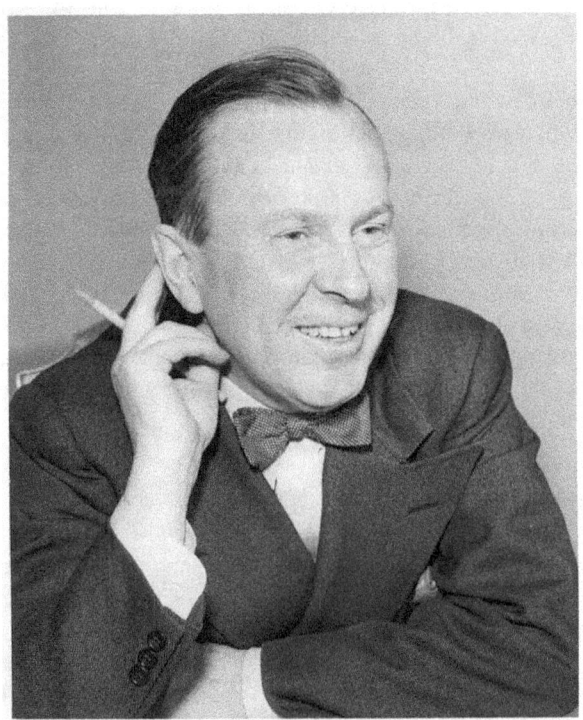

Lester B. Pearson

The HIDS Act laid the foundation for other notable developments in the Canadian health care system. One of the criticisms of the Act was that it did not cover medical

services, which in 1955 comprised approximately 40% of national healthcare costs.[3] Following the adoption of the HIDS Act, then, extending health insurance to cover additional medical services was next on the federal agenda. At the Federal-Provincial Conference in July, 1965, the decision for Medicare was made. Then, on July 1, 1967, the governing Liberals under Lester B. Pearson introduced the Medical Care Act, covering 50% of physician costs outside of a hospital.[3]

Together, the HIDS Act and Medical Care Act brought hospital and physician services to all Canadians, regardless of their ability to pay. Though criticized for imposing federal priorities on provincial jurisdiction, provincial governments were left with no option other than to meet the federal provisions or forgo supplementary funding altogether.[3] To address these concerns, the Established Programs Financing Act was passed in 1977, transferring the responsibility of the program to the provinces by decoupling the amount of the federal transfer from the provisions. Some provinces levied user charges and authorized extra-billing, which threatened universal and free access to healthcare.[8] The federal government, then, enacted the Canada Health Act in 1984 to re-instate the provisions of the HIDS Act and the Medical Care Act.

3.6.4 References

[1] Health Canada (2012). Canada's Health Care System.

[2] Archives Canada. Royal Commission on Health Services fonds.

[3] Taylor, Malcolm G. (1978). *Health Insurance and Canadian Public Policy*, McGill-Queen's University Press, Montreal.

[4] Canadian Museum of Civilization (2010). Making Medicare: The history of health care in Canada, 1914–2007.

[5] Turner, J. Gilbert (1958). The Hospital Insurance and Diagnostic Services Act: Its impact on hospital administration, *Canadian Medical Association Journal*, 78(10), 768-770.

[6] Manga, Pran, Broyles Robert W., & Angus, Douglas E. (1987). The determinants of hospital utilization under a universal public insurance program in Canada, *Medical Care*, 25(7), 658-670.

[7] Parliament of Canada. The health of Canadians – The federal role. Retrieved December 7, 2012.

[8] Madore, Odette (2005).The Canada Health Act: Overview and options.

-
-
-
-

3.7 List of countries by health insurance coverage

A **list of countries by health insurance coverage**. The table lists the percentage of the total population covered by total public and primary private health insurance, by government/social health insurance, and by primary private health insurance in the 34 Organisation for Economic Co-operation and Development (OECD) member countries in 2011.[1]

3.7.1 References

[1] OECD (June 27, 2013). "OECD Health Data: Social protection". *OECD Health Statistics (database)*. Paris: OECD. doi:10.1787/data-00544-en. Retrieved 2013-07-14.

3.8 List of countries with universal health care

See also: Health systems by country

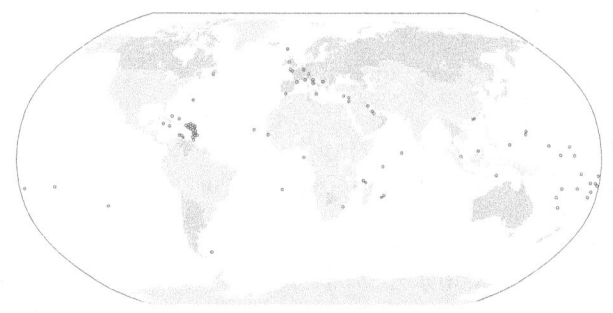

58 countries with universal health care in 2009.[1]
58 countries with legislation mandating universal health care, along with > 90% health insurance coverage, and > 90% skilled birth attendance.

Main article: Universal health care

Universal health coverage is a broad concept that has been implemented in several ways. The common denominator for all such programs is some form of government action aimed at extending access to health care as widely as possible and setting minimum standards. Most implement universal health care through legislation, regulation and taxation. Legislation and regulation direct what care must be provided, to whom, and on what basis. Usually some costs are borne by the patient at the time of consumption but the bulk of costs come from a combination of compulsory insurance and tax revenues. Some programs are paid for entirely out of tax revenues. In others tax revenues are used either to fund insurance for the very poor or for those needing long term chronic care. The UK government's National Audit Office in 2003 published an international comparison of ten different health care systems in ten developed countries, nine universal systems against one non-universal system (the U.S.), and their relative costs and key health outcomes.[2] A wider international comparison of 16 countries, each with universal health care, was published by the World Health Organization in 2004[3] In some cases, government involvement also includes directly managing the health care system, but many countries use mixed public-private systems to deliver universal health care.

The UN has adopted a resolution on universal health care. It may be the next stage after the Millennium Development Goals.[4]

3.8.1 Africa

Algeria

Algeria operates a public healthcare system. A network of hospitals, clinics, and dispensaries provide treatment to the population, with the Social Security system funding health services, although many people must still cover part of their costs due to the rates paid by the Social Security system unchanged since 1987. The poor are generally entitled to health services free of charge, while the wealthy pay for treatment according to a sliding scale.[5][6]

Botswana

Main article: Health in Botswana

Botswana operates a system of public medical centers, with 98% of health facilities in the country run by the government. All citizens are entitled to be treated in public facilities free of charge, though a nominal fee of ~70 BWP (~$6.60 USD) is typically charged for public health services except for sexual reproductive health services and antiretroviral therapy services, which are free.[7]

Burkina Faso

Burkina Faso operates a scheme called Universal Health Insurance (AMU) which provides universal healthcare to citizens. It is administered by two separate bodies, one for civilians and the other for the armed forces.[8]

Egypt

Main article: Healthcare in Egypt

Egypt operates a system of public hospitals and clinics through the Ministry of Health. Egyptian citizens can receive treatment at these facilities free of charge. However, those Egyptians who can afford it prefer to pay out of pocket for private healthcare.[9]

Ghana

Ghana operates the National Health Insurance Scheme to provide citizens with health insurance. The level of premiums citizens must pay varies according to their level of income. Most medical facilities are run directly by the Ministry of Health or Ghana Health Service.[10]

Mauritius

The Government of Mauritius operates a system of medical facilities that provide treatment to citizens free of charge.[11]

Morocco

Morocco operates a public health sector run by the government that operates 85% of the country's hospital beds. It deals mainly with the poor and rural populations, who cannot afford private healthcare. In addition, there is a nonprofit health sector operated by the National Social Security Fund which covers 16% of the population. There is also a private sector for those who can afford it.[12]

Rwanda

Rwanda operates a system of universal health insurance through the Ministry of Health called Mutuelle de Santé (Mutual Health), a system of community-based insurance where people pay premiums based on their income level into local health insurance funds, with the wealthiest paying the highest premiums and required to cover a small percentage of their medical expenses, while those at the lowest income levels are exempt from paying premiums and can still utilize the services of their local health fund. In 2012, this system insured all but 4% of the population.[13]

South Africa

Main article: Healthcare in South Africa

South Africa has a public healthcare system that provides services to the vast majority of the population, though it is chronically underfunded and understaffed, and a private system that is far better equipped, which covers the wealthier sectors of society.[14]

Tunisia

Tunisia operates a public healthcare system under the National Health Insurance Fund (*Caisse Nationale d'Assurance Maladie*). All Tunisian citizens and residents can receive treatment in state-run hospitals and clinics free of charge.[15]

3.8.2 Asia

Countries that provide public healthcare in Asia include Bhutan,[16] Bahrain,[17] China, Hong Kong, India, Iran,[18] Israel[19] (see below), Jordan,[20] Kazakhstan,[21] Macau (see below), Malaysia,[22] Mongolia,[23] Oman,[24][25] Singapore, Sri Lanka,[26] Syria,[27] Taiwan (R.O.C.)[28] (see below), Tajikistan,[29] Thailand (see below), Turkey,[30] and Turkmenistan.[31]

Bhutan

Main article: Health in Bhutan

The Royal Government of Bhutan maintains a policy of free and universal access to primary health care. As hospital facilities in the country are limited, patients with diseases that cannot be treated in Bhutan, such as cancer, are normally referred to hospitals in India for treatment. Such referral treatment is also carried out at the cost of the Royal Government.[32]

Hong Kong

Main article: Health in Hong Kong

Hong Kong has early health education, professional health services, and well-developed health care and medication system. The life expectancy is 84 for females and 78 for males,[33] which is the second highest in the world, and 2.94 infant mortality rate, the fourth lowest in the world.[34][35]

There are two medical schools in Hong Kong, and several schools offering courses in traditional Chinese medicine. The Hospital Authority is a statutory body that operates and manages all public hospitals. Hong Kong has high standards of medical practice. It has contributed to the development of liver transplantation, being the first in the world to carry out an adult to adult live donor liver transplant in 1993.[36]

India

Main article: Healthcare in India

India's healthcare system is dominated by the private sector, although there are various public healthcare systems like Rajiv Gandhi Jeevandayee Arogya Yojana in Maharashtra that provides free healthcare to those below the poverty line.[37][38] Currently, the majority of Indian citizens do not have health insurance, and must pay out of pocket for treatment. There are government hospitals that provide treatment at taxpayer expense. Some essential drugs are offered free of charge in these hospitals.

An outpatient card at AIIMS costs a one-time fee of 10 rupees (around 20 cents U.S.) and thereafter outpatient medical advice is free. In-hospital treatment costs depend on the financial condition of the patient and the facilities utilized, but are usually much less than the private sector. For instance, a patient is waived treatment costs if their income is below the poverty line. However, getting treatment at high quality government hospitals is very tough due to the high number of people needing healthcare and the lack of sufficient facilities.

Primary health care is provided by city and district hospitals and rural primary health centres (PHCs). These hospitals provide treatment free of cost, but only if they are functional. Primary care is focused on immunization, prevention of malnutrition, pregnancy, child birth, postnatal care, and treatment of common illnesses. Patients who receive specialized care or have complicated illnesses are referred to secondary (often located in district and taluk headquarters) and tertiary care hospitals (located in district and state headquarters or those that are teaching hospitals).

Now organizations like Hindustan Latex Family Planning Promotional Trust and other private organizations have started creating hospitals and clinics in India, which also provide free or subsidized health care and subsidized insurance plans.

The government-run healthcare suffers from a lack of hygiene; the rich avoid the government hospitals and go to private hospitals. With the advent of privatized healthcare, this situation has changed. India now has medical tourism for people from other countries while its own poor find high-quality healthcare either inaccessible or unaffordable.

The current Indian government is planning to unveil a national universal healthcare system called the National Health Assurance Mission, which will provide all Indian citizens with insurance coverage for serious illnesses, and free

drugs and diagnostic treatments.[39]

Israel

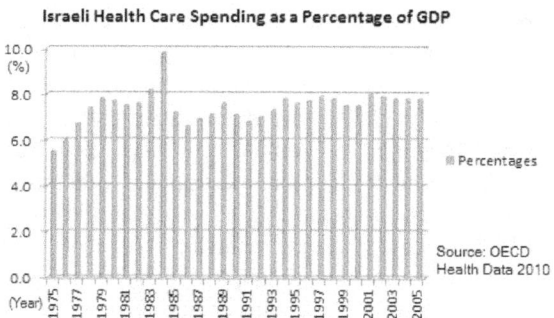

Health care in Israel as a percentage of GDP

Main article: Health care in Israel

Israel has a system of universal healthcare as set out by the 1995 National Health Insurance Law. The state is responsible for providing health services to all residents of the country, who can register with one of the four national health service funds. To be eligible, a citizen must pay a health insurance tax. Coverage includes medical diagnosis and treatment, preventive medicine, hospitalization (general, maternity, psychiatric and chronic), surgery and transplants, preventive dental care for children, first aid and transportation to a hospital or clinic, medical services at the workplace, treatment for drug abuse and alcoholism, medical equipment and appliances, obstetrics and fertility treatment, medication, treatment of chronic diseases and paramedical services such as physiotherapy and occupational therapy.[40]

In Israel, the *National Health Insurance Law* (or *National Health Insurance Act*) is the legal framework which enables and facilitates basic, compulsory universal health care. The Law was put into effect by the Knesset on January 1, 1995, and was based on recommendations put forward by a National Committee of Inquiry headed by Shoshana Netanyahu which examined restructuring the health care system in Israel in the late 1980s. Prior to the law's passage over 90% of the population was already covered by voluntarily belonging to one of four nationwide, not-for-profit sickness funds which operated some of their own medical facilities and were funded in part by employers and the government and in part by the insured by levies which varied according to income. However, there were three problems associated with this arrangement. First, membership in the largest fund, Clalit, required one to belong to the Histadrut labor organization, even if a person did not wish to (or could not) have such an affiliation while other funds restricted entry to new members based on age, pre-existing conditions or other factors. Second, different funds provided different levels of benefit coverage or services to their members and lastly was the issue mentioned above whereby a certain percentage of the population, albeit a small one, did not have health insurance coverage at all.

Before the law went into effect, all the funds collected premiums directly from members. However, upon passage of the law, a new progressive national health insurance tax was levied through Bituah Leumi (Israel's social security agency) which then re-distributes the proceeds to the sickness funds based on their membership and its demographic makeup. This ensured that *all* citizens would now have health coverage. While membership in one of the funds now became compulsory for all, free choice was introduced into movement of members between funds (a change is allowed once every six months), effectively making the various sickness funds compete equally for members among the populace. Annually, a committee appointed by the ministry of health publishes a "basket" or uniform package of medical services and prescription formulary which all funds must provide as a minimum service to all their members. Achieving this level of equality ensured that all citizens are guaranteed to receive basic healthcare regardless of their fund affiliation which was one of the principal aims of the law. An appeals process was put in place to handle rejection of treatments and procedures by the funds and evaluating cases falling outside the "basket" of services or prescription formulary.

While the law is generally considered a success and Israeli citizens enjoy a high standard of medical care comparatively, with more competition having been introduced into the field of health care in the country, and order having been brought into what was once a somewhat disorganized system, the law nevertheless does have its critics. First and foremost among the criticisms raised is that the "basket" may not provide enough coverage. To partly address this issue, the HMOs and insurance companies began offering additional "supplementary" insurance to cover certain additional services not included in the basket. However, since this insurance is optional (though usually very modestly priced, costing the equivalent of about US$10 to $20 a month), critics argue that it goes against the spirit of the new law which stressed equality among all citizens with respect to healthcare. Another criticism is that in order to provide universal coverage to all, the tax income base amount (the maximum amount of yearly earnings that are subject to the tax) was set rather high, causing many high-income taxpayers to see the amount they pay for their health premiums (now health tax) skyrocket. Finally, some complain about the constantly rising costs of copayments for certain services.

Macau

Main article: Healthcare in Macau

Macau offers universally accessible single-payer system funded by taxes. Health care is provided by the Bureau for Health.

People's Republic of China

Main article: Healthcare reform in China

Since the founding of the People's Republic of China, the goal of health care programs has been to provide care to every member of the population and to make maximum use of limited health-care personnel, equipment, and financial resources.

China is undertaking a reform on its health care system, which was largely privatized in the 1990s. The New Rural Co-operative Medical Care System (NRCMCS), is a new 2005 initiative to overhaul the healthcare system, particularly intended to make it more affordable for the rural poor. Under the NRCMCS, the annual cost of medical coverage is 50 yuan (US$7) per person. Of that, 20 yuan is paid in by the central government, 20 yuan by the provincial government and a contribution of 10 yuan is made by the patient. As of September 2007, around 80% of the whole rural population of China had signed up (about 685 million people). The system is tiered, depending on the location. If patients go to a small hospital or clinic in their local town, the scheme will cover from 70–80% of their bill. If they go to a county one, the percentage of the cost being covered falls to about 60%. And if they need specialist help in a large modern city hospital, they have to bear most of the cost themselves, the scheme would cover about 30% of the bill.[41]

On January 21, 2009, the Chinese government announced that a total of 850 billion yuan (US$127.5 billion) will be provided between 2009 and 2011 in order to improve the existing health care system.[42]

At the end of 2008, the government published its reform plan clarifying government's responsibility by saying that it would play a dominant role in providing public health and basic medical service. It declared "Both central and local governments should increase health funding. The percentage of government's input in total health expenditure should be increased gradually so that the financial burden of individuals can be reduced," The plan listed public health, rural areas, city community health services and basic medical insurance as four key areas for government investment. It also promised to tighten government control over medical fees in public hospitals and to set up a "basic medicine system" to quell public complaints of rising drug costs.[43]

The plan was passed by the Chinese Cabinet in January 2009. The long-awaited medical reform plan promised to spend 850 billion yuan by 2011 to provide universal medical service and that measures would be taken to provide basic medical security to all Chinese.[44]

Singapore

Main article: Healthcare in Singapore

Singapore has a universal health care system where government ensures affordability, largely through compulsory savings and price controls, while the private sector provides most care. Overall spending on health care amounts to only 3% of annual GDP. Of that, 66% comes from private sources.[45] Singapore currently has the second lowest infant mortality rate in the world and among the highest life expectancies from birth, according to the World Health Organization.[46] Singapore has "one of the most successful healthcare systems in the world, in terms of both efficiency in financing and the results achieved in community health outcomes," according to an analysis by global consulting firm Watson Wyatt.[47] Singapore's system uses a combination of compulsory savings from payroll deductions (funded by both employers and workers) a nationalized health insurance plan, and government subsidies, as well as "actively regulating the supply and prices of healthcare services in the country" to keep costs in check; the specific features have been described as potentially a "very difficult system to replicate in many other countries." Many Singaporeans also have supplemental private health insurance (often provided by employers) for services not covered by the government's programs.[47]

Sri Lanka

Sri Lanka provides free universal healthcare to their citizens.[48]

Taiwan

Main article: Healthcare in Taiwan

The current health care system in Taiwan, known as National Health Insurance (NHI), was instituted in 1995. NHI is a single-payer compulsory social insurance plan which centralizes the disbursement of health care dollars. The system promises equal access to health care for all citizens, and the population coverage had reached 99% by the end of 2004.[49] NHI is mainly financed through premiums, which are based on the payroll tax, and is supplemented with out-of-pocket payments and direct government funding. In the initial stage, fee-for-service predominated for both public and private providers.

NHI delivers universal coverage offered by a government-run insurer. The working population pays premiums split with their employers, others pay a flat rate with government help and the poor or veterans are fully subsidized.[50]

Under this model, citizens have free range to choose hospitals and physicians without using a gatekeeper and do not have to worry about waiting lists. NHI offers a comprehensive benefit package that covers preventive medical services, prescription drugs, dental services, Chinese medicine, home nurse visits and many more. Since NHI, the previously uninsured have increased their usage of medical services. Most preventive services are free such as annual checkups and maternal and child care. Regular office visits have co-payments as low as US $5 per visit. Co-payments are fixed and unvaried by the person's income.[51]

Thailand

Main article: Health in Thailand

Thailand introduced universal coverage reforms in 2001, becoming one of only a handful of lower-middle income countries to do so at the time. Means-tested health care for low income households was replaced by a new and more comprehensive insurance scheme, originally known as the 30 baht project, in line with the small co-payment charged for treatment. People joining the scheme receive a gold card which allows them to access services in their health district, and, if necessary, be referred for specialist treatment elsewhere. The bulk of finance comes from public revenues, with funding allocated to Contracting Units for Primary Care annually on a population basis. According to the WHO, 65% of Thailand's health care expenditure in 2004 came from the government, 35% was from private sources.[45] Although the reforms have received a good deal of critical comment, they have proved popular with poorer Thais, especially in rural areas, and survived the change of government after the 2006 military coup. The then Public Health Minister, Mongkol Na Songkhla, abolished the 30 baht co-payment and made the UC scheme free. It is not yet clear whether the scheme will be modified further under the coalition government that came to power in January 2008.[52][53][54]

3.8.3 Europe

Virtually all of Europe has either publicly sponsored and regulated universal health care or publicly provided universal healthcare. The public plans in some countries provide basic or "sick" coverage only, with their citizens being able to purchase supplemental insurance for additional coverage. Countries with universal health care include Austria,[55] Belarus,[55] Croatia, Czech Republic, Denmark, Finland, France, Germany, Greece, Iceland, Ireland, Italy, Luxembourg, Malta, Moldova,[56] the Netherlands, Norway, Portugal,[57] Romania, Russia, Serbia, Spain, Sweden, Switzerland, Ukraine,[58] and the United Kingdom.[59]

Austria

Main article: Healthcare in Austria

Healthcare in Austria is universal for residents of Austria as well as those from other EU countries.[60] Austria has a two-tier **health care system** in which many individuals receive publicly funded care; they also have the option to purchase supplementary private health insurance.

Croatia

Main article: Healthcare in Croatia

Croatia has a universal health care system that provides high quality medical services and is coordinated by the Ministry of Health. The population is covered by a basic health insurance plan provided by statute and optional insurance and administered by the Croatian Health Insurance Fund. In 2012, annual compulsory healthcare related expenditures reached 21.0 billion kunas (c. 2.8 billion euro). There are hundreds of healthcare institutions in Croatia, including 79 hospitals and clinics with 25,285 beds, caring for more than 760 thousand patients per year, 5,792 private practice offices and 79 emergency medical service units.

Czech Republic

Main article: Healthcare in the Czech Republic

Czech Republic has a universal public health system paid largely from taxation. Private health care systems do co-exist freely alongside public ones, sometimes offering better quality or faster service. Almost all medical services are covered by health insurance and insurance companies, though certain services such as prescription drugs or vision and dental care are only covered partially.

Denmark

Main article: Health care in Denmark

Denmark has a universal public health system paid largely from taxation with local municipalities delivering health care services in the same way as other Scandinavian countries. Primary care is provided by a general practitioner service run by private doctors contracting with the local municipalities with payment on a mixed per capita and fee for service basis. Most hospitals are run by the municipalities (only 1% of hospital beds are in the private sector).

Finland

Main article: Healthcare in Finland

In Finland, public medical services at clinics and hospitals are run by the municipalities (local government) and are funded 76% by taxation, 20% by patients through access charges, and 4% by others. Private provision is mainly in the primary care sector. There are a few private hospitals.[61] The main hospitals are either municipally owned (funded from local taxes) or run by the medical teaching universities (funded jointly by the municipalities and the national government). According to a survey published by the European Commission in 2000, Finland's is in the top 4 of EU countries in terms of satisfaction with their hospital care system: 88% of Finnish respondents were satisfied compared with the EU average of 41.3%.[62] Finnish health care expenditures are below the European average.[63] The private medical sector accounts for about 14 percent of total health care spending. Only 8% of doctors choose to work in private practice, and some of these also choose to do some work in the public sector.

Taxation funding is partly local and partly nationally based. The national social insurance institution KELA reimburses part of patients prescription costs and makes a contribution towards private medical costs (including dentistry) if they choose to be treated in the private sector rather than the public sector. Patient access charges are subject to annual caps. For example, GP visits cost €11 per visit with annual €33 cap; hospital outpatient treatment €22 per visit; a hospital stay, including food, medical care and medicines €26 per 24 hours, or €12 if in a psychiatric hospital. After a patient has spent €590 per year on public medical services (including prescription drugs), all treatment and medications thereafter in that year are free.

Finland has a highly decentralized three-level public system of health care and alongside this, a much smaller private health-care system.[64] Overall, the municipalities (funded by taxation, local and national) meet about two thirds of all medical-care costs, with the remaining one third paid by the national insurance system (nationally funded), and by private finance (either employer-funded or met by patients themselves).[64] Private inpatient care forms about 3–4% of all inpatient care.[64] In 1999 only 17 per cent of total funding for health care came from insurance, comprising 14.9% statutory (government) insurance and 2.1% private health insurance. Spectacles are not publicly subsidized at all, although dentistry is available as a municipal service or can be obtained privately with partial reimbursement from the state.[64] The government announced in 2009 that Kela would re-imburse the cost of private dental-hygiene work, starting in 2010.[65]

The percentage of total health expenditure financed by taxation in Finland (78%)[66] is above the OECD average and similar to the levels seen in Germany (77%) and France (80%) but below the level seen in the UK (87%). The quality of service in Finnish health care, as measured by patient satisfaction, is excellent. According to a survey published by the European Commission in 2000, Finland has one of the highest ratings of patient satisfaction with their hospital care system in the EU: 88% of Finnish respondents were satisfied compared with the EU average of 41.3%.[67]

There are caps on total medical expenses that are met out-of-pocket for drugs and hospital treatments. The National Insurance system pays all necessary costs over these caps. Public spending on health care in 2006 was 13.6 billion euros (equivalent to US$338 per person per month). The increase over 2005 at 8.2 per cent was below the OECD average of 9 percent. Household budgets directly met 18.7 per cent of all health-care costs.[68]

France

Main article: Health care in France

France has a system of universal health care largely financed by government through a system of national health insurance. It is consistently ranked as one of the best in the world.[69]

Germany

Main article: Health care in Germany

 Germany has the world's oldest national social health insurance system,[70][71][72] with origins dating back to Otto von Bismarck's Sickness Insurance Law of 1883.[73][74] The system is decentralized with private practice physicians providing ambulatory care, and independent, mostly non-profit hospitals providing the majority of inpatient care. Approximately 92% of the population is covered by a 'Statutory Health Insurance' plan, which provides a standardized level

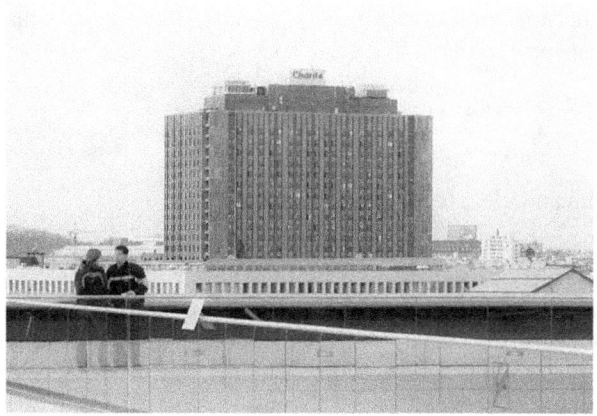

The Charité (Hospital) in Berlin

of coverage through any one of approximately 1100 public or private sickness funds. Standard insurance is funded by a combination of employee contributions, employer contributions and government subsidies on a scale determined by income level. Higher income workers sometimes choose to pay a tax and opt out of the standard plan, in favor of 'private' insurance. The latter's premiums are not linked to income level but instead to health status.[75]

Historically, the level of provider reimbursement for specific services is determined through negotiations between regional physician's associations and sickness funds. Since 1976 the government has convened an annual commission, composed of representatives of business, labor, physicians, hospitals, and insurance and pharmaceutical industries.[76] The commission takes into account government policies and makes recommendations to regional associations with respect to overall expenditure targets. In 1986 expenditure caps were implemented and were tied to the age of the local population as well as the overall wage increases. Although reimbursement of providers is on a fee-for-service basis the amount to be reimbursed for each service is determined retrospectively to ensure that spending targets are not exceeded. Capitated care, such as that provided by U.S. health maintenance organizations, has been considered as a cost containment mechanism but would require consent of regional medical associations, and has not materialized.[77] Copayments were introduced in the 1980s in an attempt to prevent overutilization and control costs. The average length of hospital stay in Germany has decreased in recent years from 14 days to 9 days, still considerably longer than average stays in the U.S. (5 to 6 days).[78][79] The difference is partly driven by the fact that hospital reimbursement is chiefly a function of the number of hospital days as opposed to procedures or the patient's diagnosis. Drug costs have increased substantially, rising nearly 60% from 1991 through 2005. Despite attempts to contain costs, overall health care expenditures rose to 10.7% of GDP in 2005, comparable to other western European nations, but substantially less than that spent in the U.S. (nearly 16% of GDP).[80]

Greece

Main article: Healthcare in Greece

The Greek healthcare system provides high quality medical services to insured citizens and is coordinated by the Ministry for Health and Social Solidarity. Public health services are provided by the National Healthcare Service, or ESY (Greek: Εθνικό Σύστημα Υγείας, ΕΣΥ). In 2010 there were 35,000 hospital beds and 131 hospitals in the country.

The Greek healthcare system has received high rankings by the World Health Organization, ranked 14th in the overall assessment and 11th in quality of service in a 2000 report by the WHO.

Guernsey / Jersey

The medical care system in the Channel Islands is very similar to that of the UK in that many of the doctors and nurses have been trained from the UK health perspective. There is universal health care for residents of the islands.[81]

Iceland

Main article: Healthcare in Iceland

Iceland has a universal public health system paid largely from taxation with local municipalities delivering health care services in the same way as other Scandinavian countries. Iceland's entire population has equal access to health care services.

Ireland

Main article: Healthcare in the Republic of Ireland

The public health care system of the Republic of Ireland is governed by the Health Act 2004,[82] which established a new body to be responsible for providing health and personal social services to everyone living in Ireland – the Health Service Executive. The new national health service came into being officially on January 1, 2005; however the new structures are currently in the process of being established as the reform program continues. In addition to the public-sector, there is also a large private health care market.

Isle of Man

The Isle of Man provides universal public health coverage to its residents.[83]

Italy

Main article: Healthcare in Italy

Italy has a public health care service for all the residents called "Servizio Sanitario Nazionale" or SSN (National Health Service) which is similar to the UK National Health Service. It is publicly run and funded mostly from taxation: some services requires small co-pays, while other services (like the emergency medicine and the general doctor) are completely free of charge. Like the UK, there is a small parallel private health care system, especially in the field of Dental Medicine.

Luxembourg

Luxembourg provides universal health care coverage to all residents (Luxembourgers and foreigners) by the National Health Insurance (CNS - *Caisse nationale de santé* (French) or *National Gesondheetskeess* (Luxembourgish)) which is funded by mandatory contributions of employers and the workforce and by government subsidies for insuring jobseekers, the poor and for financing medical infrastructure. It exists as well a mandatory public long-term care insurance.[84][85]

Netherlands

Main article: Healthcare in the Netherlands

The Netherlands has a dual-level system. All primary and curative care (i.e. the family doctor service and hospitals and clinics) is financed from private compulsory insurance. Long term care for the elderly, the dying, the long term mentally ill etc. is covered by social insurance funded from taxation. According to the WHO, the health care system in the Netherlands was 62% government funded and 38% privately funded as of 2004.[45]

Insurance companies must offer a core universal insurance package for the universal primary, curative care which includes the cost of all prescription medicines. They must do this at a fixed price for all. The same premium is paid whether young or old, healthy or sick. It is illegal in The Netherlands for insurers to refuse an application for health insurance, to impose special conditions (e.g. exclusions, deductibles, co-pays etc., or refuse to fund treatments which a doctor has determined to be medically necessary). The system is 50% financed from payroll taxes paid by employers to a fund controlled by the Health regulator. The government contributes an additional 5% to the regulator's fund. The remaining 45% is collected as premiums paid by the insured directly to the insurance company. Some employers negotiate bulk deals with health insurers and some even pay the employees' premiums as an employment benefit. All insurance companies receive additional funding from the regulator's fund. The regulator has sight of the claims made by policyholders and therefore can redistribute the funds its holds on the basis of relative claims made by policy holders. Thus insurers with high payouts will receive more from the regulator than those with low payouts. Thus insurance companies have no incentive to deter high cost individuals from taking insurance and are compensated if they have to pay out more than might be expected. Insurance companies compete with each other on price for the 45% direct premium part of the funding and try to negotiate deals with hospitals to keep costs low and quality high. The competition regulator is charged with checking for abuse of dominant market positions and the creation of cartels that act against the consumer interests. An insurance regulator ensures that all basic policies have identical coverage rules so that no person is medically disadvantaged by his or her choice of insurer.

Hospitals in the Netherlands are also regulated and inspected but are mostly privately run and not for profit, as are many of the insurance companies. Patients can choose where they want to be treated and have access to information on the internet about the performance and waiting times at each hospital. Patients dissatisfied with their insurer and choice of hospital can cancel at any time but must make a new agreement with another insurer.

Insurance companies can offer additional services at extra cost over and above the universal system laid down by the regulator, e.g. for dental care. The standard monthly premium for health care paid by individual adults is about €100 per month. Persons on low incomes can get assistance from the government if they cannot afford these payments. Children under 18 are insured by the system at no additional cost to them or their families because the insurance company receives the cost of this from the regulator's fund. There is a fixed yearly threshold of €375 for each adult person, excluding first visits for diagnosis to general physicians.

Norway

Main article: Healthcare in Norway

Norway has a universal public health system paid largely

from taxation in the same way as other Scandinavian countries. Norway's entire population has equal access to health care services. The Norwegian health care system is government-funded and heavily decentralized. The health care system in Norway is financed primarily through taxes levied by county councils and municipalities. Dental care is included for children until 18 years old, and is covered for adults for some ailments.[86]

Norway regularly comes top or close to the top of worldwide healthcare rankings.

Portugal

Main article: Health in Portugal

Portugal's National Healthcare Service, known nationally as Serviço Nacional de Saúde (SNS), is a universal and free healthcare service, provided nationwide since 1979, and is available to both Portuguese and foreigner residents. In 2014, Portugal SNS ranked 13th best healthcare service in Europe.[87] The National Medical Emergency Institute (INEM) is the main emergency medical serviced and can be activated by calling 112.

Romania

Main article: Healthcare in Romania

According to Article 34 of the Constitution of Romania, the state is obliged "to guarantee the protection of healthcare". Romania has a fully universal health care system, which covers up medical check-ups, any surgical interventions, and any post-operator medical care, as well as free or subsidized medicine for a range of diseases. The state is also obliged to fund public hospitals and clinics. Dental care is not funded by the state, although there are public dental clinics in some hospitals, which treat patients free of charge. However, due to inadequate funding and corruption, it is estimated that a third of medical expenses are, in some cases, supported by the patient.[88] Furthermore, Romania spends, per capita, less than any other EU state on medical care.

Russia and Soviet Union

Main article: Healthcare in Russia

In the Soviet Union, the preferred term was "socialist medicine"; the Russian language has no term to distinguish between "socialist" and "socialized" (other than "public", Rus: *obshchestvenniy/общественный*, sometimes "collectivized" or "nationalized", Rus: *obobshchestvlenniy/обобществленный*).[89][90]

Russia in Soviet times (between 1917 and the early 1990s) had a totally socialist model of health care with a centralised, integrated, hierarchically organised with the government providing free health care to all citizens. Initially successful at combating infectious diseases, the effectiveness of the socialized model declined with underinvestment. Despite a doubling in the number of hospital beds and doctors per capita between 1950 and 1980, the quality of care began to decline by the early 1980s and medical care and health outcomes were below western standards.

The new mixed economy Russia has switched to a mixed model of health care with private financing and provision running alongside state financing and provision. The OECD reported that unfortunately, none of this has worked out as planned and the reforms have in many respects made the system worse.[91] The population's health has deteriorated on virtually every measure. The resulting system is overly complex and very inefficient. It has little in common with the model envisaged by the reformers. Although there are more than 300 private insurers and numerous public ones in the market, real competition for patients is rare leaving most patients with little or no effective choice of insurer, and in many places, no choice of health care provider either. The insurance companies have failed to develop as active, informed purchasers of health care services. Most are passive intermediaries, making money by simply channelling funds from regional OMS funds to healthcare providers.

Main source: OECD: Health care reforms in Russia

Article 41 of the Constitution of the Russian Federation confirms a citizen's right to state healthcare and medical assistance free of charge.[92] This is achieved through state compulsory medical insurance (OMS) which is free to Russian citizens, funded by obligatory medical insurance payments made by companies and government subsidies.[93][94] Introduction in 1993 reform of new free market providers in addition to the state-run institutions intended to promote both efficiency and patient choice. A purchaser-provider split help facilitate the restructuring of care, as resources would migrate to where there was greatest demand, reduce the excess capacity in the hospital sector and stimulate the development of primary care. Russian Prime Minister Vladimir Putin announced a new large-scale health care reform in 2011 and pledged to allocate more than 300 billion rubles ($10 billion) in the next few years to improve health care in the country.[95] He also said that obligatory medical insurance tax paid by companies will increase from current 3.1% to 5.1% starting from 2011.[95]

Serbia

Main article: Healthcare in Serbia

The Constitution of the Republic of Serbia states that it is a right of every citizen to seek medical assistance free of charge.[96] This is achieved by mutual contribution to the Compulsory Social Healthcare Fund of RZZO (Republički Zavod za Zdravstveno Osiguranje or National Health Insurance Institution). The amount of contribution depends on the amount of money the person is making. During the 1990s, Serbia's healthcare system has been of a poor quality due to severe underfunding. In the recent years, however, that has changed and the Serbian government has invested heavily in new medical infrastructure, completely remodeling existing hospitals and building two new hospitals in Novi Sad and Kragujevac.

Sweden

Main article: Healthcare in Sweden

Sweden has a universal public health system paid largely from taxation in the same way as other Scandinavian countries. Sweden's entire population has equal access to health care services. The Swedish public health system is funded through taxes levied by the county councils, but partly run by private companies. Government-paid dental care for children under 21 years old is included in the system, and dental care for adults is somewhat subsidised by it.

Sweden also has a smaller private health care sector, mainly in larger cities or as centers for preventive health care financed by employers.

Sweden regularly comes in top in worldwide healthcare rankings.[97]

Switzerland

Main article: Healthcare in Switzerland

Healthcare in Switzerland is universal and is regulated by the Federal Health Insurance Act of 1994. Basic health insurance is mandatory for all persons residing in Switzerland (within three months of taking up residence or being born in the country). Insurers are required to offer insurance to everyone, regardless of age or medical condition. They are not allowed to make a profit off this basic insurance, but can on supplemental plans.[98]

United Kingdom

Main article: Healthcare in the United Kingdom

Each of the Countries of the United Kingdom has a National Health Service that provides public healthcare to all UK permanent residents that was originally designed to be free at the point of need and paid for from general taxation; but changes included introducing charging for prescription medicines and dentistry (those below 16 and those on certain benefits may still get free treatment). However, since Health is now a devolved matter, considerable differences are developing between the systems in each of the countries as for example Scotland abolished prescription charges.[99] Private healthcare companies are free to operate alongside the public one.

England   Main article: Healthcare in England
The National Health Service (NHS), created by the

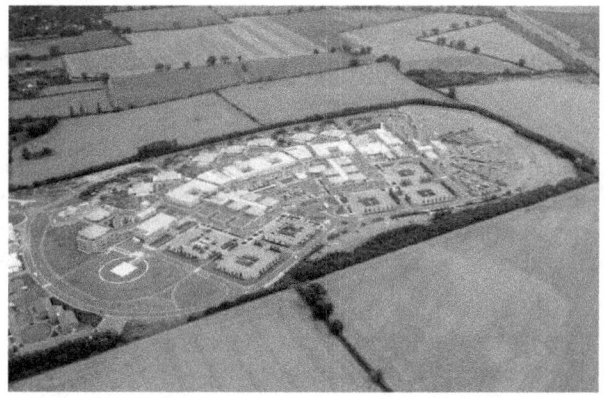

Norfolk and Norwich University Hospital, a National Health Service hospital.

National Health Service Act 1946, has provided the majority of healthcare in England since its launch on 5 July 1948.

The NHS Constitution for England documents, at high level, the objectives of the NHS, the legal rights and responsibilities of the various parties (patients, staff, NHS trust boards), and the guiding principles which govern the service.[100] The NHS constitution makes it clear that it provides a comprehensive service, available to all irrespective of age, gender, disability, race, sexual orientation, religion, or belief; that access to NHS services is based on clinical need and not an individual's ability to pay; and that care is never refused on unreasonable grounds. Patient choice in terms of doctor, care, treatments, and place of treatment is an important aspect of the NHS's ambition, and in some cases patients can elect for treatment in other European countries at the NHS's expense. Waiting times are low,

with most people able to see their primary care doctor on the same day or the following day.[101] Only 36.1% of hospital admissions are from a waiting list, with the remainder being either emergencies admitted immediately or else pre-booked admissions or the like (e.g., child birth).[102] One of the main goals of care management is to ensure that patients do not experience a delay of more than 18 weeks from initial hospital referral to final treatment, inclusive of time for all associated investigative tests and consultations.[103] At present, two-thirds of patients are treated in under 12 weeks.[104]

Although centrally funded, the NHS is not managed by a large central bureaucracy. Responsibility is highly devolved to geographical areas through Strategic Health Authorities and even more locally through NHS primary care trusts, NHS hospital trusts and increasingly to NHS foundation trusts which are providing even more decentralized services within the NHS framework, with more decision making taken by local people, patients, and staff. The central government office, the Department of Health, is not involved in day-to-day decision making in either the Strategic Health Authorities or the individual local trusts (primarily health, hospital, or ambulance) or the national specialist trusts such as NHS Blood and Transplant, but it does lay down general guidelines for them to follow. Local trusts are accountable to their local populations, whilst government ministers are accountable to Parliament for the service overall.

The NHS provides, among other things, primary care, inpatient care, long-term healthcare, psychiatric care and treatments, ophthalmology, and dentistry. All treatment is free with the exception of certain charges for prescriptions, dentistry and ophthalmology (which themselves are free to children, certain students in full-time education, the elderly, the unemployed and those on low incomes). Around 89 pc of NHS prescriptions are obtained free of charge, mostly for children, pensioners, and pregnant women. Others pay a flat rate of £8.20,[105] and others may cap their annual charges by purchasing an NHS Prescription Prepayment Certificate. Private health care has continued parallel to the NHS, paid for largely by private insurance. Private insurance accounts for only 4 percent of health expenditure and covers little more than a tenth of the population.[106] Private insurers in the UK only cover acute care from specialists. They do not cover generalist consultations, pre-existing conditions, medical emergencies, organ transplants, chronic conditions such as diabetes, or conditions such as pregnancy or HIV.[107]

Most NHS general practitioners are private doctors who contract to provide NHS services, but most hospitals are publicly owned and run through NHS Trusts. A few NHS medical services (such as "surgicentres") are sub-contracted to private providers[108] as are some non-medical services (such as catering). Some capital projects such as new hospitals have been funded through the Private Finance Initiative, enabling investment without (in the short term) increasing the public sector borrowing requirement, because long-term contractually obligated PFI spending commitments are not counted as government liabilities.

Northern Ireland Main article: Health and Social Care in Northern Ireland

Health and Social Care in Northern Ireland is the designation of the national public health service in Northern Ireland.

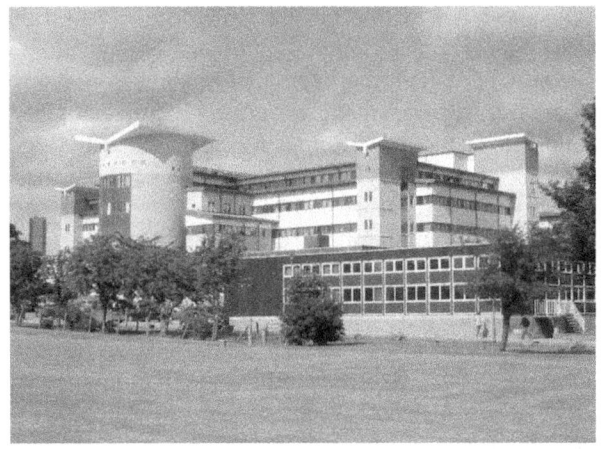

The Royal Aberdeen Children's Hospital is a specialist children's hospital within NHS Scotland.

Scotland Main article: Healthcare in Scotland

NHS Scotland, created by the National Health Service (Scotland) Act 1947, was also launched on 5 July 1948, although it has always been a separate organization. Since devolution, NHS Scotland has followed the policies and priorities of the Scottish Government, including the phasing out of all prescription charges by 2011.

Wales Main article: Healthcare in Wales

NHS Wales was originally formed as part of the same NHS structure created by the National Health Service Act 1946 but powers over the NHS in Wales came under the Secretary of State for Wales in 1969,[109] in turn being transferred under devolution to what is now the Welsh Government.

3.8.4 North America

The Bahamas, Barbados, Canada, Costa Rica, Cuba, Mexico, Panama, and Trinidad and Tobago all provide some level of universal health coverage.

The Bahamas

The Bahamas approved the National Health Insurance Act in August 2016. The legislation allows for the establishment of a universal health coverage system that will begin with universal coverage of primary health care services and later expand to include a wide set of benefits including all specialized care. The system will allow for universal coverage of a basic benefit package and for voluntary insurance to be purchased as a top up policy to cover services or amenities that are not included in the government plan.[110]

Canada

Main article: Health care in Canada

In 1984, the Canada Health Act was passed, which prohibited extra billing by doctors on patients while at the same time billing the public insurance system. In 1999, the prime minister and most premiers reaffirmed in the Social Union Framework Agreement that they are committed to health care that has "comprehensiveness, universality, portability, public administration and accessibility."[111]

The system is for the most part publicly funded, yet most of the services are provided by private enterprises or private corporations, although most hospitals are public. Most doctors do not receive an annual salary, but receive a fee per visit or service.[112] About 29% of Canadians' health care is paid for by the private sector or individuals.[113] This mostly goes towards services not covered or only partially covered by Medicare such as prescription drugs, dentistry and vision care.[114] Many Canadians have private health insurance, often through their employers, that cover these expenses.[115]

The Canada Health Act of 1984 "does not directly bar private delivery or private insurance for publicly insured services," but provides financial disincentives for doing so. "Although there are laws prohibiting or curtailing private health care in some provinces, they can be changed," according to a report in the New England Journal of Medicine.[116][117] The legality of the ban was considered in a decision of the Supreme Court of Canada which ruled in *Chaoulli v. Quebec* that "the prohibition on obtaining private health insurance, while it might be constitutional in circumstances where health care services are reasonable as to both quality and timeliness, is not constitutional where the public system fails to deliver reasonable services." The appellant contended that waiting times in Quebec violated a right to life and security in the Quebec Charter of Human Rights and Freedoms. The Court agreed, but acknowledged the importance and validity of the Canada Health Act, and at least four of the seven judges explicitly recognized the right of governments to enact laws and policies which favour the public over the private system and preserve the integrity of the public system.

Costa Rica

Universal healthcare and pensions are run by the Caja Costarricense de Seguro Social (CCSS). In 1941, Costa Rica established Caja Costarricense de Seguro Social (CCSS), a social security insurance system for wage-earning workers. In 1961, coverage was expanded to include workers' dependents and from 1961 to 1975, a series of expansions extended coverage for primary care and out-patient and inpatient specialized services to people in rural areas, the low-income population, and certain vulnerable populations. Further expansions during the late 1970s extended insurance coverage to farmers, peasants, and independent contract workers. Additionally, CCSS mandates free health service provision to mothers, children, indigenous people, the elderly, and people living with disabilities, regardless of insurance coverage. By 2000, 82 percent of the population was eligible for CCSS, which has continued to expand in the ensuing period. By covering all population groups through the same system, Costa Rica has avoided social insurance stratification and inequity common in many other countries in the region.[118]

CCSS is funded by a 15 percent payroll tax, as well as payments from retiree pensions [6]. Taxes on luxury goods, alcohol, soda, and imported products also help to cover poor households who do otherwise pay into the system. All CCSS funds are merged into a single pool, which is managed by the central financial administration of CCSS. In 1973, the Ministry of Health decided to move away from direct service provision and adopt a steering role. Responsibility for the provision of most care was transferred to the CCSS, although the Ministry retained responsibility for disease control, food and drug regulation, environmental sanitation, child nutrition, and primary care for the poor. Through the CCSS, health care is now essentially free to nearly all Costa Ricans. Private health care is also widely available and INS offers private health insurance plans to supplement CCSS insurance.[119]

Cuba

Main article: Healthcare in Cuba

The Cuban government operates a national health system and assumes fiscal and administrative responsibility for the health care of all its citizens. There are no private hospitals or clinics as all health services are government-run. The present Minister for Public Health is Roberto Morales Ojeda. However, although the coverage is wide, the system is underfunded and recently also understaffed. The government organized medical missions in other countries has taken a very significant amount of doctors and other personal. In 2005 there were 25,000 Cuban doctors in Venezuela.

Mexico

Main article: Healthcare in Mexico

Public health care delivery is accomplished via an elaborate provisioning and delivery system instituted by the Mexican Federal Government. Public health care is provided to all Mexican citizens as guaranteed via Article 4 of the Constitution. Public care is either fully or partially subsidized by the federal government, depending on the person's (Spanish: derechohabiente's) employment status. All Mexican citizens are eligible for subsidized health care regardless of their work status via a system of health care facilities operating under the federal Secretariat of Health (formerly the Secretaria de Salubridad y Asistencia, or SSA) agency. Employed citizens and their dependents, however, are further eligible to use the health care program administered and operated by the Instituto Mexicano del Seguro Social (IMSS) (English: Mexican Social Security Institute). The IMSS health care program is a tripartite system funded equally by the employee, its private employer, and the federal government. The IMSS does not provide service to employees of the public sector. Employees in the public sector are serviced by the Instituto de Seguridad y Servicios Sociales de los Trabajadores del Estado (ISSSTE) (English: Institute for Social Security and Services for State Workers), which attends to the health and social care needs of government employees. This includes local, state, and federal government employees. The government of the states in Mexico also provide health services independently of those services provided by the federal government programs. In most states, the state government has established free or subsidized healthcare to all their citizens.

On December 1, 2006, the Mexican government created the Health Insurance for a New Generation also known as "life insurance for babies".[120][121][122] On May 16, 2009,

Mexico to Achieve Universal Health Coverage by 2011.[123] On May 28, 2009, Mexico announced Universal Care Coverage for Pregnant Women.[124] On August 2012 Mexico installed a universal healthcare system.[125]

Trinidad and Tobago

Main article: Healthcare in Trinidad and Tobago

A universal health care system is used in Trinidad and Tobago and is the primary form of health-care available in the country. It is used by the majority of the population seeking medical assistance, as it is free for all citizens.

United States

Main article: Patient Protection and Affordable Care Act
See also: Health care reform in the United States and Health care in the United States

The United States does not have a universal health care system. However, the Patient Protection and Affordable Care Act (PPACA) as amended by the Health Care and Education Reconciliation Act of 2010, seeks to have expanded insurance coverage to legal residents by 2014. It provides for federally mandated health insurance to be implemented in the United States during the 2010–2019 decade with the Federal government subsidizing legal resident households with income up to 400% of the Federal poverty level.[126] This threshold varies according to State and household size, but for an average family of four, subsidies would be available for families whose income was about $88,000 or lower.[127] In June 2010 adults with pre-existing conditions became eligible to join a temporary high-risk pool.[128] In 2014, applicants of the same age began to be able to obtain health insurance at the same published rate regardless of health status — the first time in U.S. history that insurers no longer had the right to load the premium or deny coverage prior to contract, or cancel a policy after contract due to an adverse health condition, or test result indicating that one may be imminent. The law prohibits insurers from capping their liability for a person's health care needs, a move which is expected to rectify medically induced bankruptcy. As of April 13, 2015, the U.S. uninsured rate fell to 11.9% from the 17.1% recorded at the end of the fourth quarter of 2013. This is the lowest quarterly average recorded since Gallup and Healthways began tracking the percentage of uninsured Americans in 2008. Gallup attributed this sharp decline to the Affordable Care Act's requirements for most Americans to have healthcare in the beginning of the first quarter of 2014.[129]

The Congressional Budget Office and related government agencies scored the cost of a universal health care system several times since 1991, and have uniformly predicted cost savings,[130] partly from the elimination of insurance company overhead costs.[131] In 2009, a universal health care proposal was pending in Congress, the United States National Health Care Act (H.R. 676, formerly the "Medicare for All Act").

The Congressional Budget Office (CBO) estimated that the bill would reduce the number of nonelderly people who are uninsured by about 32 million, leaving about 23 million nonelderly residents uninsured (about one-third of whom would be illegal immigrants). Under the legislation, the share of legal nonelderly residents with insurance coverage would rise from about 83 percent in 2010 to about 94 percent by 2019.[132]

In May 2011, the state of Vermont became the first state to pass legislation establishing a single-payer health care system. The legislation, known as Act 48, establishes health care in the state as a "human right" and lays the responsibility on the state to provide a health care system which best meets the needs of the citizens of Vermont. The proposal was shelved not long after the main provisions of the law took effect in 2014.[133] A revised estimate in July 2012 by the CBO stated 30 million people would gain access to health insurance under the law.[134]

Discussion in the United States commonly uses the term socialized medicine to impart a pejorative meaning to the idea of universal health care.

3.8.5 South America

Argentina, Brazil, Chile, Colombia, Peru, Uruguay, and Venezuela all have public universal health care provided.

Argentina

Main article: Health care in Argentina

Health care is provided through a combination of employer and labor union-sponsored plans (Obras Sociales), government insurance plans, public hospitals and clinics and through private health insurance plans. It costs almost 10% of GDP and is available to anyone regardless of ideology, beliefs, race or nationality.

Brazil

Main article: Healthcare in Brazil

The universal health care system was adopted in Brazil in

1988 after the end of the military regime's rule. However, universalized/socialized health care was available many years before, in some cities, once the 27th amendment to the 1969 Constitution imposed the duty of applying 6% of their income in healthcare on the municipalities.[135]

Chile

Main article: Healthcare in Chile

Health care in Chile is provided by the government (via Fonasa) and by private insurers (via Isapre). All workers and pensioners are mandated to pay 7% of their income for health care insurance (the poorest pensioners are exempt from this payment). Workers who choose not to join an Isapre, are automatically covered by Fonasa. Fonasa also covers unemployed people receiving unemployment benefits, uninsured pregnant women, insured worker's dependant family, people with mental or physical disabilities and people who are considered poor or indigent.

Fonasa costs vary depending on income, disability or age. Attention at public health facilities via Fonasa is free for low-income earners, people with mental or physical disabilities and people over the age of 60. Others pay 10% or 20% of the costs, depending on income and number of dependants. Fonasa beneficiaries may also seek attention in the private sector, for a designated fee.

Additionally, there are a number of high-mortality illnesses (currently 69) that have special attention guarantees for both Isapre and Fonasa affiliates, in relation to access to treatment, waiting times, maximum costs and quality of service.

Colombia

Main article: Health care in Colombia

In 1993 a reform transformed the health care system in Colombia, trying to provide a better, sustainable, health care system and to reach every Colombian citizen.

Peru

Main article: Healthcare in Peru

On April 10, 2009, the Government of Peru published the Law on Health Insurance to enable all Peruvians to access quality health services, and contribute to regulate the financing and supervision of these services. The law enables all population to access diverse health services to prevent illnesses, and promote and rehabilitate people, under a

Health Basic Plan (PEAS).[136][137]

On April 2, 2010, President Alan Garcia Perez on Friday signed a supreme ordinance approving the regulations for the framework law on the Universal Health Insurance, which seeks to provide access to quality health care for all Peruvian citizens.

Peru's Universal Health Insurance law aims to increase access to timely and quality health care services, emphasizes maternal and child health promotion, and provides the poor with protection from financial ruin due to illness.[138]

The regulation states that membership of the Universal Health Insurance (AUS for its Spanish acronym) is compulsory for the entire population living in the country. To that end, the Ministry of Health will approve, by supreme ordinance, the mechanisms leading to compulsory membership, as well as escalation and implementation.[139]

3.8.6   Oceania

Australia and New Zealand have universal health care.

Australia

Main articles: Medicare (Australia) and Health care in Australia
In Australia, Medibank — as it was then known — was

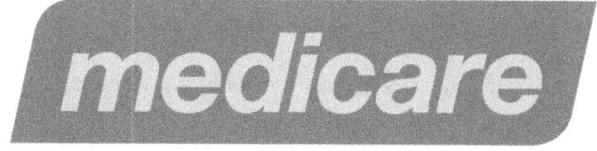

Medicare logo

introduced, by the Whitlam Labor government on July 1, 1975, through the Health Insurance Act 1973. The Australian Senate rejected the changes multiple times and they were passed only after a joint sitting after the 1974 double dissolution election. However, Medibank was supported by the subsequent Fraser Coalition (Australia) government and became a key feature of Australia's public policy landscape. The exact structure of Medibank/Medicare, in terms of the size of the rebate to doctors and hospitals and the way it has administered, has varied over the years. The original Medibank program proposed a 1.35% levy (with low income exemptions) but these bills were rejected by the Senate, and so Medibank was funded from general taxation. In 1976, the Fraser Government introduced a 2.5% levy and split Medibank in two: a universal scheme called Medibank Public and a government-owned private health insurance company, Medibank Private.

During the 1980s, Medibank Public was renamed Medicare by the Hawke Labor government, which also changed the funding model, to an income tax surcharge, known as the Medicare Levy, which was set at 1.5%, with exemptions for low income earners.[140] The Howard Coalition government introduced an additional levy of 1.0%, known as the Medicare Levy Surcharge, for those on high annual incomes ($70,000) and do not have adequate levels of private hospital coverage.[141] This was part of an effort by the Coalition to encourage take-up of private health insurance. According to WHO, government funding covered 67.5% of Australia's health care expenditures in 2004; private sources covered the remaining 32.5% of expenditures.[45]

New Zealand

Main article: Health care in New Zealand

As with Australia, New Zealand's healthcare system is funded through general taxation. According to the WHO, government sources covered 77.4% of New Zealand's health care costs in 2004; private expenditures covered the remaining 22.6%.[45]

3.8.7 See also

- Health system

- Health systems by country

- List of countries by health insurance coverage

3.8.8 References

[1] Stuckler, David; Feigl, Andrea B.; Basu, Sanjay; McKee, Martin (November 2010). "The political economy of universal health coverage. Background paper for the First Global Symposium on Health Systems Research, 16–19 November 2010, Montreaux, Switzerland" (PDF). *Pacific Health Summit.* Seattle: National Bureau of Asian Research. p. 16. Figure 2. Global Prevalence of Universal Health Care in 2009; 58 countries: Andorra, Antigua, Argentina, Armenia, Australia, Austria, Azerbaijan, Bahrain, Belarus, Belgium, Bosnia and Herzegovina, Botswana, Brunei Darussalam, Bulgaria, Canada, Chile, Costa Rica, Croatia, Cuba, Cyprus, Czech Republic, Denmark, Estonia, Finland, France, Germany, Greece, Hungary, Iceland, Ireland, Israel, Italy, Japan, Kuwait, Luxembourg, Moldova, Mongolia, Netherlands, New Zealand, Norway, Oman, Panama, Portugal, Romania, Singapore, Slovakia, Slovenia, South Korea, Spain, Sweden, Switzerland, Taiwan, Thailand, Tunisia, UAE, Ukraine, United Kingdom, Venezuela.

[2] "International Health Comparisons: A Compendium of published information on healthcare systems, the provision of health care and health achievement in 10 countries". Retrieved October 15, 2013.

[3] "Snapshots of Health Systems: The state of affairs in 16 countries in summer 2004 WHO" (PDF). Archived from the original (PDF) on 2010-01-25.

[4] Tran, Mark (December 13, 2012), "Global development,Health (Society),Society,United Nations (News),World news", *The Guardian*, London

[5] "Algeria – Health And Welfare". Countrystudies.us. Retrieved November 14, 2011.

[6] http://www.marines.mil/Portals/59/Publications/Algeria%20Profile.pdf

[7] "Botswana:The Health System - AHO". Retrieved November 30, 2016.

[8] JLN. "Burkina Faso adopts universal health insurance system - Joint Learning Network". Retrieved November 30, 2016.

[9] "Insurance". Retrieved November 30, 2016.

[10] "NHIS - Your Access to Healthcare". Retrieved November 30, 2016.

[11] "Tiny African Island Has Soaring GDP, Free Healthcare and Free Higher Education - The Utopianist". Retrieved November 30, 2016.

[12] "International Journal for Equity in Health | Full text | Social inequalities and health inequity in Morocco". Equity-healthj.com. Retrieved November 14, 2011.

[13] "In Rwanda, Health Care Coverage That Eludes the U.S.". *Opinionator* (blog of *The New York Times*). Archived from the original on 2014-02-03.

[14] "Health care in South Africa". SouthAfrica.info. Retrieved November 14, 2011.

[15] "The healthcare system in Tunisia". Retrieved November 30, 2016.

[16] "National Health Policy: Ministry of Health" (PDF).

[17] "Introduction to healthcare in Bahrain". Justlanded.com. Retrieved November 14, 2011.

[18] Health care in Iran

[19] *The Health Care System in Israel- An Historical Perspective* Israel Ministry of Foreign Affairs. Retrieved June 7, 2006.

[20] "Embassy of Jordan (Washington, D.C.) – Jordan Information Bureau". Jordanembassyus.org. Retrieved November 14, 2011.

[21] "Kazakhstan Health System – Flags, Maps, Economy, History, Climate, Natural Resources, Current Issues, International Agreements, Population, Social Statistics, Political System". Photius.com. Retrieved November 14, 2011.

[22] "Malaysia Health System Review" (PDF).

[23] "Mongolia Health-Care Systems – Flags, Maps, Economy, History, Climate, Natural Resources, Current Issues, International Agreements, Population, Social Statistics, Political Sy". Photius.com. Retrieved November 14, 2011.

[24] "Oman Guide: Introduction, An introduction to health care in Oman: Oman offers high quality health care equal". Just-landed.com. Retrieved November 14, 2011.

[25] "WHO | Primary Health Care in Action". Who.int. September 26, 2008. Retrieved November 14, 2011.

[26] ""Ministry of Health and Nutrition, Sri Lanka"". Health.gov.lk. Retrieved November 14, 2011.

[27] Obaida Hamad (February 2011). "Health system reforms: Better services at what cost?". *Forward Magazine*.

[28] ""Bureau of National Health Insurance, Taiwan"". Nhi.gov.tw. September 28, 2011. Retrieved November 14, 2011.

[29] "Tajikistan Health Care System – Flags, Maps, Economy, History, Climate, Natural Resources, Current Issues, International Agreements, Population, Social Statistics, Political S". Photius.com. Retrieved November 14, 2011.

[30] "Health Care in Turkey". All About Turkey. November 20, 2006. Retrieved November 14, 2011.

[31] "Turkmenistan Structure of Health Care – Flags, Maps, Economy, History, Climate, Natural Resources, Current Issues, International Agreements, Population, Social Statistics, Pol". Photius.com. Retrieved November 14, 2011.

[32] "Country Health System Profile: Bhutan". World Health Organization. Archived from the original on 2012-06-01.

[33] "Healthy life expectancy in Hong Kong". World Health Organization. Retrieved June 7, 2008.

[34] "Rank Order – Life expectancy at birth". The World Factbook, Central Intelligence Agency. January 24, 2008. Retrieved February 1, 2008.

[35] "World Population Prospects: The 2006 Revision" (PDF). United Nations. 2007. Retrieved February 1, 2008.

[36] "Live Donor Liver Transplantation: Current Status" (PDF). Springerlink.com. Retrieved November 14, 2011.

[37] "Modi's ambitious health policy may dwarf Obamacare". Retrieved November 30, 2016.

[38] "Rajiv Gandhi Jeevandayee Arogya Yojana". *Government of Maharashtra*. 16 January 2016. Retrieved 16 January 2016.

[39] Kalra, Aditya. "India's universal healthcare rollout to cost $26 billion". Retrieved November 30, 2016.

[40] "history of Israel health care".

[41] Carrin G, Ron A, Hui Y, et al. (April 1999). "The reform of the rural cooperative medical system in the People's Republic of China: interim experience in 14 pilot counties". *Soc Sci Med*. **48** (7): 961–72. doi:10.1016/S0277-9536(98)00396-7. PMID 10192562.

[42] 3☐☐☐☐☐☐8500☐. Retrieved January 21, 2009.

[43] Staff (October 14, 2008). "Medical Reform Draft Open to Public Debate". Xinhua News Agency (via the China Internet Information Center). Retrieved April 10, 2014.

[44] Staff (January 21, 2009). "China Passes New Medical Reform Plan". xinhuanet.com. Retrieved April 10, 2014.

[45] "World Health Organization Statistical Information System: Core Health Indicators". Who.int. Retrieved November 14, 2011.

[46] World Health Organization, "World Health Statistics 2007: Mortality", based on 2005 data.

[47] John Tucci, "The Singapore health system – achieving positive health outcomes with low expenditure", Watson Wyatt Healthcare Market Review, October 2004. Archived April 19, 2010, at the Wayback Machine.

[48] http://workinsrilanka.lk/living/healthcare-in-sri-lanka/

[49] Fanchiang, Cecilia (January 2, 2004). "New IC health insurance card expected to offer many benefits" Archived June 6, 2008, at the Wayback Machine.. *Taiwan Journal*. Retrieved March 28, 2008.

[50] "Taiwan Takes Fastrack to Universal Health Care". All Things Considered, NPR. April 15, 2008. Retrieved October 5, 2008.

[51] Jui-Fen Rachel Lu; William C. Hsiao (2003). "Does Universal Health Insurance Make Health Care Unaffordable? Lessons From Taiwan". *Health Affairs*. **22** (3): 77–88. doi:10.1377/hlthaff.22.3.77. PMID 12757274.

[52] G20 Health Care: "Health Care Systems and Health Market Reform in the G20 Countries." Prepared for the World Economic Forum by Ernst & Young. January 3, 2006.

[53] ""The Universal Coverage Policy of Thailand: An Introduction"". Unescap.org. Retrieved November 14, 2011.

[54] Hughes D, Leethongdee S (2007). "Universal coverage in the land of smiles: lessons from Thailand's 30 baht health reforms". *Health Affairs*. **26** (4): 999–1008. doi:10.1377/hlthaff.26.4.999. PMID 17630443.

[55] Belarus. "Health in Belarus. Healthcare system of Belarus". Europe-cities.com. Retrieved November 14, 2011.

[56] Moldova Healthcare Archived January 25, 2010, at the Wayback Machine.

[57] Portugal: Bentes M, Dias CM, Sakellarides C, Bankauskaite V. *Health Care Systems in Transition: Portugal.* WHO are Regional Offices for Europe on behalf of the European Observatory on Health Systems and Policies, 2004.

[58] Constitution of Ukraine Chapter 2, Article 49. Adopted at the Fifth Session of the Verkhovna Rada of Ukraine on June 28, 1996.

[59] Physicians for a National Health Program "International Health Systems".

[60] Staff (undated). "The Austrian healthcare system Overview of how it works". justlanded.com. Retrieved October 16, 2011.

[61] "KELA – Use of European Health Insurance Card in Finland". Kela.fi. Retrieved November 14, 2011.

[62] "European Commission: Health and long-term care in the European Union" (PDF). Retrieved November 14, 2011.

[63] "Health Systems in Transition Vol. 10 No. 4 2008; Finland health system review" (PDF). Retrieved January 9, 2015. line feed character in |title= at position 29 (help)

[64] Järvelin, Jutta (2002). "Health Care Systems in Transition" (PDF). The European Observatory on Health Care Systems. Retrieved February 25, 2009.

[65] Kela publication to all households 2009.

[66] http://www.oecd.org/dataoecd/52/33/38976604.pdf

[67] http://ec.europa.eu/public_opinion/archives/ebs/ebs_283_en.pdf European Commission: Health and long-term care in the European Union

[68] "News item on healthcare costs in 2006 (in Finnish)".

[69] "World Health Organization Assesses the World's Health Systems". Who.int. 8 December 2010. Retrieved 6 January 2012.

[70] Bump, Jesse B. (October 19, 2010). "The long road to universal health coverage. A century of lessons for development strategy" (PDF). Seattle: PATH. Retrieved March 11, 2013. Carrin and James have identified 1988—105 years after Bismarck's first sickness fund laws—as the date Germany achieved universal health coverage through this series of extensions to minimum benefit packages and expansions of the enrolled population. Bärnighausen and Sauerborn have quantified this long-term progressive increase in the proportion of the German population covered by public and private insurance. Their graph is reproduced below as Figure 1: German Population Enrolled in Health Insurance (%) 1885–1995.

[71] Carrin, Guy; James, Chris (January 2005). "Social health insurance: Key factors affecting the transition towards universal coverage" (PDF). *International Social Security Review.* **58** (1): 45–64. doi:10.1111/j.1468-246x.2005.00209.x. Retrieved March 11, 2013. Initially the health insurance law of 1883 covered blue-collar workers in selected industries, craftspeople and other selected professionals.[6] It is estimated that this law brought health insurance coverage up from 5 to 10 per cent of the total population.

[72] Bärnighausen, Till; Sauerborn (May 2002). "One hundred and eighteen years of the German health insurance system: are there any lessons for middle- and low income countries?" (PDF). *Social Science & Medicine.* **54** (10): 1559–1587. doi:10.1016/S0277-9536(01)00137-X. PMID 12061488. Retrieved March 11, 2013. As Germany has the world's oldest SHI [social health insurance] system, it naturally lends itself to historical analyses. |first3= missing |last3= in Authors list (help)

[73] Leichter, Howard M. (1979). *A comparative approach to policy analysis: health care policy in four nations.* Cambridge: Cambridge University Press. p. 121. ISBN 0-521-22648-1. The Sickness Insurance Law (1883). Eligibility. The Sickness Insurance Law came into effect in December 1884. It provided for compulsory participation by all industrial wage earners (i.e., manual laborers) in factories, ironworks, mines, shipbuilding yards, and similar workplaces.

[74] Hennock, Ernest Peter (2007). *The origin of the welfare state in England and Germany, 1850–1914: social policies compared.* Cambridge: Cambridge University Press. p. 157. ISBN 978-0-521-59212-3.

[75] GmbH, Finanztip Verbraucherinformation gemeinnützige. "Finanztip : Finanztip – Das gemeinnützige Verbraucherportal". Retrieved November 30, 2016.

[76] Kirkman-Liff BL (1990). "Physician Payment and Cost-Containment Strategies in West Germany: Suggestions for Medicare Reform". *Journal of Health Care Politics, Policy and Law (Duke University).* **15** (1): 69–99. doi:10.1215/03616878-15-1-69. PMID 2108202.

[77] Henke KD (May 2007). "[External and internal financing in health care]". *Med. Klin. (Munich)* (in German). **102** (5): 366–72. doi:10.1007/s00063-007-1045-0. PMID 17497087.

[78] "Length of hospital stay, Germany". Groupeconomics.allianz.com. July 25, 2005. Retrieved November 14, 2011.

[79] "Length of hospital stay, U.S". Cdc.gov. Retrieved November 14, 2011.

[80] Borger C, Smith S, Truffer C, et al. (2006). "Health spending projections through 2015: changes on the horizon". *Health Aff (Millwood).* **25** (2): w61–73. doi:10.1377/hlthaff.25.w61. PMID 16495287.

[81] "Expat Guernsey". Retrieved August 7, 2011.

[82] "Health Act 2004". *Irish Statute Book*. Office of the Attorney General. Retrieved October 5, 2010.

[83] <Please add first missing authors to populate metadata.>. "Department of Health Service Delivery Plan 2011" (PDF). Retrieved August 7, 2011.

[84] "Life rsciences & health care in Luxembourg".

[85] "Législation-Code de la sécurité sociale & Statuts de la Caisse nationale de santé".

[86] "Who Pays Your Dental Bill?". *Helsenorge*.

[87] http://www.healthpowerhouse.com/files/EHCI_2014/EHCI_2014_report.pdf

[88] "Bribes in hospitals: "tariff" for a surgery or a C-cut".

[89] Zhuraleva *et al.*, Teaching History of Medicine in Russia.

[90] Yandex Lingvo

[91] "Search Official Documents - OECD" (PDF). Retrieved November 30, 2016.

[92] "The Constitution of the Russian Federation".

[93] "О МЕДИЦИНСКОМ СТРАХОВАНИИ ГРАЖДАН В РОССИЙСКОЙ ФЕДЕРАЦИИ".

[94] "Russia – Unified Social Tax replaced by insurance contributions". Archived from the original on June 28, 2010.

[95] "Putin says Russia needs major health care reform".

[96] "Ustav Republike Srbije (The Constitution of the Republic of Serbia)".

[97] "How the NHS could learn from Sweden". BBC News. November 28, 2005. Retrieved September 15, 2009.

[98] Schwartz, Nelson D. (October 1, 2009). "Swiss health care thrives without public option". *The New York Times*. p. A1.

[99] NHS now four different systems BBC January 2, 2008

[100] "NHS Constitution for England". Dh.gov.uk. Retrieved 2011-11-14.

[101] Cathy Schoen and Robin Osborn (2004). "The Commonwealth Fund 2004 International Health Policy Survey of Primary Care in Five Countries" (PDF).

[102] Kingdom, NHS Digital, 1 Trevelyan Square, Boar Lane, Leeds, LS1 6AE, United. "Hospital Episode Statistics" (PDF). Retrieved November 30, 2016.

[103] "18 weeks patient pathway". Retrieved November 30, 2016.

[104] "18 weeks patient pathway" (PDF). Retrieved November 30, 2016.

[105] "NHS charges to rise in England". BBC News. 5 March 2009. Retrieved 2011-11-14.

[106] Smee, Clive (October 2000). "Department of Health Special Section: Reconsidering the Role of Competition in Health Care Markets". *Journal of Health Politics, Policy and Law*. **25** (5): 945–951.

[107] Are you buying private medical insurance? Association of British Insurers

[108] "N. generation surgery-centers to carry out thousands more NHS operations every year". Department of Health. 3 December 2002. Retrieved 2006-09-15.

[109] Introduction to NHS Wales 1960's www.wales.nhs.uk

[110] "NHI Bahamas -". Retrieved November 30, 2016.

[111] Government of Canada, Social Union, News Release, "A Framework to Improve the Social Union for Canadians: An Agreement between the Government of Canada and the Governments of the Provinces and Territories, February 4, 1999." Retrieved December 20, 2006.

[112] Public vs. private health care. *CBC*, December 1, 2006.

[113] Press release, "Health care spending to reach $160 billion this year", Canadian Institute for Health Information, November 13, 2007. Retrieved November 19, 2007.

[114] National Health Expenditure Trends, 1975–2007, Canadian Institute for Health Information, November 13, 2007. Retrieved November 19, 2007.

[115] The OECD Health Project (2004). *Private Health Insurance In OECD Countries*. Organisation for Economic Cooperation and Development. ISBN 92-64-00668-0.

[116] Kraus, Clifford (February 26, 2006). "As Canada's Slow-Motion Public Health System Falters, Private Medical Care Is Surging". *The New York Times*. Retrieved July 16, 2007.

[117] Steinbrook, R. (April 2006). "Private health care in Canada". *New England Journal of Medicine*. **354** (16): 1661–4. doi:10.1056/NEJMp068064. PMID 16625005.

[118] "Health System Innovations in Central America". The World Bank. July 1, 2005. doi:10.1596/978-0-8213-6278-5. Retrieved November 30, 2016 – via elibrary.worldbank.org (Atypon).

[119] Toward Universal Health Coverage and Equity in Latin America and the Caribbean http://dx.doi.org/10.1596/978-1-4648-0454-0

[120] Message to the Nation from the President of Mexico, Felipe Calderón Hinojosa, on the occasion of his first State of the Union Address Archived December 8, 2009, at the Wayback Machine.

[121] President Calderón during First National Week of Affiliation to Medical Insurance for a New Generation Archived January 10, 2011, at the Wayback Machine.

[122] President Calderón at Launching of Affiliation to Medical Insurance for a New Generation Archived June 22, 2009, at the Wayback Machine.

[123] Mexico to Achieve Universal Health Coverage by 2011 Archived June 22, 2009, at the Wayback Machine.

[124] International Women's Day Archived June 22, 2009, at the Wayback Machine.

[125] "Mexico achieves universal health coverage, enrolls 52.6 million people in less than a decade". Harvard School of Public Health. August 15, 2012. Retrieved September 16, 2013.

[126] "5 key things to remember about health care reform". CNN. March 25, 2010.

[127] "2009 Poverty Guideline Computations". Aspe.hhs.gov. Retrieved November 14, 2011.

[128] Grier, Peter (March 24, 2010). "Health care reform bill 101: rules for preexisting conditions". *The Christian Science Monitor*. Retrieved March 25, 2010.

[129] "In U.S., Uninsured Rate Dips to 11.9% in First Quarter". *Gallup*.

[130] Physicians for a National Health Program (January, 2008) "Single Payer System Cost?" *pnhp.org*

[131] Levy A.R., et al. (2010). "International comparison of comparative effectiveness research in five jurisdictions: insights for the US". *PharmacoEconomics*. **28** (10): 813–30. doi:10.2165/11536150-000000000-00000. PMID 20831289.

[132] "Cost Estimate for Pending Health Care Legislation". CBO Director's Blog. Retrieved March 21, 2010.

[133] "Why single payer died in Vermont". Retrieved November 30, 2016.

[134] http://www.cbo.gov/sites/default/files/cbofiles/attachments/43471-hr6079.pdf

[135] "Emc1". Planalto.gov.br. Retrieved November 14, 2011.

[136] "Law on Health Insurance published today". Andina.com.pe. Retrieved November 14, 2011.

[137] "President Garcia: Law on Health Insurance marks major reform". Andina.com.pe. Retrieved November 14, 2011.

[138] "Aseguramiento Universal de Salud – Perú". Ausperu.blogspot.com. February 24, 2004. Retrieved November 14, 2011.

[139] "President Garcia signs regulations for Universal Health Insurance law". Andina.com.pe. Retrieved November 14, 2011.

[140] Australian Taxation Office (June 19, 2007). "What is the Medicare levy?". Archived from the original on October 22, 2007. Retrieved February 15, 2008.

[141] "Medicare Levy Surcharge". Ato.gov.au. Retrieved November 14, 2011.

3.9 Massachusetts health care reform

The Commonwealth of **Massachusetts passed a health care reform law** in 2006 with the aim of providing health insurance to nearly all of its residents. The law mandated that nearly every resident of Massachusetts obtain a minimum level of insurance coverage, provided free health care insurance for residents earning less than 150% of the federal poverty level (FPL) and mandated employers with more than 10 "full-time" employees to provide healthcare insurance. The law was amended significantly in 2008 and twice in 2010 to make it consistent with the federal Affordable Care Act. Major revisions related to health care industry price controls were passed in August 2012, and the employer mandate was repealed in 2013 in favor of the federal mandate (even though enforcement of the federal mandate was delayed until January 2015).[1] Because Mitt Romney was the governor of Massachusetts at the time, the law has colloquially been called **Romneycare**, a reference to the nicknaming of the Patient Protection and Affordable Care Act as "Obamacare".[2]

Among its many effects, the law established an independent public authority, the Commonwealth Health Insurance Connector Authority, also known as the **Massachusetts Health Connector**. The Connector acts as an insurance broker to offer free, highly subsidized and full-price private insurance plans to residents, including through its web site. As such it is one of the models of the Affordable Care Act's health insurance exchanges. The 2006 Massachusetts law successfully covered approximately two-thirds of the state's then-uninsured residents, half via federal-government-paid-for Medicaid expansion (administered by MassHealth) and half via the Connector's free and subsidized network-tiered health care insurance for those not eligible for expanded Medicaid. Relatively few Massachusetts residents used the Connector to buy full-priced insurance.

3.9.1 Background

The healthcare insurance reform law was enacted as **Chapter 58 of the Acts of 2006** of the Massachusetts General Court; its long form title is **An Act Providing Access to Affordable, Quality, Accountable Health Care**. In October 2006, January 2007, and November 2007, bills were enacted that amended and made technical corrections to the statute (Chapters 324 and 450 of the Acts of 2006, and chapter 205 of the Acts of 2007).[3]

The movement to reform Massachusetts healthcare insurance regulations and market between 2004 and 2006 was driven by multiple issues, not all of which were clearly an issue or directly related to then and now most critical issues of rising costs:

1. A six-year-old federal-government waiver as to how Massachusetts administered its Medicaid program was expiring. Unless the waiver was extended or amended, a large number of people would lose Medicaid coverage as the state reverted to Federal regulations.[4]

2. Reforms made in 1997 to the portion of the insurance market that related to the individual purchase of insurance had failed. In 2000, over 100,000 Massachusetts residents (about 1.5% of the population) were covered by individually purchased insurance but the number had dropped to under 50,000 by the time of the reform debate.[5]

3. As illustrated in the state report referenced in the previous sentence, the price of insurance that covered about 600,000 people in the small group market (about 10% of the population) was rising faster than the prices for the vast majority of the non-senior-citizen population, most of which were – and still are – covered by self-insured group insurance from large employers (self-insured plans are not subject to state regulation).

4. There was a widespread feeling that emergency rooms were misused for non-emergency medical care (the misuse was and is undeniable, not unique to Massachusetts, and continues; the relation to healthcare insurance or lack of it was less clear and apparently did/does not exist).

5. The taxes that fed the state's "free care pool",[6] which covered uninsured emergency room visits as well as uninsured hospital admissions (as well as funding community health centers), consistently underfunded the pool and had to be raised almost annually (with differences made up by appropriations from general revenue). The combination of issues four and five was dubbed by Romney and others the free-rider problem although subsequent to the passage of the law, it is argued that the free-rider problem did not really exist. Almost all people who did not have insurance could not afford it, but since they were still using the good it is considered free riding.

6. Advocacy groups wanted a long list of non-traditionally covered (e.g., vision care) or under-covered (e.g., mood-altering pharmaceuticals) healthcare procedures and goods mandated.[7]

7. Large employers—even large employers that were self-insured—were increasingly dropping health insurance as an employee benefit and/or restricting it to "full-time employees such that the "take up rate" of healthcare insurance by employees was dropping. However, the drop in take-up rate actually accelerated after passage of the law although there is no demonstrable relationship between the law's passage and the accelerated drop.[8][9]

Allegedly because of their lack of health insurance, uninsured Massachusetts residents commonly utilize emergency rooms as a source of primary care.[10] The United States Congress passed the Emergency Medical Treatment and Active Labor Act (EMTALA) in 1986. EMTALA requires hospitals and ambulance services to provide care to anyone needing emergency treatment regardless of citizenship, legal status or ability to pay. EMTALA applies to virtually all hospitals in the U.S but includes no provisions for reimbursement. EMTALA is therefore considered an "unfunded safety net program" for patients seeking care at the nation's emergency rooms.[11][12] As a result of the 1986 EMTALA legislation, hospitals across the country faced unpaid bills and mounting expenses to care for the uninsured.[13]

In Massachusetts, a pool of over $1 billion in 2004/2005, funded by a tax on paying hospital customers and insurance premiums, known as the Uncompensated Care Pool (or "free care pool"), was used to partially reimburse hospitals and health centers for these ED expenses. A much larger portion of the pool was used for non-ED hospital care for the uninsured and for other care at Community Health Centers.[14] It was predicted that implementation of the 2006 Massachusetts healthcare insurance reform law would result in almost complete elimination of the need for this fund. In 2006, an MIT economics professor Jonathan Gruber predicted that the amount of money in the "free care pool" would be sufficient to pay for reform legislation without requiring additional funding or taxes.[15]

3.9.2   Reform coalitions

In November 2004, political leaders began advocating major reforms of the Massachusetts health care insurance system to expand coverage. First, the Senate President Robert Travaglini called for a plan to reduce the number of uninsured by half. A few days later, Governor Romney announced that he would propose a plan to cover virtually all the uninsured.[16]

At the same time, the ACT (Affordable Care Today) Coalition introduced a bill that expanded MassHealth (Medicaid and SCHIP) coverage and increased health coverage subsidy programs and required employers to either provide coverage or pay an assessment to the state. The coalition began gathering signatures to place their proposal on the ballot in November 2006 if the legislature did not enact comprehensive health care reform, resulting in the collection of over 75,000 signatures on the MassACT ballot proposal. The Blue Cross Blue Shield Foundation sponsored a study, "Roadmap to Coverage," to expand coverage to everyone in the Commonwealth.[17]

Attention focused on the House when then-Massachusetts House Speaker Salvatore DiMasi, speaking at a Blue Cross Blue Shield Foundation Roadmap To Coverage forum in October 2005, pledged to pass a bill through the House by the end of the session. At the forum, the Foundation issued a series of reports on reform options, all of which included an individual mandate. At the end of the month, the Joint Committee on Health Care Financing approved a reform proposal crafted by House Speaker DiMasi, Committee co-chair Patricia Walrath, and other House members.[18] The state faced pressure from the federal government to make changes to the federal waiver that allows the state to operate an expanded Medicaid program. Under the existing waiver, the state was receiving $385 million in federal funds to reimburse hospitals for services provided to the uninsured. The free care pool had to be restructured so that individuals, rather than institutions, received the funding.[19] Then-U.S. Senator Edward Kennedy (D-MA) made a special effort to broker a compromise between the Republican Governor and the Democratic State Legislature.

3.9.3   Legislation

In Fall 2005, the House and Senate each passed health care insurance reform bills. The legislature made a number of changes to Governor Romney's original proposal, including expanding MassHealth (Medicaid and SCHIP) coverage to low-income children and restoring funding for public health programs. The most controversial change was the addition of a provision which requires firms with 11 or more workers that do not provide "fair and reasonable" health coverage to their workers to pay an annual penalty. This contribution, initially $295 annually per worker, is intended to equalize the free care pool charges imposed on employers who do and do not cover their workers.

On April 12, 2006, Governor Romney signed the health legislation.[20] He vetoed eight sections of the health care legislation, including the controversial employer assessment.[21] He vetoed provisions providing dental benefits to poor residents on the Medicaid program, and providing health coverage to senior and disabled legal immigrants not eligible for federal Medicaid.[22] The legislature promptly overrode six of the eight gubernatorial sec-

tion vetoes, on May 4, 2006, and by mid-June 2006 had overridden the remaining two.[23]

3.9.4   Statute

The enacted statute, Chapter 58 of the Acts of 2006, established a system to require individuals, with a few exceptions, to obtain health insurance.[24]

Chapter 58 had several key provisions: the creation of the Health Connector; the establishment of the subsidized Commonwealth Care Health Insurance Program; the employer Fair Share Contribution and Free Rider Surcharge; and a requirement that each individual must show evidence of coverage on their income tax return or face a tax penalty, unless coverage was deemed unaffordable by the Health Connector.[24]

The statute expanded MassHealth (Medicaid and SCHIP) coverage for children of low income parents and restores MassHealth benefits like dental care and eyeglasses. The legislation included a merger of the individual (non-group) insurance market into the small group market to allow individuals to get lower group insurance rates. The process of merging the two markets also froze the market for such insurance for a short period in April–May 2010 as the current government tried to keep the leading non-profit insurers, which insure over 90% of the residents, in the state from raising premiums for small businesses and individuals. Eventually the state's non-partisan insurance board ruled that the government did not have the actuarial data or right to freeze the premiums. Five of the non-profit insurers then settled for slightly lower premium increases than they had initially requested rather than litigate further. The sixth litigated and won the right to implement all its original increases retroactively. Payment rates were supposed to be increased to hospitals and physicians under the statute but that has not happened. The statute also formed a *Health Care Quality and Cost Council* to issue quality standards and publicize provider performance.[25]

Commonwealth Health Insurance Connector Authority

The Health Connector is designed as a clearinghouse for insurance plans and payments. It performed the following functions:

- It administers the Commonwealth Care program for low-income residents (up to 300% of the FPL) who do not qualify for MassHealth[26] and who meet certain eligibility guidelines.

- It offers for purchase health insurance plans for individuals who:

- are not working,

- are employed by a small business (less than 50 employees) that uses the Connector to offer health insurance. These residents will purchase insurance with pre-tax income.[27]

- are not qualified under their large employer plan,

- are self-employed, part-time workers, or work for multiple employers,

- It sets premium subsidy levels for Commonwealth Care.

- It defines "affordability" for purposes of the individual mandate.

Employer taxes

Employers with more than ten full-time equivalent employees (FTEs) must provide a "fair and reasonable contribution" to the premium of health insurance for employees.[28] Employers who do not will be assessed an annual fair share contribution that will not exceed $295 per employee per year.[28] The fair share contribution will be paid into the Commonwealth Care Trust Fund to fund Commonwealth Care and other health reform programs.[25]

The Division of Health Care Finance and Policy defined by regulation what contribution level meets the "fair and reasonable" test in the statute. The regulation imposes two tests. First, employers are deemed to have offered "fair and reasonable" coverage if at least 25% of their full-time workers are enrolled in the firm's health plan. Alternatively, a company meets the standard if it offers to pay at least 33% of the premium cost of an individual health plan. For employers with 50 or more FTEs, both standards must be met, or 75% of full-time workers must be enrolled in the firm's health plan. Regulatory and analytic information is available on the Division's website.

There was an additional Free Rider Surcharge assessible to the employer.[29] This surcharge is different from the fair share contribution. The surcharge is applied when an employer does not arrange for a pre-tax payroll deduction system for health insurance (a Section 125 plan, or a "cafeteria plan"), and has employees who receive care that is paid from the uncompensated care pool, renamed in October 2007 as the Health Safety Net.[26]

Individual taxes

Residents of Massachusetts must have health insurance coverage under Chapter 58.[30] Residents must indicate on their tax forms if they had insurance on December 31 of that tax year, had a waiver for religious reasons, or had a waiver

from the Connector. The Connector waiver can be obtained if the resident demonstrates that there is no available coverage that is defined by the Connector as affordable.[25] In March 2007, the Connector adopted an affordability schedule that allows residents to seek a waiver. If a resident does not have coverage and does not have a waiver, the Department of Revenue will enforce the insurance requirement by imposing a penalty. In 2007, the penalty was the loss of the personal exemption. Beginning in 2008, the penalty is half the cost of the lowest available yearly premium which will be enforced as an assessed addition to the individual's income tax.[31]

Young adult coverage

Beginning July 2007, the Connector offered reduced benefit plans for young adults up to age 26 who do not have access to employer-based coverage.[32]

Changes to the law

In 2008 and 2010, much more substantive changes were made to the law, one of the most important of which was to begin an open enrollment period for those receiving subsidized health insurance and anyone buying insurance, including those paying full price, as an individual.[33] Prior to that 2010 change, under the Massachusetts law, residents buying healthcare insurance individually could do so at any time, even—theoretically—as being admitted to a hospital or entering an emergency room. This led to a gaming of the system and research by the state said this gaming added 1%–2% to premium costs,[34] which were continuing to rise for other reasons as well. Given the continuing overall rise in premiums post Massachusetts 2006 healthcare insurance reform,[35] the major goal of the 2012 amendment was to introduce price controls on health care itself; it is not directly related to healthcare insurance as are the earlier legislative actions.

Starting in 2014, Commonwealth Care insurance (and Commonwealth Choice insurance for those not receiving subsidies) has been replaced by insurance compatible with the federal Patient Protection and Affordable Care Act. Among other differences, consistent with PPACA, the out of pocket spending limits and deductibles are higher under similarly priced (after a PPACA tax credit) PPACA-consistent insurance than the superseded Massachusetts insurance law. To try to compensate for these higher limits and deductibles, the Commonwealth funded an additional insurance program called Connectorcare, by which residents who previously would have qualified for Commonwealth Care can get very similar benefits for about the same price.

3.9.5 Implementation

The implementation of healthcare insurance reform began in June 2006, with the appointment of members of the Connector board and the naming of Jon Kingsdale, a Tufts Health Plan official, as executive director of the Connector. On July 1, MassHealth began covering dental care and other benefits, and began enrolling children between 200% and 300% of the poverty level. The federal Centers for Medicare and Medicaid Services approved the state's waiver application on July 26, 2006, allowing the state to begin enrolling 10,500 people from the waitlist for the MassHealth Essential program, which provides Medicaid coverage to long-term unemployed adults below the poverty line.[36] In 2006, the Division of Health Care Finance and Policy issued regulations defining "fair and reasonable" for the fair share assessment. The regulations provide that companies with 11 or more full-time equivalent employees will meet the "fair and reasonable" test if at least 25 percent of those employees are enrolled in that firm's health plan and the company is making a contribution toward it. A business that fails that test may still be deemed to offer a "fair and reasonable" contribution if the company offers to pay at least 33 percent of an individual's health insurance premium.[37]

Also effective in 2006, the Connector Board set premium levels and copayments for the state subsidized Commonwealth Care plans. Premiums will vary from $18 per month, for individuals with incomes 100%–150% of the poverty line, to $106 per month for individuals with incomes 250%–300% of poverty. The Connector approved two copayment schemes for plans for people 200%–300% of poverty. One plan will have higher premiums and lower copayments, while a second choice will have lower premiums and higher copayments.[38] Four managed care plans began offering Commonwealth Care on November 1, 2006. Coverage for people above 100% of poverty up to 300% of poverty began on February 1, 2007. As of December 1, 2007, around 158,000 people had been enrolled in Commonwealth Care plans. Initial bids received by the Connector showed a likely cost for the minimum insurance plan of about $380 per month. The Connector rejected those bids, and asked insurers to propose less expensive plans. New bids were announced on March 3, 2007. The Governor announced that "the average uninsured Massachusetts resident will be able to purchase health insurance for $175 per month."[39] But plan costs will vary greatly depending on the plan selected, age and geographic location, ranging from just over $100 per month for plans for young adults with high copayments and deductibles to nearly $900 per month for comprehensive plans for older adults with low deductibles and copayments. Copayments, deductibles and out-of-pocket contributions may vary among plans. The proposed minimum creditable coverage plan would have

a deductible no higher than $2,000 per individual, $4,000 per family, and would limit out-of-pocket expenses to a $5,000 maximum for an individual and $7,500 for a family. Before the deductible applies, the proposed plan includes preventive office visits with higher copayments, but would not include emergency room visits if the person was not admitted.[40]

The new plan covered abortions (both elective and medically necessary) in the heavily Catholic state.[41]

Health care plans provided through Commonwealth Health Insurance Connector Authority in 2014

With the implementation of PPACA in 2014, those citizens acquiring insurance through currently available Massachusetts Health Connector plans, will need to re-enroll or select a new plan, given the new guidelines stipulated by PPACA. Approximately 100,000 Massachusetts residents who received free or highly subsidized CommonWealth Care insurance, will be moved to Medicaid. The number of available plans under the Affordable Care Act that will offer service beginning on January 1, 2014, rose to more than 100 from just under 100 in 2013. The open enrollment period of the insurance marketplace, during which citizens may re-enroll or purchase, lasted from 1 October 2013 to 31 March 2014, but those who did not re-enroll by December 15, were to have no insurance coverage in January 2014 (unless they were among the 100,000 moved to Medicaid).

Health plans are to be offered by the following providers: Ambetter from CeltiCare, Blue Cross Blue Shield of Massachusetts (which did not participate in the prior Massachusetts health care insurance program), Boston Medical Center HealthNet, Fallon Community Health Plan, Harvard Pilgrim Health Care, Health New England, Minuteman Health, Neighborhood Health Plan (a new plan following the co-op model introduced with PPACA), Network Health, and Tufts Health Plan.

The primary features of each plan are illustrated in this table based on the data provided at the Summary of Benefits & Coverage located within the Plan Information section of the Individuals and Families portal.[42] The source to the below list of available plans is via the Massachusetts Health Connector —[43]

By comparison, Commonwealth Care insurance had either zero or $250 deductibles (depending on which of three types of Commonwealth Care insurance it was) and zero or very low co-pays as compared to the PPACA-consistent insurance (not illustrated in the table). "Not applicable" in the table above means the subscriber (a) cannot go out of network at all or (b) can go out of network but will be responsible for all charges incurred; it does not mean the deductible does not apply. Both Commonwealth Care and PPACA-consistent insurance is networked and almost all versions of both insurances offered gym memberships.

3.9.6 Outcomes

From 2006, the number of uninsured Massachusetts residents dropped from about 6% to about 2% in 2010 according to the Massachusetts Department of Healthcare Finance and Policy (DHCFP), depending on the methodology used,[44] According to the Massachusetts Center on Health Information and Analsysis (CHIA), which replaced the DHCFP in 2012, the percentage of uninsured rose back to between 3–4% in 2012. The United States Census Department shows a higher percentage of uninsured for the same years but a similar trend line. Both trend lines mirror—from different baselines—the approximately 400,000 Massachusetts residents added to the rolls of the insured in 2006/2007 via an expansion in Medicaid eligibility rules and the subsidization of the Commonwealth Care insurance program.

A 2011 view of the data, released by the state in 2013, shows the number of people receiving employer-sponsored insurance (ESI) in Massachusetts has decreased by approximately 500,000 people (about 8% of the state population) since the enactment of the Massachusetts health insurance law in 2006. (The state of Massachusetts stopped putting out regular information on various types of insurance enrollment altogether between 2011 and 2013; prior to 2011, it released such data quarterly. In 2013, the state released 2011 data.) The latest U.S. Census data on health care insurance types in Massachusetts was released in September 2012, and also illustrates the long-term decrease in ESI, and an increase in public, free and subsidized insurance.

In the early years of the implementation of the law, approximately 2% of those eligible were determined not to have had access to affordable insurance, and a small number opted for a religious exemption to the mandate.[45] Approximately 1% of taxpayers were determined by the Commonwealth to have had access to affordable insurance during tax year 2009 (latest data available), and had to pay an income tax penalty instead.

Comparing the first half of 2007 to the first half of 2009, spending from the Health Safety Net Fund dropped 38%–40%, as more people became insured.[45] The Fund—which replaced the Uncompensated Care Pool or Free Care—pays for medically necessary health care for those who do not have access to health insurance, and pays for the underinsured.[46] According to the DHCFP in a report dated September 2011, "Total Health Safety Net (HSN) payments increased by 7% in the first six months of Health Safety Net fiscal year 2011 (HSN11) compared to the same period in the prior year[,] while demand increased by 10%.

Demand represents the amount that providers would have been paid in the absence of a funding shortfall. Because HSN11 demand is expected to exceed HSN11 funding, hospital providers experienced a $38 million shortfall during the first six months of HSN11." Versus the same period two years earlier, HSN spending plus demand has increased 20%

The reduced state HSN payments anticipated (but not realized), that by reducing the number of uninsured people, Commonwealth Care would reduce the amount of charity care provided by hospitals.[47] In a subsequent story that same month, the Boston Globe reported, that Commonwealth Care faced a short-term funding gap of $100 million and the need to obtain a new three-year funding commitment from the federal government of $1.5 billion.[48] By June 2011, enrollment was projected to grow to 342,000 people at an annual expense of $1.35 billion. The original projections were for the program to ultimately cover approximately 215,000 people at a cost of $725 million.[49]

Enrollment in the full-price Commonwealth Choice Plans, offered through the Commonwealth Health Insurance Connector, fluctuates between 15,000-20,000 according to the state. According to the DHCFP's quarterly Key Indicator reports, 89,000 people bought healthcare insurance directly as of June 2009, up from 40,000 in June 2006. The number of people with group insurance in Massachusetts has held steady at around 4,400,000 since passage of the health care reform law, according to the DHCFP's quarterly Key Indicators reports available on its website. One outcome has been the unavailability of coverage by many insurers previously doing business in Massachusetts.

A study published in *The American Journal of Medicine*, "Medical Bankruptcy in Massachusetts: Has Health Reform Made a Difference?", compared bankruptcy filers from 2007, before reforms were implemented, to those filing in the post-reform 2009 environment to see what role medical costs played. The study found that: 1) From 2007 to 2009, the total number of medical bankruptcies (defined as due to unpaid medical bills or to loss of income due to illness, with no distinction between those causes) in Massachusetts increased by more than one third, from 7,504 to 10,093; and 2) Illness and medical costs contributed to 59.3% of bankruptcies in 2007 and 52.9% in 2009. The researchers note that the financial crisis beginning in 2008 likely contributed to the increased number of bankruptcies, and Massachusetts' increase in medical bankruptcies over the 2007–2009 period was nevertheless below the national average rate of increase. Still, the researchers explain that health costs continued to go up over the period in question, and their overall findings are "incompatible with claims that health reform has cut medical bankruptcy filings significantly."[50]

During the week of April 5, 2010, the *Boston Globe* reported that more than a thousand people in Massachusetts had "gamed" the mandate/penalty provision of the law since implementation by choosing to be insured only a few months a year, typically when in need of a specific medical procedure. On the average, the Globe reported, these part-time enrolees were paying $1,200–$1,600 in premiums over a few months and receiving $10,000 or more in healthcare services before again dropping coverage.[51]

A study conducted by the Urban Institute and released in December 2010 by the Massachusetts Division of Health Care Finance and Policy stated that as of June 2010, 98.1 percent of state residents had coverage. This compared to 97.3 percent having coverage in the state in 2009 and 83.3 percent having coverage nationwide. Among children and seniors the 2010 coverage rate was even higher, at 99.8 percent and 99.6 percent respectively. The breakdown of insurance coverage consisted of that 65.1 percent of state residents being covered by employers, 16.4 percent by Medicare, and 16.6 percent via public plans such as Commonwealth Care. The state's Secretary of Health and Human Services, JudyAnn Bigby, said, "Massachusetts' achievements in health care reform have been nothing short of extraordinary. With employers, government and individuals all sharing the responsibility of reform, we continue to have the highest insurance rate in the nation."[52]

In June 2011, a *Boston Globe* review concluded that the healthcare overhaul "has, after five years, worked as well as or better than expected."[53] A study by the fiscally conservative Beacon Hill Institute was of the view that the reform was "responsible for a dramatic increase in health care spending," however.[54]

In March 2012, the National Bureau of Economic research released a working paper stating "that health care reform in Massachusetts led to better overall self-assessed health... [and] improvements in several determinants of overall health, including physical health, mental health, functional limitations, joint disorders, body mass index, and moderate physical activity." [55]

In 2012, the Blue Cross Foundation of Massachusetts funded and released in April research that showed that the 2006 law and its subsequent amendments – simply in terms of measuring the state-budget effect on the uncompensated care pool and funding subsidized insurance (see Background section above) had cost approximately $2 billion in fiscal year 2011 versus approximately $1 billion in fiscal year 2006. Some of this doubling in cost was funded by temporary grants and waivers from the United States federal government. The Blue Cross funded research did not address the increased costs in premiums for employers and individuals or other market dynamics – such as increased providers' costs and increased co-pays/deductibles

– necessary to meet minimum creditable coverage standards that were introduced in Massachusetts by other parts of the 2006 legislature and its resulting regulations. Separate research on Premiums and Expenditures released by the Massachusetts DHCFP in May 2012 found that fully adjusted premiums per member per month (PPMPM) for Massachusetts residents covered by comprehensive private insurance policies (approximately two thirds of the state population) increased approximately 9% in both 2009 and 2010 (latest data available) for subscribers in the "merged market", 7% in the midsized group market, and 5.4% in the large group market. These premium increase do not reflect actual resident experience particularly in the merged market because Massachusetts regulations allow age and other rating factors (e.g., even if premiums were held flat for 55-year-olds living on Cape Cod in construction work from year to year, the 55-year-old in 2009 would pay 10% more in 2010 for the same policy, possibly with lesser benefits).

During the years before the changes in the state law related to the enactment of the federal PPACA, the state still used the free care pool—renamed the Health Safety Net—both as originally intended and to fund the subsidies for free (under 150% of FPL) and almost free (151–300% of FPL) networked health care insurance. In addition the state spent a substantial amount of general revenue on the insurance reform. Based on the combination of the increased Health Safety Net tax, general revenue (state income and sales taxes were increased 20%) and smaller additional taxes, the cost of the reform reached about 2% of the state's annual budget in fiscal year 2013, which ended June 30, 2013, up from 1.5% in fiscal 2011.[56]

Data following enactment of mandatory insurance showed total emergency visits and spending continued to increase, and low-severity emergency visits decreased less than 2%; researchers concluded, "To the extent that policymakers expected a substantial decrease in overall and low-severity ED visits, this study does not support those expectations."[57] Other analysis concluded that preventable ED visits were reduced 5-8% for non-urgent or primary care ED visits relative to other states.[58] A more complete report released in January 2012 found between 2006 and 2010 emergency department visits and non-urgent visits had dropped 1.9 and 3.8% respectively.[59] A 2014 study found that the reform was associated with "significant reductions in all-cause mortality and deaths from causes amenable to health care."[60]

According to a 2016 study in the *American Economic Journal*, the reform "reduced the amount of debt that was past due, improved credit scores, reduced personal bankruptcies and reduced third-party collections."[61] The authors note that the "results show that health care reform has implications that extend well beyond the health of those who gain insurance coverage."[61]

3.9.7 Legal challenges

Fountas v. Dormitzer

A legal challenge was filed in the Superior Court of Essex County, contesting the fine imposed for a citizen's failure to get health insurance as well as the fine imposed for a failure to provide information on a tax return as to whether that citizen had health insurance. The judge dismissed the case upon a motion filed by an assistant to Attorney General Martha Coakley for failure to state a case upon which relief can be granted. A petition for a writ of mandamus to the Massachusetts Supreme Judicial Court (SJC), ordering Essex Superior Court to vacate this dismissal on procedural grounds, the failure to provide trial by jury in a dispute over property as requested by the plaintiff, was denied by Associate Justice Spina. An appeal was then filed with the Massachusetts Appeals Court. A later petition for a writ of mandamus with the SJC was also denied, this time by Chief Justice Ireland.[62] The Appeals Court then heard the appeal and declined to send the case back to Essex Superior Court for trial by jury based on their belief that no facts needed to be determined and therefore trial by jury in this case was not a protected right under either the US or Massachusetts Constitutions.[63] The SJC declined to hear any further appeals.

3.9.8 References

[1] Matt Dunning (2013). "Mass. health care reform law's employer mandate repealed". Business Insurance.

[2] Taylor, Jessica (23 October 2015). "Mitt Romney Finally Takes Credit For Obamacare". *NPR*. Retrieved 18 March 2016.

[3] For text of the laws, provided by *The General Court of The Commonwealth of Massachusetts*

  • "Summary of the Massachusetts Health Reform Law" (PDF). *The Official Website of the Commonwealth of Massachusetts*. Boston: Commonwealth of Massachusetts. 2011.

  • "Chapter 58 of the Acts of 2006, An Act Providing Access to Affordable, Quality Accountable Health Care". *The Official Website of the Commonwealth of Massachusetts*. Boston: Commonwealth of Massachusetts. 2011.

  • "Chapter 324 of the Acts of 2006, An Act Relative to Health Care Access". *The Official Website of the Commonwealth of Massachusetts*. Boston: Commonwealth of Massachusetts. 2011.

  • "Chapter 450 of the Acts of 2006, An Act Further Regulating Health Care Access". *The Official Website of the Commonwealth of Massachusetts*. Boston: Commonwealth of Massachusetts. 2011.

  • "Chapter 205 of the Acts of 2007, An Act Further Regulating Health Care Access". *The Official Website of the Commonwealth of Massachusetts*. Boston: Commonwealth of Massachusetts. 2011.

[4] "Massachusetts Health Waiver Renewal".

[5] "Impact of Merging the Massachusetts Non-Group and Small Group Health Insurance Markets" (PDF).

[6] "Uncompensated Care Pool PFY05 Utilization Report".

[7] "CHIA Publications".

[8] "Annual Report on the Massachusetts Health Care Market" (PDF).

[9] "Massachusetts Employer Survey 2010" (PDF).

[10] "In Massachusetts, Health Care for All?". Retrieved 2011-07-11.

[11] American College of Emergency Physicians (2006). "American College of Emergency Physicians Survey of Emergency Department Directors". American College of Emergency Physicians. Retrieved 2011-07-11.

[12] "How To Access Health Care – Massachusetts Uncompensated (Free) Care Pool". *Boston Public Health Commission*. Retrieved 2011-07-11.

[13] "Romney's Mission: Massachusetts Health Care". *NPR*. Retrieved 2011-07-11.

[14] "Uncompensated Care Pool PFY05 Utilization Report". *The Official Website of the Commonwealth of Massachusetts*. Boston: Commonwealth of Massachusetts. 2011. Retrieved 2011-07-11.

[15] Lieberman, Trudy (January 28, 2010). "A Tale of Two Jonathans". *Columbia Journalism Review*. Retrieved 2013-12-19.

[16] "My plan for Massachusetts health insurance reform".

[17] "Research on providing health coverage for the uninsured in Massachusetts". *Roadmap to Coverage*. Retrieved 2011-07-11.

[18] "ACT Health Care Reform". Retrieved 2011-07-11.

[19] "Health Care Reform in Massachusetts". Worcester, Massachusetts: University of Massachusetts Medical School. Retrieved 2011-07-11.

[20] "Landmark Health Bill Signed". The Seattle Times. Los Angeles Times and Associated Press. April 13, 2006.

[21] Greenberger, Scott S. (November 4, 2005). "House approves healthcare overhaul". *The Boston Globe*. Retrieved 2011-07-11.

[22] "Romney signs health care bill". *North Adams Transcript*. Retrieved 2011-07-11.

[23] "Chapter 58 of the Acts of 2006, An Act Providing Access to Affordable, Quality Accountable Health Care". *The Official Website of the Commonwealth of Massachusetts*. Boston, MA: Commonwealth of Massachusetts. 2011. Retrieved 2011-07-11. The six prompt overrides were noted at the foot of the chapter: Approved (in part) April 12, 2006. Disapproved sections 5, 27, 29, 47, 112, 113, 134 and 137. Sections 5, 29, 47, 113, 134 and 137, overridden on May 4, 2006; see chapter 58 text for overrides.

[24] "Chapter 58 of the Acts of 2006, An Act Providing Access to Affordable, Quality Accountable Health Care". *The Official Website of the Commonwealth of Massachusetts*. Boston: Commonwealth of Massachusetts. 2011. Retrieved 2011-07-11.

[25] Report from Massachusetts Secretary of Health and Human Services, Timothy Murphy, to the Massachusetts General Court, "Chapter 58 Implementation Update" (June 12, 2006).

[26] "Health Care FAQ" (PDF). Boston: Massachusetts General Court, Committee on Health Care Financing. April 4, 2006. Retrieved 2011-07-11.

[27] Mitt Romney (April 11, 2006). "Health Care for Everyone?". *Wall Street Journal*. Retrieved 2011-07-11.

[28] 2006 Mass. Act Chp. 58, sec. 47

[29] 2006 Mass. Acts Chp. 58, sec. 44

[30] 2006 Mass. Acts Chp. 58, sec. 12

[31] "Massachusetts's Health Care Reform Law Fact Sheet" (PDF). Boston: HCFAMA. Retrieved 2011-07-11.

[32] Blue Cross Foundation (2010). "Massachusetts Health Care Reform Bill Summary" (PDF). *The Massachusetts Law and its History*. Boston: Blue Cross Foundation. Retrieved 2011-07-11.

[33] "Open enrollment set in Massachusetts for health care".

[34] "Analysis of Individual Health Coverage In Massachusetts Before and After the July 1, 2007 Merger of the Small Group and Nongroup Health Insurance Markets" (PDF).

[35] "Premium Levels and Trends in Private Health Plans: 2007–2009" (PDF).

[36] "Press Release on waiver approval". *The Official Website of the Commonwealth of Massachusetts*. Boston: Commonwealth of Massachusetts. July 28, 2006. Retrieved 2011-07-11.

[37] "Press Release on Fair Share regulations". *The Official Website of the Commonwealth of Massachusetts*. Boston: Commonwealth of Massachusetts. September 8, 2006. Retrieved 2011-07-11.

[38] "Commonwealth Care page". Health Care For All. Retrieved 2011-07-11.

[39] "Press release on minimum creditable coverage plans" (PDF). Boston: HCFAMA. March 3, 2007. Retrieved 2011-07-11.

[40] Dembner, Alice (2007-01-19). "Outline for new insurance plan proposed". *The Boston Globe*. Retrieved 2011-07-11.

[41] Allison, Wes. "PolitiFact | Indeed, abortions are covered". PolitiFact. Retrieved October 8, 2012.

[42] "Summary of Benefits and Coverage". *The Massachusetts Health Connector*. Boston, MA: Commonwealth of Massachusetts. November 8, 2013. Retrieved 2013-11-08.

[43] "Massachusetts Health Connector". Commonwealth of Massachusetts. n.d.

[44] "Estimate of Uninsured" (PDF). *The Official Website of the Commonwealth of Massachusetts*. Boston: Commonwealth of Massachusetts. 2011. Retrieved 2011-07-11.

[45] "Week Beginning March 9, 2008: Facts and Figures" (MS Word Document). *Current Updates*. Boston: Massachusetts Health Connector. Retrieved 2011-07-11.

[46] Massresources.org (2011). "Health Safety Net – HSN (Free Care): an overview". *Health Care Programs: General – in Massachusetts*. Boston: Community Resources Information, Inc. Retrieved 2011-07-11.

[47] Krasner, Jeffrey (March 18, 2008). "Safety net hospitals strained by reform". *The Boston Globe*. Retrieved 2011-07-11.

[48] Dembner, Alice (2008-03-26). "Healthcare cost increases dominate Mass. budget debate". *The Boston Globe*. Retrieved 2011-07-11.

[49] Dembner, Alice (2008-02-03). "Subsidized care plan's cost to double: Enrollment is outstripping state's estimate". *The Boston Globe*. Retrieved 2011-07-11.

[50] "Medical Bankruptcy in Massachusetts: Has Health Reform Made a Difference?". Journalist's Resource.org. Retrieved 2011-07-11.

[51] Lazar, Kay (April 4, 2010). "Short-Term Customers Boosting Health Costs". *The Boston Globe*. Retrieved 2011-07-11.

[52] Geisel, Jerry (December 14, 2010). "Massachusetts' insured rate hits 98.1%: Analysis". *Business Insurance*. Retrieved 2011-07-11.

[53] Brian C. Mooney 'RomneyCare' – a revolution that basically worked *Boston Globe* June 26, 2011

[54] BHI Study: Massachusetts Health Care Reform drives up insurance costs both public and private *Beacon Hill Institute July 2011*

[55] Courtemanche, Charles J.; Daniela Zapata (March 2012). "Does Universal Coverage Improve Health? The Massachusetts Experience (NBER Working Paper No. 17893)". Retrieved 12 March 2012.

[56] "Massachusetts Health Reform Spending, 2006–2011: An Update on the "Budget Buster" Myth" (PDF). *Massachusetts Taxpayer Foundation.* Boston: Massachusetts Taxpayer Foundation. 2011. Retrieved 2012-06-30.

[57] http://www.sciencedaily.com/releases/2011/06/ 110606142555.htm http://www.boston.com/news/local/ massachusetts/articles/2010/07/04/emergency_room_ visits_grow_in_mass/

[58] Miller, Sarah (June 2012). "The Effect of Insurance on Emergency Room Visits: An Analysis of the 2006 Massachusetts Health Reform)" (PDF). Retrieved 11 July 2012.

[59] Long, Sharon K; Karen Stockley; Heather Dahlen (January 2012). "Massachusetts Health Reforms: Uninsurance Remains Low, Self-Reported Health Status Improves As State Prepares To Tackle Costs". Retrieved 19 December 2013.

[60] Sommers, Benjamin D.; Long, Sharon K.; Baicker, Katherine (6 May 2014). "Changes in Mortality After Massachusetts Health Care Reform". *Annals of Internal Medicine.* **160** (9): 585. doi:10.7326/M13-2275.

[61] Mazumder, Bhashkar; Miller, Sarah (2016-08-01). "The Effects of the Massachusetts Health Reform on Household Financial Distress". *American Economic Journal: Economic Policy.* **8** (3): 284–313. doi:10.1257/pol.20150045. ISSN 1945-7731.

[62] Supreme Judicial Court for Suffolk County (2009). "GEORGE FOUNTAS vs. COMMISSIONER OF THE MASS. DEPARTMENT OF REVENUE (SJ-2009-0146)". *Public Case Information.* Boston: Supreme Judicial Court and Appeals Court of the Commonwealth of Massachusetts. Retrieved 2011-07-11.

[63] APPEALS COURT OF MASSACHUSETTS. "GEORGE FOUNTAS vs. COMMISSIONER OF THE MASS. DEPARTMENT OF REVENUE" (PDF). Retrieved 2012-05-23.

3.9.9 Further reading

- "Access to Health Care in Massachusetts" (PDF). *The Official Website of the Commonwealth of Massachusetts.* Boston: Commonwealth of Massachusetts, Division of Health Care Finance and Policy (DHCFP). 2004. Archived from the original (PDF) on 2007-09-29.

- Lyons, Ed (August 26, 2014). The Health Connector Autopsy Report (Report).

- Pulos, Vicky, *MassHealth Advocacy Guide*, Massachusetts Law Reform Institute (MLRI) and Massachusetts Continuing Legal Education, Inc. (MCLE), Massachusetts Legal Services, 2009 edition, updated again in 2010 (3/18/2010)

3.9.10 External links

- Massachusetts Health Connector - official site

3.10 National health insurance

National health insurance (NHI) – sometimes called **statutory health insurance (SHI)** – is a legally enforced scheme of health insurance that insures a national population against the costs of health care. It may be administered by the public sector, the private sector, or a combination of both. Funding mechanisms vary with the particular program and country. National or Statutory health insurance does not equate to government-run or government-financed health care, but is usually established by national legislation. In some countries, such as Australia's Medicare system or the UK's National Health Service, contributions to the system are made via general taxation and therefore are not optional even though use of the health scheme it finances is. In practice, of course, most people paying for NHI will join the insurance scheme. Where the NHI scheme involves a choice of multiple insurance funds, the rates of contributions may vary and the person has to choose which insurance fund to belong to.

3.10.1 History

Germany has the world's oldest national social health insurance system,[1] with origins dating back to Otto von Bismarck's Sickness Insurance Law of 1883.[2][3] In Britain, the National Insurance Act 1911 included national social health insurance for primary care (not specialist or hospital care), initially for about one third of the population—employed working class wage earners, but not their dependents.[4] This system of health insurance continued in force until the creation of the National Health Service in 1948 which created a universal service, funded out of general taxation rather than on an insurance basis, and providing health services to all legal residents.

3.10.2 Types of programs

See also: Health care systems, Single-payer health care, and Universal health care

National healthcare insurance programs differ both in how the money is collected, and in how the services are provided. In countries such as Canada, payment is made by the government directly from tax revenue. The collection is administered by government. In France a similar system of compulsory contributions is made, but the collection is administered by non-profit organisations set up for the purpose. This is known in the United States as single-payer health care. The provision of services may be through either publicly or privately owned health care providers.

An alternative funding approach is where countries implement national health insurance by legislation requiring compulsory contributions to competing insurance funds. These funds (which may be run by public bodies, private for-profit companies, or private non-profit companies), must provide a minimum standard of coverage and are not allowed to discriminate between patients by charging different rates according to age, occupation, or previous health status. To protect the interest of both patients and insurance companies, the government establishes an equalization pool to spread risks between the various funds. The government may also contribute to the equalization pool as a form of health care subsidy. This is the model used in the Netherlands.

Other countries are largely funded by contributions by employers and employees to sickness funds. With these programs, funds come from neither the government nor direct private payments. This system operates in countries such as Germany and Belgium. These funds are usually not for profit institutions run solely for the benefit of their members. Usually characterization is a matter of degree: systems are mixes of these three sources of funds (private, employer-employee contributions, and national/subnational taxes).

In addition to direct medical costs, some national insurance plans also provide compensation for loss of work due to ill-health, or may be part of wider social insurance plans covering things such as pensions, unemployment, occupational retraining, and financial support for students.

National schemes have the advantage that the pool or pools tend to be very very large and reflective of the national population. Health care costs, which tend to be high at certain stages in life such as during pregnancy and childbirth and especially in the last few years of life can be paid into the pool over a lifetime and be higher when earnings capacity is greatest to meet costs incurred at times when earnings capacity is low or non existent. This differs from the private insurance schemes that operate in some countries which tend to price insurance year on year according to health risks such as age, family history, previous illnesses, and height/weight ratios. Thus some people tend to have to pay more for their health insurance when they are sick and/or are least able to afford it. These factors are not taken into consideration in NHI schemes. In private schemes in competitive insurance markets, these activities by insurance companies tend to act against the basic principles of insurance which is group solidarity.

3.10.3 National health insurance schemes

See also: Universal health coverage by country

- Health care in Australia - Medicare (Australia)
- Healthcare in Belgium - Sickness and Invalidity Insurance
- Healthcare in Germany
- Health care in Ghana - National Health Insurance Scheme (NHIS)
- Health care in Colombia - Law 100 - National Health Insurance Scheme: Contributory Vs. Subsidized coverage (NHIS)
- Health care in Japan - People without insurance through employers can participate in a national health insurance program administered by local governments.
- Health care in France
- Healthcare in South Korea
- Healthcare in Switzerland - A compulsory health insurance covers a range of treatments which are set out in detail in the Federal Act.
- Healthcare in Taiwan - National Health Insurance (NHI)
- Healthcare in Nigeria - National Health Insurance Scheme (NHIS)
- Health care in Canada
- Healthcare in the Philippines - Social Health Insurance Program, a resource pooling, risk sharing health care program that provides quality health care financing not only to the employed but to the sick, elderly, and indigents, as well

This list is incomplete; you can help by expanding it.

3.10.4 See also

- Health care compared - tabular comparisons of the US, Canada, and other countries not shown above.
- Health care politics
- Publicly funded health care
- Single-payer health care
- Universal health care

3.10.5   References

[1] Bump, Jesse B. (October 19, 2010). "The long road to universal health coverage. A century of lessons for development strategy" (PDF). Seattle: PATH. Retrieved March 10, 2013. Carrin and James have identified 1988—105 years after Bismarck's first sickness fund laws—as the date Germany achieved universal health coverage through this series of extensions to minimum benefit packages and expansions of the enrolled population. Bärnighausen and Sauerborn have quantified this long-term progressive increase in the proportion of the German population covered by public and private insurance. Their graph is reproduced below as Figure 1: German Population Enrolled in Health Insurance (%) 1885–1995.
Carrin, Guy; James, Chris (January 2005). "Social health insurance: Key factors affecting the transition towards universal coverage" (PDF). *International Social Security Review.* **58** (1): 45–64. doi:10.1111/j.1468-246x.2005.00209.x. Retrieved March 10, 2013. Initially the health insurance law of 1883 covered blue-collar workers in selected industries, craftspeople and other selected professionals.[6] It is estimated that this law brought health insurance coverage up from 5 to 10 per cent of the total population.
Bärnighausen, Till; Sauerborn (May 2002). "One hundred and eighteen years of the German health insurance system: are there any lessons for middle- and low income countries?" (PDF). *Social Science & Medicine.* **54** (10): 1559–1587. doi:10.1016/S0277-9536(01)00137-X. PMID 12061488. Retrieved March 10, 2013. As Germany has the world's oldest SHI [social health insurance] system, it naturally lends itself to historical analyses. |first3= missing |last3= in Authors list (help)

[2] Leichter, Howard M. (1979). *A comparative approach to policy analysis: health care policy in four nations.* Cambridge: Cambridge University Press. p. 121. ISBN 0-521-22648-1. The Sickness Insurance Law (1883). Eligibility. The Sickness Insurance Law came into effect in December 1884. It provided for compulsory participation by all industrial wage earners (i.e., manual laborers) in factories, ironworks, mines, shipbuilding yards, and similar workplaces.

[3] Hennock, Ernest Peter (2007). *The origin of the welfare state in England and Germany, 1850–1914: social policies compared.* Cambridge: Cambridge University Press. p. 157. ISBN 978-0-521-59212-3.

[4] Leathard, Audrey (2000). "Health care in Britain: pre-war provision, 1900–1939". *Health care provision: past, present, and into the 21st century* (2nd ed.). Cheltenham: Stanley Thornes. pp. 3–4. ISBN 9780748733545.

3.10.6   Further reading

• Nicholas Laham: *Why the United States lacks a national health insurance program*, Westport, Conn. [u.a.] : Greenwood Press, 1993

• Barona, B., Plaza, B., and Hearst, N. (2001) Managed Competition for the poor or poorly managed: Lessons from the Colombian health reform experience. Oxford University Press

• Ronald L. Numbers (ed.): *Compulsory Health Insurance: The Continuing American Debate*, Westport, Conn. : Greenwood Press, 1982.

• Saltman, R.B., Busse, R. and Figueras, J. (2004) *Social health insurance systems in western Europe*, Berkshire/New York: Open University Press/McGraw-Hill. ISBN 0-335-21363-4

• Saltman, R.B. and Dubois, H.F.W. (2004) Individual incentive schemes in social health insurance systems, 10(2): 21-25. Full text

• Van de Ven, W.P.M.M., Beck, K., Buchner, F. et al. (2003) Risk adjustment and risk selection on the sickness fund market in five European countries, Health Policy, 65(1=: 75-98.

• Saltman, R.B. and Dubois, H.F.W. (2005) Current reform proposals in social health insurance countries, Eurohealth, 11(1): 10-14. Full text

3.10.7   External links

• Health Care for America NOW!. An advocacy group that supports a public health insurance option for universal health care.

• Health Care Issues & Resources Barack Obama Website

• Health Debate Pros and Cons Family Doctor Magazine Website

3.11   Primary healthcare

This article is about an approach to providing universal health care. For the sector of the health care system, see Primary care.

Primary healthcare (PHC) refers to "essential health care" that is based on scientifically sound and socially acceptable methods and technology, which make universal health care accessible to all individuals and families in a community. It is through their full participation and at a cost that the community and the country can afford to maintain at every stage of their development in the spirit of self-reliance and self-determination".[1] In other words, PHC is an approach to health beyond the traditional health care system that focuses on health equity-producing social policy.[2][3] PHC includes all areas that play a role in

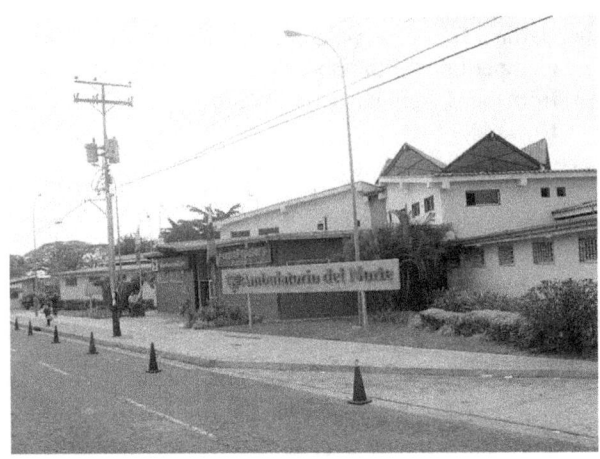

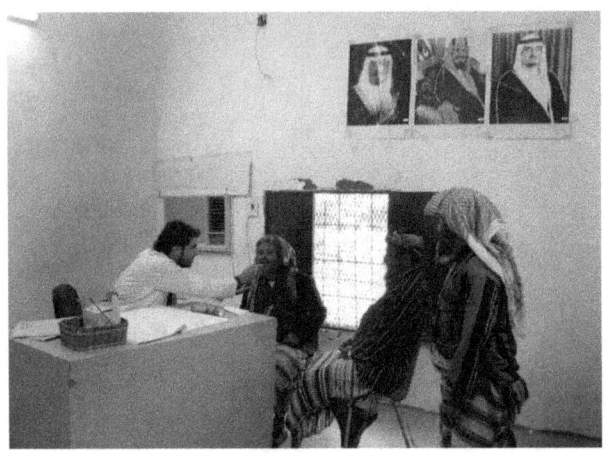

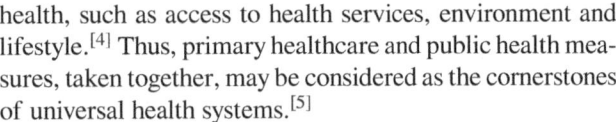

Public ambulatory care facility in Maracay, Venezuela, providing primary care for ambulatory care sensitive conditions.

A primary health care worker in Saudi Arabia, 2008

health, such as access to health services, environment and lifestyle.[4] Thus, primary healthcare and public health measures, taken together, may be considered as the cornerstones of universal health systems.[5]

This ideal model of healthcare was adopted in the declaration of the International Conference on Primary Health Care held in Alma Ata, Kazakhstan in 1978 (known as the "Alma Ata Declaration"), and became a core concept of the World Health Organization's goal of *Health for all*.[6] The Alma-Ata Conference mobilized a "Primary Health Care movement" of professionals and institutions, governments and civil society organizations, researchers and grassroots organizations that undertook to tackle the "politically, socially and economically unacceptable" health inequalities in all countries. There were many factors that inspired PHC; a prominent example is the Barefoot doctors of China.[4][7][8]

3.11.1 Goals and principles

The ultimate goal of primary healthcare is the attainment of better health services for all. It is for this reason that World Health Organization (WHO), has identified five key elements to achieving this goal:[9]

- reducing exclusion and social disparities in health (universal coverage reforms);

- organizing health services around people's needs and expectations (service delivery reforms);

- integrating health into all sectors (public policy reforms);

- pursuing collaborative models of policy dialogue (leadership reforms); and

- increasing stakeholder participation.

Behind these elements lies a series of basic principles identified in the Alma Ata Declaration that should be formulated in national policies in order to launch and sustain PHC as part of a comprehensive health system and in coordination with other sectors:[1]

- Equitable distribution of health care – according to this principle, primary care and other services to meet the main health problems in a community must be provided equally to all individuals irrespective of their gender, age, caste, color, urban/rural location and social class.

- Community participation – in order to make the fullest use of local, national and other available resources. Community participation was considered sustainable due to its grass roots nature and emphasis on self-sufficiency, as opposed to targeted (or vertical) approaches dependent on international development assistance.[4]

- Health workforce development – comprehensive healthcare relies on adequate number and distribution of trained physicians, nurses, allied health professions, community health workers and others working as a health team and supported at the local and referral levels.

- Use of appropriate technology – medical technology should be provided that is accessible, affordable, feasible and culturally acceptable to the community. Examples of appropriate technology include refrigerators for vaccine cold storage. Less appropriate could include, in many settings, body scanners or heart-lung machines, which benefit only a small minority concentrated in urban areas. They are generally not accessible to the poor, but draw a large share of resources.[4]

- Multi-sectional approach – recognition that health cannot be improved by intervention within just the formal health sector; other sectors are equally important in promoting the health and self-reliance of communities. These sectors include, at least: agriculture (e.g. food security); education; communication (e.g. concerning prevailing health problems and the methods of preventing and controlling them); housing; public works (e.g. ensuring an adequate supply of safe water and basic sanitation); rural development; industry; community organizations (including Panchayats or local governments, voluntary organizations, etc.).

In sum, PHC recognizes that healthcare is not a short-lived intervention, but an ongoing process of improving people's lives and alleviating the underlying socioeconomic conditions that contribute to poor health. The principles link health and development, advocating political interventions, rather than passive acceptance of economic conditions.[4]

3.11.2 Approaches

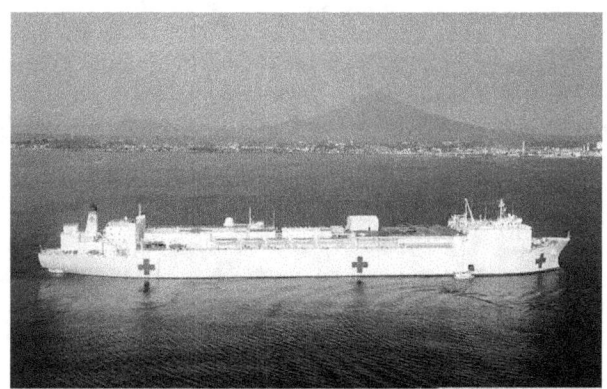

The hospital ship USNS Mercy *(T-AH-19) in Manado, Indonesia, during Pacific Partnership 2012.*

The primary health care approach has seen significant gains in health were applied even when adverse economic and political conditions prevail.[10]

Although the declaration made at the Alma-Ata conference deemed to be convincing and plausible in specifying goals to PHC and achieving more effective strategies, it generated numerous criticisms and reactions worldwide. Many argued the declaration did not have clear targets, was too broad, and was not attainable because of the costs and aid needed. As a result, PHC approaches have evolved in different contexts to account for disparities in resources and local priority health problems; this is alternatively called the Selective Primary Health Care (SPHC) approach.

Selective PHC

After the year 1978 Alta Alma Conference, the Rockefeller Foundation held a conference in 1979 at its Bellagio conference center in Italy to address several concerns. Here, the idea of Selective Primary Health Care was introduced as a strategy to complement comprehensive PHC. It was based on a paper by Julia Walsh and Kenneth S. Warren entitled "Selective Primary Health Care, an Interim Strategy for Disease Control in Developing Countries".[11] This new framework advocated a more economically feasible approach to PHC by only targeting specific areas of health, and choosing the most effective treatment plan in terms of cost and effectiveness. One of the foremost examples of SPHC is "GOBI" (growth monitoring, oral rehydration, breastfeeding, and immunization),[4] focusing on combating the main diseases in developing nations.

GOBI-FFF

Selective PHC approach consists of techniques known collectively under the acronym "GOBI-FFF". It focuses on severe population health problems in certain developing countries, where a few diseases are responsible for high rates of infant and child mortality. Health care planning is employed to see which diseases require most attention and, subsequently, which intervention can be most effectively applied as part of primary care in a least-cost method. The targets and effects of Selective PHC are specific and measurable. The approach aims to prevent most health and nutrition problems before they begin:[12][13]

- **G**rowth monitoring: the monitoring of how much infants grow within a period, with the goal to understand needs for better early nutrition.[4]

- **O**ral rehydration therapy: to combat dehydration associated with diarrhea

- **B**reastfeeding

- **I**mmunization

- **F**amily planning (birth spacing)

- **F**emale education

- **F**ood supplementation: for example, iron and folic acid fortification/supplementation to prevent deficiencies in pregnant women.

PHC and population aging

Given global demographic trends, with the numbers of people age 60 and over expected to double by 2025, PHC approaches have taken into account the need for countries to address the consequences of population ageing. In particular, in the future the majority of older people will be living in developing countries that are often the least prepared to confront the challenges of rapidly ageing societies, including high risk of having at least one chronic non-communicable disease, such as diabetes and osteoporosis.[14] According to WHO, dealing with this increasing burden requires health promotion and disease prevention intervention at community level as well as disease management strategies within health care systems.

PHC and mental health

Some jurisdictions apply PHC principles in planning and managing their healthcare services for the detection, diagnosis and treatment of common mental health conditions at local clinics, and organizing the referral of more complicated mental health problems to more appropriate levels of mental health care.[15]

3.11.3 Background and controversies

Barefoot Doctors

The "Barefoot doctors" of China were an important inspiration for PHC because they illustrated the effectiveness of having a healthcare professional at the community level with community ties. Barefoot doctors were a diverse array of village health workers who lived in rural areas and received basic healthcare training. They stressed rural rather than urban healthcare, and preventive rather than curative services. They also provided a combination of western and traditional medicines. They had close community ties, were relatively low-cost, and perhaps most importantly they encouraged self-reliance through advocating prevention and hygiene practices.[4] The program experienced a massive expansion of rural medical services in China, with the number of barefoot doctors increasing dramatically between the early 1960s and the Cultural Revolution (1964-1976).

Criticisms

Although many countries were keen on the idea of primary healthcare after the Alma Ata conference, the Declaration itself was criticized for being too "idealistic" and "having an unrealistic time table".[4] More specific approaches to prevent and control diseases - based on evidence of prevalence, morbidity, mortality and feasibility of control (cost-effectiveness) - were subsequently proposed. The best known model was the Selective PHC approach (described above). Selective PHC favoured short-term goals

and targeted health investment, but it did not address the social causes of disease. As such, the SPHC approach has been criticized as not following Alma Ata's core principle of everyone's entitlement to healthcare and health system development.[4]

In Africa, the PHC system has been extended into isolated rural areas through construction of health posts and centers that offer basic maternal-child health, immunization, nutrition, first aid, and referral services.[16] Implementation of PHC is said to be affected after the introduction of structural adjustment programs by the World Bank.[16]

3.11.4 See also

3.11.5 References

[1] World Health Organization. Declaration of Alma-Ata. Adopted at the International Conference on Primary Health Care, Alma-Ata, USSR, 6–12 September 1978.

[2] Starfield, Barbara. "Politics, primary healthcare and health." *J Epidemiol Community Health* 2011;65:653–655 doi:10.1136/jech.2009.102780

[3] Public Health Agency of Canada. About Primary Health Care. Accessed 12 July 2011.

[4] Marcos, Cueto (2004). "The ORIGINS of Primary Health Care and SELECTIVE Primary Health Care.". *Am J Public Health*. 22. **94**: 1864–1874. doi:10.2105/ajph.94.11.1864.

[5] White F. Primary health care and public health: foundations of universal health systems. Med Princ Pract 2015 doi:10.1159/000370197

[6] Secretariat, WHO. "International Conference on Primary Health Care, Alma-Ata: twenty-fifth anniversary" (PDF). *Report by the Secretariat*. WHO. Retrieved 28 March 2011.

[7] Bulletin of the World Health Organization (October 2008). "Consensus during the Cold War: back to Alma-Ata". World Health Organization.

[8] Bulletin of the World Health Organization (December 2008). "China's village doctors take great strides". World Health Organization.

[9] "Health topics: Primary health care". World Health Organisation. Retrieved 28 March 2011.

[10] Braveman, Paula; E. Tarimo (1994). *Screening in Primary Health Care: Setting Priorities With Limited Resources.* World Health Organization. p. 14. ISBN 9241544732. Retrieved 4 November 2012.

[11] Walsh, Julia A., and Kenneth S. Warren. 1980. Selective primary health care:An interim strategy for disease control in developing countries. Social Science & Medicine. Part C: Medical Economics 14 (2):145-163

[12] Rehydration Project. *UNICEF's GOBI-FFF Programs*. Accessed 16 June 2011.

[13] World Health Organization. *World Health Report 2005*, Chapter 5: Choosing Interventions to Reduce Specific Risks. Geneva, WHO Press.

[14] World Health Organization. *Older people and Primary Health Care (PHC)*. Accessed 16 June 2011.

[15] Department of Health, Provincial Government of the Western Cape. *Mental Health Primary Health Care (PHC) Services*. Accessed 16 June 2011.

[16] Pfeiffer, J. 2003. International NGOs and primary health care in Mozambique: the need for a new model of collaboration. Social Science & Medicine 56(4):725-738.

3.11.6 Further reading

- WHO (1978). "Alma Ata 1978: Primary Health Care". *HFA Sr.* (1).

- WHO (2008). *The World Health Report 2008: Primary Health Care, Now More Than Ever.*

- McGilvray, James C. (1981). "The Quest for Health and Wholeness". Tübingen: German Institute for Medical Missions. ISBN 0-7289-0014-9.

- Socrates Litsios (2002). "The Long and Difficult Road to Alma-Ata: A Personal Reflection". *International Journal of Health Services.* **32** (4): 709–732. doi:10.2190/RP8C-L5UB-4RAF-NRH2. PMID 12456122.

- Socrates Litsios (November 1994). "The Christian Medical Commission and the Development of WHO's Primary Health Care Approach". *American Journal of Public Health.* **94** (11): 1884–1893. doi:10.2105/AJPH.94.11.1884. PMC 1448555. PMID 15514223.

- Gatrell, A.C. (2002) *Geographies of Health: an Introduction*, Oxford: Blackwell.

3.11.7 External links

- Declaration of Alma-Ata.

- WHO European Observatory on Health Systems and Policies.

3.12 Rajiv Gandhi Jeevandayee Arogya Yojana

Rajiv Gandhi Jeevandayee Arogya Yojana (RGJAY) is a Universal health care scheme run by the Government of Maharashtra for the poor people of the state of Maharashtra who holds one of the 4 cards issued by the government; Antyodaya card, Annapurna card, yellow ration card or orange ration card. The scheme was first launched in 8 districts of the Maharashtra state in July 2012 and then across all 35 districts of the state in November 2013. It provides free access to medical care in government empanelled 488 hospitals for 971 types of diseases, surgeries and therapies costing up to Rs.1,50,000 per year per family (Rs.2,50,000 only for renal transplant). As of 17 January 2016, around 11.81 lakh procedures amounting to Rs.1827 crore have been performed on patients from 7.13 lakh beneficiary families which includes over 7.27 lakh surgeries and therapies. The scheme is called successful amid some allegations of hospitals directly or indirectly causing patients to incur out-of-pockets expenses on some part of the treatment.

3.12.1 History

In 1997, the then Chief Minister of Maharashtra Manohar Joshi started 'Jeevandayee Yojana' for the poor people which covered cost of treatment of very serious illnesses. But this scheme had shortcomings.[1] This scheme was used to cover only 4 procedures related to brain, heart, kidney and cancer. Also Rashtriya Swasthya Bima Yojana (RSBY) launched by the Government of India in 2008 had largely failed, while the Aarogyasri health insurance scheme of neighbouring Andra Pradesh state had become very successful. So the Maharashtra government closed the RSBY scheme, revamped the old 1997 'Jeevandayee Yojana' and modelled it on the 'Aarogyasri' scheme of the Andra Pradesh to cover 971 types of surgeries, therapies, procedures.[2][3] It was renamed as 'Rajiv Gandhi Jeevandayee Arogya Yojana' after the former Prime Minister Rajiv Gandhi and it was launched as pilot project on 2 July 2012 over eight districts of the Maharashtra state and it covered 52.37 lakh families. These districts were Mumbai, Thane, Dhule, Nanded, Amravati, Gadchiroli, Solapur and Raigad. Under this scheme, more than 1 lakh procedures were carried out between July 2012 and October 2013. Following the success of this pilot scheme, government of Maharashtra decided to launch this scheme in all 35 districts of the state.[4][5]

3.12.2 Overview

Introduction

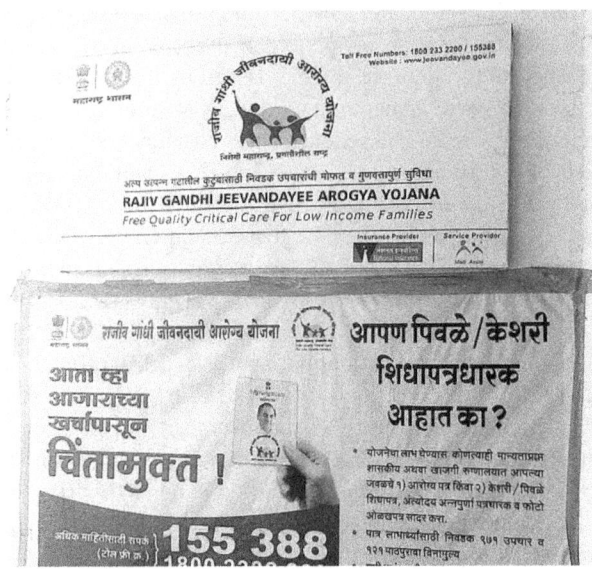

RGJAY information board in an empanelled hospital

The scheme was launched in all 35 districts of the Maharashtra on 21 November 2013 at Nagpur by the Indian National Congress president Sonia Gandhi in the presence of Maharashtra Chief Minister Prithviraj Chavan, Maharashtra Health Minister Suresh Shetty, Union Agriculture Minister Sharad Pawar, and others. The scheme now covers around 2.11 crore families from 35 districts of the Maharashtra state.[4]

Under this scheme, Maharashtra govt pays insurance premium of Rs.333 plus taxes per year per one beneficiary family to the public sector National Insurance Company towards Rs.1,50,000 health insurance policy and the beneficiary family gets medical access for 971 surgeries, therapies and procedures in the government empanelled hospitals. The scheme covers pre-existing diseases and ailments. The scheme is launched on floater basis; that means a single member of family can get free medical access costing up to Rs.150,000 in one year or whole family can get free medical access costing up to Rs.150,000 in one year. Renal transplant is treated exceptional case and government offers up to Rs.250,000 per year for this operation.[4][6][7] In December 2015 Maharashtra govt announced increase in limit on kidney transplant expenses from Rs 2.50 lakh to Rs 3 lakh which includes medical check-up of kidney donor and receiver. Govt also announced separate funds for poor patients to undergo dialysis.[8]

Statistics

As per RGJAY society, 6,61,333 surgeries or procedures were carried out throughout Maharashtra under this scheme until 15 November 2015 which amounted to 1641.10 crore rupees.[5] Until December 2015, RGJAY Society had empanelled 476 hospitals across the Maharashtra state out of which 76 were government hospitals. Out of 6.62 lakh surgeries, 3.5 lakh were major surgeries and cancer surgeries ranked first followed by kidney and heart surgeries.[9]

The TISS report observed that in public hospitals 53% beneficiaries were yellow ration card holders (BPL beneficiaries) while 47% beneficiaries were orange ration card holders (non-BPL beneficiaries). The report further observed that in private hospitals, 63% beneficiaries were orange ration card holders and 37% beneficiaries were yellow ration card holders.[5][10]

Statistics of beneficiaries are daily updated on RGJAY Society website which reflects data since 2 July 2012 i.e. since the commencement of the scheme. As per these statistics available as of 17 January 2016, 12,48,970 patients (from 7,22,703 beneficiary families) were enrolled across the Maharashtra state out of which 11,81,066 patients were registered. The govt has incurred 1827.7 Crore rupees until 17 January 2016 for the treatment of these patients. Out of 11,81,066 patients, surgeries and therapies were carried out on 7,27,437 patients. 14,210 death cases have occurred; 5,300 patients died in govt hospitals while 8,910 patients died in private hospitals. 6169 health camps were organized across the Maharashtra state.[11]

3.12.3 Eligibility

Below Poverty Line families having income less than one lakh rupees per annum and who holds either Antyodaya card or Annapurna card or Yellow or orange ration card are eligible for free medical access under this scheme. The scheme does not cover Above Poverty Line families which holds white ration card. Data from valid card coupled with Aadhar card is used to issue 'Rajiv Gandhi Jeevandayee Arogya Yojana Health Card' to the beneficiary family which bears names, ages and photos of family members. Until this health card is issued, valid ration card and Aadhar card (or driving license, voter's ID card issued by the Election Commission of India) can be used to gain access to free medical care under this scheme.[4][6]

3.12.4 Benefits

The scheme covers 971 surgeries, therapies and procedures which falls under following 30 categories:

- 1 General surgery

- 2 ENT surgery

- 3 Ophthalmology surgery

- 4 Gynaecology and obstetrics surgery

- 5 Orthopedic surgery and procedures

- 6 Surgical gastroenterology

- 7 Cardiac and cardiothoracic surgery

- 8 Pediatric surgery

- 9 Genitourinary system

- 10 Neurosurgery

- 11 Surgical oncology

- 12 Medical oncology

- 13 Radiation oncology

- 14 Plastic surgery

- 15 Burns

- 16 Poly trauma

- 17 Prostheses

- 18 Critical care

- 19 General medicine

- 20 Infectious diseases

- 21 Pediatrics medical management

- 22 Cardiology

- 23 Nephrology

- 24 Neurology

- 25 Pulmonology

- 26 Dermatology

- 27 Rheumatology

- 28 Endocrinology

- 29 Gastroenterology

- 30 Interventional radiology

Out of 971 procedures, 131 procedures are performed only in government hospitals.[6] Illnesses which can be treated in primary health center or any other ordinary hospital are not covered under this scheme. Pneumonia is not covered, but advanced and serious forms of this disease and other lung related procedures like lobar pneumonia, bronchopneumonia, aspiration pneumonia, pneumoconiosis, pneumothorax, pneumonectomy, etc. are covered in this scheme. Diarrhea is not covered, but various surgical and medical gastroenterology procedures are included in this scheme. diabetes is not covered, but advanced and complicated stages of diabetes like diabetic retinopathy, diabetic ketoacidosis, uncontrolled diabetes with infectious emergencies etc. are covered under this scheme. Snakebite without ventilation support is not covered, but snakebite with ventilation support is covered under this scheme.[3][12][13] Hernia and appendicitis are not covered, but Diaphragmatic hernia and appendicular perforation are covered. In emergency case of appendicitis, hospital may admit the patient and RGJAY Society may approve the package mentioned in the policy.[14]

In the original scheme knee replacement and hip replacement surgeries were not included. In July 2015 it was reported that the government was considering to include these surgeries in the scheme and roll out the same from November 2015.[15]

3.12.5   System

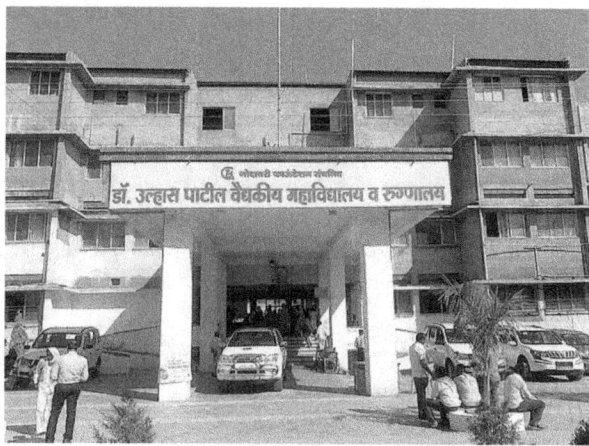

Dr. Ulhas Patil Medical College And Hospital at Jalgaon - one of the RGJAY empanelled network hospital

Maharashtra govt has formed 'Rajiv Gandhi Jeevandayee Arogya Yojana Society' (RGJAY Society) to implement and monitor this scheme in coordination with the National Insurance Company (NIC).[16] RGJAY Society and NIC has identified eligible hospitals throughout the Maharashtra and has empanelled them to implement this scheme. As of January 2016, 488 hospitals are empanelled at 35 district places. NIC and RGJAY Society has connected all of these hospitals through a computer network with dedicated database of beneficiary families. These hospitals are referred as 'Network Hospitals'.[17]

The beneficiary patient can directly approach the network hospital. Or the patient can be referred to the network hospital by a doctor in nearby govt hospital (run by the Zilla Parishad) or by a doctor in health camp.

Network hospital

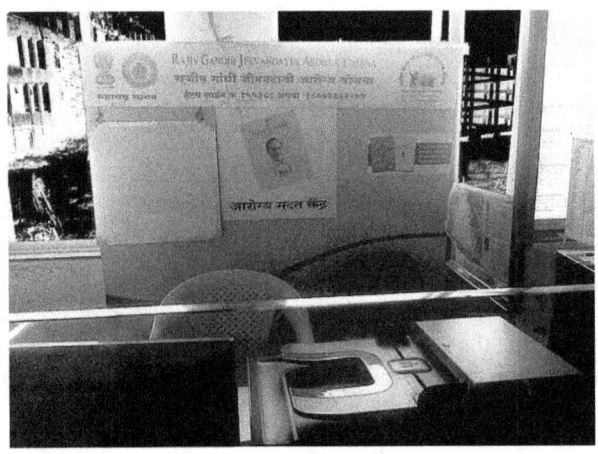

RGJAY Aarogyamitra help center in one of the RGJAY empanelled network hospital

The govt has appointed 'Aarogyamitra' (Health Friend) in all network hospitals. This Aarogyamitra checks referral card, health card or any other necessary documents. If all documents are in order, the network hospital admits the patient and sends online pre-authorization request to the insurer NIC which can also be reviewed by the RGJAY Society. The preauthorization request is processed within 24 hours. In emergency cases, network hospital can give telephonic intimation to the NIC and approval can be granted immediately.

Once the patient is admitted, all expenses pertaining to the patient are borne by the hospital and thereafter the hospital sends bill to the insurer NIC for reimbursement. These expenses include bed charges in general ward, nursing and boarding charges, fees of doctors involved in the treatment (surgeons, anaesthetists, medical practitioner etc.), consultants fees, cost of anaesthesia, blood bottles, oxygen, operating theater charges, cost of surgical appliances, medicines and drugs, cost of prosthetic devices, implants, X-Ray and diagnostic tests, food to inpatient, one side transport cost (from Hospital to residence of patient only by bus or railway. The scheme does not cover ambulance charges for transporting patient from home to

hospital or from one hospital to another hospital.) etc. That means, the patient can walk in hospital without a single rupee in his pocket and come out after full treatment of his ailment without paying any money for anything related to his treatment. The insurer has identified 125 procedures for free follow-up consultation and medicine. If the illness of the patient falls under these 125 procedures, then the hospital also covers cost of follow-up consultation and free medicine for one year from the date of discharge of the patient. [6][14][18][19]

NABH audit of network hospitals is mandatory. Government hospitals which have A1 grade gets full reimbursement of expenses incurred on the patients. Other government hospitals which have grades below A1 receives more than 10% cuts in the refund.[20]

Health camp

The process of health camps organizations is coordinated by the RGJAY Society and NIC and MDIndia Healthcare seNices acts as the third-party administrator. The venue of the health camp is identified by the district collector (or by the additional commissioner in case of BMC). Thereafter district coordinator of NIC, TPA and district health officer organizes the health camp in consultation with the network hospital and the district collector. Local NGOs can also participate in the organization of health camp. Organization of health camp is publicised through newspaper advertisements, pamphlets, local cable network, public address system etc. At least 6 MBBS doctors - 3 male and 3 female - are required to attend the patients along with 10 Aarogyamitras (5 male and 5 female).

Objectives of the health camp includes identifying beneficiary families and creating awareness about the scheme among them, training generalist medical officers of primary health centers (PHCs) about 971 types of procedures so that they can refer the patients from PHCs to network hospitals after proper screening, training Aarogyamitras of PHCs about helping patients in proper documentary work etc. Basic amenities -like shade, fans, chairs, water, snacks etc. - are provided to the patients attending the camp.

Network hospital is required to carry screening equipments like stethoscope, sphygmomanometer, glucometer, thermometer, ECG machine, fundoscope, pseudoscope, weigh machine, height scale, otoscope, tuning fork etc. Network hospital is also required to carry common drugs which includes ibuprofen, paracetamol, aspirin, diclofenac sodium, metronidazole, albendazole, norfloxacin, ciprofloxacin, ampicillin, ranitidine, B-complex etc. Doctors in health camp are required to carry out following investigations on the patients - hemogram, ESR, BSL, blood group, routine microscopic X-ray, fundoscopy, otoscopy, radiological ECG, USG, vision test, hearing test etc.

After proper screening, if the illness of patient does not fall within 971 predefined procedures, then only free consultation is provided to the patient. If the illness falls within predefined 971 procedures, then free treatment and medicine is given to the patient in the health camp. If the patient can be treated only in the network hospital, then doctors give 'Health Camp Referral Card' to the patient which mentions all the details and date of appointment.[21]

3.12.6 Updates

In February 2016, it was reported that the Maharashtra govt has decided to remove 130 procedures and add new 270 procedures in the scheme when it will sign fresh MOU with the insurance company in November 2016. Senior citizens will be the focus of new amended scheme. Govt may modify criteria of 'minimum 30 beds' to accommodate smaller hospitals in the interior area of Maharashtra.[22]

3.12.7 Grievances

Under this scheme, full treatment of the beneficiary patient is supposed to be free and cashless, but as per Tata Institute of Social Sciences, 63% beneficiary patients had incurred out-of-pocket expenses for diagnostics, treatment or consumables. As per TISS, the reasons included lack of time to do paperwork, unawareness about the benefits of the scheme, lack of cooperation from the hospital staff etc. RGJAY Society denied this claim by stating that 6.62 lakh procedures were carried out, but only 6232 grievances were received which amounts to only 0.94%. The Society further said that out of 6232 grievances, 82.22% grievances were resolved. The Society has cancelled empanelment of 102 hospitals and 7 hospitals were suspended from the scheme.[5][10]

3.12.8 References

[1] "RGJAY jay or parajay". *The Financial Express (India)*. 7 September 2013. Retrieved 18 January 2016.

[2] "'Health scheme for poor a non-starter'". *The Times of India*. 8 July 2014. Retrieved 18 January 2016.

[3] "'RGJAY formulated after a lot of research'". *The Times of India*. 21 November 2013. Retrieved 23 January 2016.

[4] "Sonia Gandhi to roll out health scheme". *Daily News and Analysis*. 20 November 2013. Retrieved 17 January 2016.

[5] "Rajiv Gandhi Jeevandayee Arogya Yojana: 82.22% grievances resolved till Nov 15, says Maharashtra govt". *The*

Indian Express. 3 December 2015. Retrieved 17 January 2016.

[6] "Rajiv Gandhi Jeevandayee Arogya Yojana". *Government of Maharashtra*. 16 January 2016. Retrieved 16 January 2016.

[7] "Jeevandayee Arogya scheme to be extended to whole state". *The Indian Express*. 14 May 2013. Retrieved 17 January 2016.

[8] "Amravati: State raises aid for kidney transplant under RGJAY to Rs 3 lakh". *The Economic Times*. 13 December 2015. Retrieved 24 January 2016.

[9] "Cancer tops list of surgeries for poor under state's RGJAY". *The Indian Express*. 26 December 2015. Retrieved 18 January 2016.

[10] "Despite state-run mediclaim, 60% forced to pay cash: TISS -". *The Economic Times*. 22 November 2015. Retrieved 17 January 2016.

[11] "Explore-Statistics". *Government of Maharashtra*. 18 January 2016. Retrieved 18 January 2016.

[12] "Rajiv Gandhi Jeevandayee Arogya yojana". *Government of Maharashtra*. 2 July 2012. Retrieved 25 January 2016.

[13] "Maharashtra government to include joint replacements, physiotherapy in Rajiv Gandhi yojana". *Daily News and Analysis*. 5 July 2015. Retrieved 24 January 2016.

[14] "FAQs - Rajiv Gandhi Jeevandayee Arogya yojana". *Government of Maharashtra*. 2 July 2012. Retrieved 14 February 2016.

[15] "State caps knee, hip implant prices". *Mumbai Mirror*. 15 July 2015. Retrieved 20 January 2016.

[16] "RGJAY Society - Rajiv Gandhi Jeevandayee Arogya Yojana". *Government of Maharashtra*. 17 January 2016. Retrieved 17 January 2016.

[17] "Network Hospitals - Rajiv Gandhi Jeevandayee Arogya Yojana". *Government of Maharashtra*. 17 January 2016. Retrieved 17 January 2016.

[18] "Eligibility Criteria - RGJAY". *Government of Maharashtra*. 18 January 2016. Retrieved 18 January 2016.

[19] "Emergency Telephonic Intimation" (PDF). *Government of Maharashtra*. 2 July 2012. Retrieved 26 January 2016.

[20] "Hospitals must have top grade to get full refund under RGJAY". *The Times of India*. 25 June 2015. Retrieved 14 February 2016.

[21] "Health Camp Policy" (PDF). *Government of Maharashtra*. 2 July 2012. Retrieved 24 January 2016.

[22] "Jeevandayee to add 270 procedures, drop 130". *The Hindu*. 9 February 2016. Retrieved 14 February 2016.

3.12.9 External links

- List of 971 illnesses/surgeries etc. covered under RG-JAY

- Detailed analysis of RGJAY scheme up to Sept 2013 by The Financial Express

3.13 Rashi Fein

Rashi Fein (February 6, 1926 – September 8, 2014) was an American health economist termed 'a father of Medicare' in the United States[2] and 'an architect of Medicare',[3] was Professor of Economics of Medicine, Emeritus, in the Department of Global Health and Social Medicine at Harvard Medical School, and the author of the book *Medical Care, Medical Costs: The Search for a Health Insurance Policy*[4] (Harvard University Press, 1986, 1989).[5][6]

His work has included: benefit-cost analysis, health care financing, health care workforce policy, health equity, cost containment, the financing of medical education, and health care reform.

He was the brother of Leonard J. Fein, also known as Leibel Fein, an American activist, writer, who had taught political science at MIT and was Deputy Director of the Harvard–MIT Joint Center for Urban Studies, and who specialized in Jewish social themes.[7] Fein served on the Advisory Committee of the Jewish Alliance for Law and Social Action.[8] Fein died in 2014 of melanoma at Massachusetts General Hospital in Boston.[9]

3.13.1 Education

- B.A., Johns Hopkins University, Baltimore, MD (1948)

- Ph.D. (political economy), Johns Hopkins University, Baltimore, MD (1956)

- M.A., Harvard University (1976)

- (Hon) D. Litt., State University of New York (1996)[10]

3.13.2 Professional and academic career

- Staff, President Harry S. Truman's Commission on the Health Needs of the Nation, 1952

- Lecturer to Associate Professor, Economics Department, University of North Carolina, Chapel Hill, 1952-1961

- Project Director, Economics of Mental Illness, Joint Commission on Mental Illness and Health, Cambridge, MA, 1957-1958

- Statistician, U.S. Bureau of the Census, Suitland, MD, 1958-1959

- Senior Staff, President John F. Kennedy's Council of Economic Advisors, 1961-1963

- Senior Fellow, Economics Study Program, The Brookings Institution, 1963-1968

- Professor of Economics of Medicine, Department of Social Medicine, Harvard Medical School, 1968 - 1999

- Professor of Economics of Medicine, Harvard Kennedy School of Government, 1968 - 1999

- Professor of Economics of Medicine Emeritus, Department of Social Medicine, Harvard Medical School, 1995 - 2014

3.13.3 Career

Rashi Fein began his service to the United States during World War II, in the United States Navy.[11] He spent much of his time after that thinking and writing about health care reform. He was a member of the Truman Commission on the Health Care Needs of the Nation, which as early as 1952 had supported national health insurance and regionalization of health care delivery. Later, he served on President John F. Kennedy's Council of Economic Advisors as a senior staff member (1961-1963). There, he helped to develop the initial legislation for Medicare, a healthcare model he continued to advocate throughout his life.[12][13] Professor Fein had also served on the Board of the Committee for National Health Insurance under the leadership of former United Auto Workers President Douglas Fraser and under Walter Reuther on a Board investigating malnutrition in the United States.[14][15] He was a charter member of the Institute of Medicine (IOM), had received numerous honors for service in medical economics, and sat on boards of a number of not-for-profit health care institutions. He had authored nine books, the most recent of which was *Lessons Learned: Medicine, Economics and Public Policy*,[16] published in November 2009.[17]

He joined the Harvard faculty of the school of medicine and the John F. Kennedy School of Government in 1968. He also served as senior fellow in the economics program at the Brookings Institution in Washington, D.C.

His 1982 "What Is Wrong with the Language of Medicine?"[18] in the New England Journal of Medicine began:

A new language is infecting the culture of American medicine. It is the language of the marketplace, of the tradesman, and of the cost accountant. It is a language that depersonalizes both patients and physicians and describes medical care as just another commodity. It is a language that is dangerous.

He concluded that paper:

A decent medical-care system that helps all the people cannot be built without the language of equity and care. If this language is permitted to die and is completely replaced by the language of efficiency and cost control, all of us — including physicians — will lose something precious.

He served as chair of the National Advisory Committee (NAC) for the Robert Wood Johnson Foundation's Scholars in Health Policy Research Program from 1994 to 2002 and was its Chair Emeritus until his death. His work has included: benefit-cost analysis, health care financing, health care workforce policy, cost containment, the financing of medical education, and health care reform. His first book was Economics of Mental Illness (1958). His most recent (2010) book, Lessons Learned: Medicine, Economics and Public Policy, was built on various lessons and stories that, as Chair of the NAC, he presented over the years at the Scholars' Annual Meeting in Aspen.

As an invited speaker, he presented his then-forthcoming 2009 book at the "Health Care Reform 2009:Politics and Paranoia" in Boston, on October 21, 2009, sponsored by the Boston Democratic Socialists of America and Mass-Care.[19]

Among colleagues, Fein was admired for his wry, often-humorous anecdotes drawn from Jewish culture and over fifty years of experience in the policy arena, which he brought together in his final book, *Learning Lessons: Medicine, Economics, and Public Policy* (Transaction Publishers, 2010).[20]

He also had served as a Director at Newbridge on the Charles, a senior living facility, an affiliate of the Harvard Medical School.[21][22]

3.13.4   Recognitions and awards

- Rashi Fein was a charter (founding) member of the Institute of Medicine (IOM), a nonprofit NGO founded in 1970.[23]

- Founding Member, National Academy of Social Insurance

- He received numerous honors for his writings in medical economics.

- Traveling Fellowship, World Health Organization, 1971

- John M. Russell Medal, Markle Scholars (Markle Fund) for "Advancement of Knowledge in Medicine", 1971[24]

- Martin E. Rehfuss Medal and Lectureship "For Distinguished Service to Medicine"

- Theobald Smith Lectureship, Albany Medical College, "For Teaching", Albany, NY, 1976

- Heath Clark Lecturer, London School of Hygiene and Tropical Medicine, 1980, delivered paper "Social and economic attitudes shaping American health policy" on March 24 and 26, 1980[25]

- Johns Hopkins University Alumni Association, 1999

- Lifetime Achievement Award "For Fearlessly Promoting the Rights of All to Health Care", Health Care, 2000

- Adam Yarmolinsky Medal from the Institute of Medicine, 2000[26]

- On June 30, 2009, he received the Debs-Thomas-Bernstein Awards, sponsored by Boston Democratic Socialists of America, in Boston.[27]

3.13.5   Publications

- *Economics of Mental Illness*, Basic Books, 1958.

- *The Doctor Shortage: An Economic Diagnosis*, The Brookings Institution, 1967.

- *Financing Medical Education: An Analysis of Alternative Policies and Mechanisms* (with Gerald I. Weber), McGraw Hill, 1971.

- A *Right to Health: The Problem of Access to Primary Medical Care* (with Charles Lewis and David Mechanic), John Wiley & Sons, 1976.

- *Employment Impacts of Health Policy Developments* (with Christine Bishop), Special Report No.11, National Commission for Manpower Policy, 1976.

- *Alcohol in America: The Price We Pay*. California: Care Institute, 1984.

- *Medical Care, Medical Costs: The Search for a Health Insurance Policy*, Harvard University Press, 1986, 1989.

- *The Health Care Mess: How We Got Into It and What It Will Take To Get Out* (with Julius B. Richmond), Harvard University Press, 2005.

- *Learning Lessons: Medicine, Economics, and Public Policy*, Transaction Publishers, 2010.

3.13.6 See also

- Link to journal publications, 1954-2010, and downloadable abstracts

- Harvard Catalyst profile for Rashi Fein

- Google Scholar search for Rashi Fein: read portions of Rashi Fein's writings, and citations of Rashi Fein's work

- Social Security Administration

3.13.7 References

[1] Legacy.com obituary: Rashi Fein

[2] Rashi Fein, a 'father of Medicare,' dies, September 9, 2014, 11:52am, in *JTA*

[3] Boston Globe obituary for Rashi Fein

[4] brief review of Medical Care, Medical Costs: The Search for a Health Insurance Policy

[5] Rashi Fein Faculty Profile page, Department of Global Health and Social Medicine, Harvard Medical School

[6] Listing for Rashi Fein in The International Who's Who: 1990-91, page 491, gives date of birth and full encyclopedia bibliography and CV/bio

[7] A brother's tribute to Leonard Fein, MAZON: A Jewish Response to Hunger, October 26, 2010

[8] Rashi Fein, a 'father of Medicare,' dies, September 9, 2014, 11:52am, in *JTA*

[9] https://www.nytimes.com/2014/09/14/us/ rashi-fein-economist-who-urged-medicare-dies-at-88. html?ref=obituaries

[10] SUNY Honorary Degrees, Awarded and Pending, website of State University of New York, Albany

[11] "Rashi Fein" article in KeyWiki

[12] History of SSA During the Johnson Administration 1963-1968; Rashi Fein was a Members of the 1968-1969 Advisory Committee

[13] Papers of Wilbur J. Cohen, notes Rashi Fein's role as member of the Advisory Council on Research Development, which provided assistance to the Social Security Administration for its research program

[14] National Health Insurance—A Brief History of Reform Efforts in the U.S., March 2009, in Focus on Health Reform, blog of the Henry K. Kaiser Family Foundation

[15] Index of Archives of Committee for National Health Insurance Collection in the Walter P. Reuther Library of Wayne State University

[16] JAMA book review for Lessons Learned: Medicine, Economics and Public Policy

[17] Profile Page for Rashi Fein, Scholars in Health Policy Research, Robert Wood Johnson

[18] Fein, R., 1982, "What Is Wrong with the Language of Medicine?", N Engl J Med 1982; 306:863-864April 8, 1982DOI: 10.1056/NEJM198204083061409

[19] OpenMedia's review of Health Care Reform 2009: Politics and Paranoia

[20] A brother's tribute to Leonard Fein, MAZON: A Jewish Response to Hunger, October 26, 2010

[21] Continuum of Care, Newbridge on the Charles website

[22] Trustees and Associates, Newbridge on the Charles

[23] ReachMD profile for Rashi Fein

[24] Rashi Fein profile, Publishers of Record in International Social Science

[25] Fein, R., Social and economic attitudes shaping American health policy, Milbank Quarterly, Vol. 58, No. 3, Summer, 1980

[26] List of Adam Yarmolinsky Award Recipients, IOM website

[27] TYR, June 2009

3.14 Right to health

The **right to health** is the economic, social and cultural right to a universal minimum standard of health to which all individuals are entitled. The concept of a right to health has been enumerated in international agreements which include the Universal Declaration of Human Rights, International Covenant on Economic, Social and Cultural Rights and the Convention on the Rights of Persons with Disabilities. However, there remains some international variation in the interpretation and application of the right to health due to considerations such as how health is defined, what minimum entitlements are encompassed in a right to health, and which institutions are responsible for ensuring a right to health.

3.14.1   Definition

Constitution of the World Health Organization

The preamble of the 1946 World Health Organization (WHO) Constitution defines health broadly as "a state of complete physical, mental and social well-being and not merely the absence of disease or infirmity."[1] The Constitution defines the right to health as "the enjoyment of the highest attainable standard of health," and enumerates some principles of this right as healthy child development; equitable dissemination of medical knowledge and its benefits; and government-provided social measures to ensure adequate health.

Frank P. Grad credits the WHO Constitution as "claiming ... the full area of contemporary international public health," establishing the right to health as a "fundamental, inalienable human right" that governments cannot abridge, and are rather obligated to protect and uphold.[2] The WHO Constitution, notably, marks the first formal demarcation of a right to health in international law.

Universal Declaration of Human Rights

Article 25 of the United Nations' Universal Declaration of Human Rights 1948 states that "Everyone has the right to a standard of living adequate for the health and well-being of himself and of his family, including food, clothing, housing and medical care and necessary social services." The Universal Declaration makes additional accommodations for security in case of physical debilitation or disability, and makes special mention of care given to those in motherhood or childhood.[3]

The Universal Declaration of Human Rights is noted as the first international declaration of fundamental human rights, both freedoms and entitlements alike. United Nations High Commissioner for Human Rights Navanethem Pillay writes that the Universal Declaration of Human Rights "enshrines a vision that requires taking all human rights—civil, political, economic, social, or cultural—as an indivisible and organic whole, inseparable and interdependent."[4] Likewise, Gruskin et al. contend that the interrelated nature of the rights expressed in the Universal Declaration establishes a "responsibility [that] extends beyond the provision of essential health services to tackling the determinants of health such as, provision of adequate education, housing, food, and favourable working conditions," further stating that these provisions "are human rights themselves and are necessary for health."[5]

International Convention on the Elimination of All Forms of Racial Discrimination

Health is briefly addressed in the United Nations' International Convention on the Elimination of All Forms of Racial Discrimination, which was adopted in 1965 and entered into effect in 1969. The Convention calls upon States to "Prohibit and to eliminate racial discrimination in all its forms and to guarantee the right of everyone, without distinction as to race, colour, or national or ethnic origin, to equality before the law," and references under this provision "The right to public health, medical care, social security and social services."[6]

International Covenant on Economic, Social and Cultural Rights

The United Nations further defines the right to health in Article 12 of the 1966 International Covenant on Economic, Social and Cultural Rights, which states:[7]

> The States Parties to the present Covenant recognize the right of everyone to the enjoyment of the highest attainable standard of physical and mental health. The steps to be taken by the States Parties to the present Covenant to achieve the full realization of this right shall include those necessary for:
>
> > The reduction of the stillbirth-rate and of infant mortality and for the healthy development of the child;
> >
> > The improvement of all aspects of environmental and industrial hygiene;
> >
> > The prevention, treatment and control of epidemic, endemic, occupational and other diseases;
> >
> > The creation of conditions which would assure to all medical service and medical attention in the event of sickness.

General Comment No. 14   In 2000, the United Nations' Committee on Economic, Social and Cultural Rights issued General Comment No. 14, which addresses "substantive issues arising in the implementation of the International Covenant on Economic, Social and Cultural Rights" with respect to Article 12 and "the right to the highest attainable standard of health."[8] The General Comment provides more explicit, operational language on the freedoms and entitlements included under a right to health.

The General Comment makes the direct clarification that "the *right to health* is not to be understood as a *right to be healthy.*" Instead, the right to health is articulated as a set of both freedoms and entitlements which accommodate the individual's biological and social conditions as well as the State's available resources, both of which may preclude a *right to be healthy* for reasons beyond the influence or control of the State. Article 12 tasks the State with recognizing that each individual holds an inherent right to the best feasible standard of health, and itemizes (at least in part) the 'freedoms from' and 'entitlements to' that accompany such a right; however, it does not charge the State with ensuring that all individuals, in fact, are fully healthy, nor that all individuals have made full recognition of the rights and opportunities enumerated in the right to health.

Relation to other rights   Like the Universal Declaration of Human Rights, the General Comment clarifies the interrelated nature of human rights, stating that, "the right to health is closely related to and dependent upon the realization of other human rights," and thereby underscoring the importance of advancements in other entitlements such as the rights to food, work, housing, life, non-discrimination, human dignity, and access to importance, among others, towards the recognition of the right to health. Similarly, the General Comment acknowledges that "the right to health embraces a wide range of socio-economic factors that promote conditions in which people can lead a healthy life, and extends to the underlying determinants of health." In this respect, the General Comment holds that the specific steps towards realizing the right to health enumerated in Article 12 are non-exhaustive and strictly illustrative in nature.

Health equity   The General Comment also makes additional reference to the question of health equity, a concept not addressed in the initial International Covenant. The document notes, "The Covenant proscribes any discrimination in access to health care and underlying determinants of health, as well as to means and entitlements for their procurement." Moreover, responsibility for ameliorating discrimination and its effects with regards to health is delegated to the State: "States have a special obligation to provide those who do not have sufficient means with the necessary health insurance and health-care facilities, and to prevent any discrimination on internationally prohibited grounds in the provision of health care and health services." Additional emphasis is placed upon non-discrimination on the basis of gender, age, disability, or membership in indigenous communities.

Responsibilities of states and international organizations   Subsequent sections of the General Comment detail the obligations of nations and international organizations towards a right to health. The obligations of nations are placed into three categories: obligations to respect, obligations to protect, and obligations to fulfill the right to health. Examples of these (in non-exhaustive fashion) include preventing discrimination in access or delivery of care; refraining from limitations to contraceptive access or family planning; restricting denial of access to health information; reducing environmental pollution; restricting coercive and/or harmful culturally-based medical practices; ensuring equitable access to social determinants of health; and providing proper guidelines for the accreditation of medical facilities, personnel, and equipment. International obligations include allowing for the enjoyment of health in other countries; preventing violations of health in other countries; cooperating in the provision of humanitarian aid for disasters and emergencies; and refraining from use of embargoes on medical goods or personnel as an act of political or economic influence.

Convention on the Elimination of All Forms of Discrimination Against Women

Article 12 of the 1979 United Nations Convention on the Elimination of All Forms of Discrimination against Women outlines women's protection from gender discrimination when receiving health services and women's entitlement to specific gender-related healthcare provisions. The full text of Article 12 states:[9]

> **Article 12**:
>
> 1. States Parties shall take all appropriate measures to eliminate discrimination against women in the field of health care in order to ensure, on a basis of equality of men and women, access to health care services, including those related to family planning.
>
> 2. Notwithstanding the provisions of paragraph I of this article, States Parties shall ensure to women appropriate services in connection with pregnancy, confinement and the post-natal period, granting free services where necessary, as well as adequate nutrition during pregnancy and lactation.

Convention on the Rights of the Child

Health is mentioned on several instances in the Convention on the Rights of the Child (1989). Article 3 calls upon parties to ensure that institutions and facilities for the care of children adhere to health standards. Article 17 recognizes the child's right to access information that is pertinent to his/her physical and mental health and well-being. Article

23 makes specific reference to the rights of disabled children, in which it includes health services, rehabilitation, preventive care. Article 24 outlines child health in detail, and states, "Parties recognize the right of the child to the enjoyment of the highest attainable standard of health and to facilities for the treatment of illness and rehabilitation of health. States shall strive to ensure that no child is deprived of his or her right of access to such health care services." Towards implementation of this provision, the Convention enumerates the following measures:[10]

- To diminish infant and child mortality;
- To ensure the provision of necessary medical assistance and health care to all children with emphasis on the development of primary health care;
- To combat disease and malnutrition, including within the framework of primary health care, through, inter alia, the application of readily available technology and through the provision of adequate nutritious foods and clean drinking-water, taking into consideration the dangers and risks of environmental pollution;
- To ensure appropriate pre-natal and post-natal health care for mothers;
- To ensure that all segments of society, in particular parents and children, are informed, have access to education and are supported in the use of basic knowledge of child health and nutrition, the advantages of breastfeeding, hygiene and environmental sanitation and the prevention of accidents;
- To develop preventive health care, guidance for parents and family planning education and services.

The World Health Organization website comments, "The CRC is the normative and legal framework for WHO's work across the broad spectrum of child and adolescent health."[11] Goldhagen presents the CRC as a "template for child advocacy" and proposes its use as a framework for reducing disparities and improving outcomes in child health.[12]

Convention on the Rights of Persons with Disabilities

Article 25 of the Convention on the Rights of Persons with Disabilities (2006) specifies that "persons with disabilities have the right to the enjoyment of the highest attainable standard of health without discrimination on the basis of disability." The sub-clauses of Article 25 state that States

shall give the disabled the same "range, quality, and standard" of health care as it provides to other persons, as well as those services specifically required for prevention, identification, and management of disability. Further provisions specify that health care for the disabled should be made available in local communities and that care should be geographically equitable, with additional statements against the denial or unequal provision of health services (including "food and fluids" and "life insurance") on the basis of disability.[13]

Hendriks criticizes the failure of the Convention to define specifically the term "disability"; he contends further that "the absence of a clear description [...] may prejudice the uniform interpretation, or at least place in jeopardy the consistent protection the Convention seeks to guarantee." [14] He does, however, acknowledge that the lack of a clear definition for "disability" may benefit the disabled by limiting the State's ability to limit extension of the Convention's provisions to specific populations or those with certain conditions.

Definitions in academic literature

While most human rights are theoretically framed as *negative rights,* meaning that they are areas upon which society cannot interfere or restrict by political action, Mervyn Susser contends that the right to health is a particularly unique and challenging right because it is often expressed as a *positive right,* where society bears an obligation to provide certain resources and opportunities to the general population.

Susser further sets out four provisions that he sees as covered under a right to health: equitable access to health and medical services; a "good-faith" social effort to promote equal health among different social groups; means to measure and assess health equity; and equal sociopolitical systems to give all parties a unique voice in health advocacy and promotion. He is careful to note here that, while this likely entails some minimum standard of access to health resources, it does not guarantee or necessitate an equitable state of health for each person due to inherent biological differences in health status.[15] This distinction is an important one, as some common critiques of a "right to health" are that it establishes a right to an unreachable standard and that it aspires to a state of health that is too subjectively variable from person to person or from one society to the next.[16]

While Susser's discussion centers on healthcare as a positive right, Paul Hunt refutes this view and makes the argument that the right to health also encompasses certain negative rights such as a protection from discrimination and the right to not receive medical treatment without the recipient's voluntary consent. However, Hunt does concede that some positive rights, such as the responsibility of society to pay special attention to the health needs of the underserved and vulnerable, are included in the right to health.[17]

Paul Farmer addresses the issue of unequal access to health care in his article, "The Major Infectious Diseases in the World - To Treat or Not to Treat." He discusses the growing "outcome gap" between the populations receiving health interventions and the ones that are not. Poor people are not receiving the same treatment, if any at all, as the more financially fortunate. The high costs of medicine and treatment make it problematic for poor countries to receive equal care. He states, "Excellence without equity looms as the chief human-rights dilemma of health care in the 21st century."[18]

3.14.2 Human right to health care

An alternative way to conceptualize one facet of the right to health is a "human right to health **care**." Notably, this encompasses both patient and provider rights in the delivery of healthcare services, the latter being similarly open to frequent abuse by the states.[19] Patient rights in health care delivery include: the right to privacy, information, life, and quality care, as well as freedom from discrimination, torture, and cruel, inhumane, or degrading treatment.[19][20] Marginalized groups, such as migrants and persons who have been displaced, racial and ethnic minorities, women, sexual minorities, and those living with HIV, are particularly vulnerable to violations of human rights in healthcare settings.[21][22] For instance, racial and ethnic minorities may be segregated into poorer quality wards, disabled persons may be contained and forcibly medicated, drug users may be denied addiction treatment, women may be forced into vaginal examinations and may be denied life-saving abortions, suspected homosexual men may be forced into anal examinations, and women of marginalized groups and transgender persons may be forcibly sterilized.[22][23]

Provider rights include: the right to quality standards of working conditions, the right to associate freely, and the right to refuse to perform a procedure based on their morals.[19] Healthcare providers often experience violations of their rights. For instance, particularly in countries with weak rule of law, healthcare providers are often forced to perform procedures which negate their morals, deny marginalized groups the best possible standards of care, breach patient confidentiality, and conceal crimes against humanity and torture.[24][25] Furthermore, providers who do not oblige these pressures are often persecuted.[24] Currently, especially in the United States, much debate surrounds the issue of "provider consciousness", which retains the right of providers to abstain from performing pro-

cedures that do not align with their moral code, such as abortions.[26][27]

Legal reform as a mechanism to combat and prevent violations of patient and provider rights presents a promising approach. However, in transitional countries (newly formed countries undergoing reform), and other settings with weak rule of law, may be limited.[19] Resources and tools for lawyers, providers, and patients interested in improving human rights in patient care have been formulated.[19]

3.14.3 Criticism

Some scholars have questioned or criticized the concept of a right to health. Philip Barlow writes that health care should not be considered a human right because of the difficulty of defining what it entails and where the 'minimum standard' of entitlements under the right ought to be established. Additionally, Barlow contends that rights establish duties upon others to protect or guarantee them, and that it is unclear who holds the social responsibility for the right to health.[28] John Berkeley, in agreement with Barlow, critiques further that the right to health does not consider adequately the responsibility that an individual has to uphold his or her own health.[29]

Richard D Lamm vehemently argues against making healthcare a right. He defines a right as one that is to be defended at all costs, and a concept that is defined and interpreted by the judicial system. Making healthcare a right would require governments to spend a large portion of its resources to provide its citizens with it. He asserts that the healthcare system is based on the erroneous assumption of unlimited resources. Limited resources inhibits governments from providing everyone with adequate healthcare, especially in the long term. Attempting to provide "beneficial" healthcare to all people utilizing limited resources could lead to economical collapse. Lamm asserts that access to healthcare but a small part in producing a healthy society, and to create a healthy society, resources should also be spent on social resources.[30]

Another criticism of the right to health is that it is not feasible. Imre J.P. Loefler argues that the financial and logistical burdens of ensuring health care for all are unattainable, and that resource constraints make it unrealistic to justify a right towards prolonging life indefinitely. Instead, Loefler suggests that the goal of improving population health is better served through socioeconomic policy than a formal right to health.[31]

3.14.4 See also

- Health and Human Rights journal

- Universal health care

3.14.5 References

[1] *Constitution of the World Health Organization* (PDF). Geneva: World Health Organization. 1948.

[2] Grad, Frank P. (Jan 2002). "The Preamble of the Constitution of the World Health Organization" (PDF). *Bulletin of the World Health Organization.* **80** (12): 981.

[3] *Universal Declaration of Human Rights,* United Nations, 1948

[4] Pillai, Navanethem (Dec 2008). "Right to Health and the Universal Declaration of Human Rights" (PDF). *The Lancet.* **372** (9655): 2005–2006. doi:10.1016/S0140-6736(08)61783-3. Retrieved 14 Oct 2013.

[5] Gruskin, Sofia; Edward J. Mills; Daniel Tarantola (August 2007). "History, Principles, and Practice of Health and Human Rights". *The Lancet.* **370** (9585): 449–455. doi:10.1016/S0140-6736(07)61200-8.

[6] *International Convention on the Elimination of All Forms of Racial Discrimination,* United Nations, 1965

[7] *International Covenant on Economic, Social and Cultural Rights,* United Nations, 1966

[8] *General Comment No. 14.* Geneva: UN Committee on Economic, Social and Cultural Rights. 2000.

[9] *Convention on the Elimination of All Forms of Discrimination against Women.* New York: United Nations. 1979.

[10] *Convention on the Rights of the Child.* New York: United Nations. 1989.

[11] "Child Rights". World Health Organization. Retrieved 5 November 2013.

[12] Goldhagen, Jeffrey (Sep 2003). "Children's Rights and the United Nations Convention on the Rights of the Child". *Pediatrics.* **112** (Supp. 3): 742–745. PMID 12949339. Retrieved 5 November 2013.

[13] "Convention on the Rights of Persons with Disabilities". Un.org. 2007-03-30. Retrieved 2013-11-07.

[14] Hendriks, Aart (Nov 2007). "UN Convention on the Rights of Persons with Disabilities". *European Journal of Health Law.* **14** (3): 273–298. doi:10.1163/092902707X240620.

[15] Susser, Mervyn (Mar 1993). "Health as a Human Right: An Epidemiologist's Perspective on the Public Health" (PDF). *American Journal of Public Health.* **83** (3): 418–426. doi:10.2105/ajph.83.3.418. PMC 1694643. PMID 8438984. Retrieved 14 November 2013.

[16] Toebes, Brigit (Aug 1999). "Towards an Improved Understanding of the International Human Right to Health". *Human Rights Quarterly.* **21** (3): 661–679. doi:10.1353/hrq.1999.0044. JSTOR 762669.

[17] Hunt, Paul (Mar 2006). "The Human Right to the Highest Attainable Standard of Health: New Opportunities and Challenges" (PDF). *Transactions of the Royal Society of Tropical Medicine and Hygiene.* **100**: 603–607. doi:10.1016/j.trstmh.2006.03.001. Retrieved 14 November 2013.

[18] Farmer, Paul. 2001. The Major Infectious Diseases in the World -- To Treat or Not to Treat? N Engl J Med 345 (3):208-210.

[19] Beletsky L, Ezer T, Overall J, Byrne I, Cohen J (2013). "Advancing human rights in patient care: the law in seven transitional countries". *Open Society Foundations.*

[20] Open Society Institute. (2013). "Health and human rights: a resource guide". *Open Society Foundations.*

[21] Ezer T. (May 2013). "making laws work for patients". *Open Society Foundations.*

[22] J Amon. (2010). "Abusing patients: health providers' complicity in torture and cruel, inhuman or degrading treatment". *World Report 2010, Human Rights Watch.*

[23] Ezer T. (May 2013). "Making Laws Work for Patients". *Open Society Foundations.*

[24] International Dual Loyalty Working Group. (1993). "Dual Loyalty & Human Rights in Health Professional Practice: Proposed Guidelines & Institutional Mechanisms" (PDF).

[25] F Hashemian; et al. (2008). "Broken laws, broken lives: medical evidence of torture by US personnel and its impact" (PDF). *Physicians for Human Rights.*

[26] CNN. (2008). "Rule aims to protect health providers' right of conscience". *CNNHealth.com.*

[27] T Stanton Collett. (2004). "Protecting the healthcare provider's right of conscience". *Trinity International University, the Center for Bioethics and Human Dignity.*

[28] Barlow, Philip (31 Jul 1999). "Health Care Is Not a Human Right". *British Medical Journal.* **319** (7205): 321. doi:10.1136/bmj.319.7205.321. PMC 1126951. PMID 10426762.

[29] Berkeley, John (4 Aug 1999). "Health Care Is Not a Human Right". *British Medical Journal.* **319** (7205): 321. doi:10.1136/bmj.319.7205.321. PMC 1126951. PMID 10426762. Retrieved 14 November 2013.

[30] Lamm, R. (1998), "The case against making healthcare a "right."", *American Bar Association: Defending Liberty Pursuing Justice,* **25** (4), pp. 8–11, JSTOR 27880117

[31] Loefler, Imre J.P. (26 Jun 1999). ""Health Care Is a Human Right" Is a Meaningless and Devastating Manifesto". *British Medical Journal.* **318** (7200): 1766. doi:10.1136/bmj.318.7200.1766a. PMC 1116108. PMID 10381735.

3.14.6   External links

- Joint Fact Sheet WHO/OHCHR/323

- The Right to Health cartoon

- Right to health on the Children's Rights Portal

- General Comment No. 14. The right to the highest attainable standard of health CESCR, 2000

- The right to health and the European Social Charter Secretariat of ESC, 2009

- The Right to Health: Fact Sheet No. 31 WHO and UN HCHR

- 25 Questions & Answers on Health and Human Rights, WHO

3.14.7   Bibliography

- Andrew Clapham, Mary Robinson (eds), Realizing the Right to Health, Zurich: rüffer & rub, 2009.

- Bogumil Terminski, Selected Bibliography on Human Right to Health, Geneva: University of Geneva, 2013.

- Judith Paula Asher, The Right to Health: A Resource Manual for Ngos, Dordrecht: Martinus Nijhoff Publishers, 2010. I

3.15   Two-tier healthcare

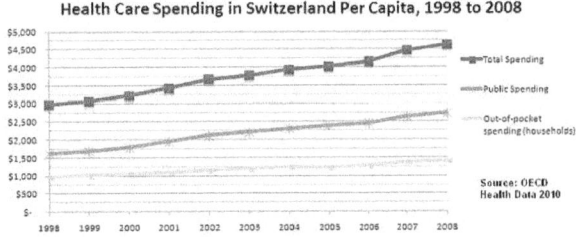

This graph contrasts total health care spending with public spending, in US dollars adjusted for purchasing power parity in Switzerland.

Two-tier healthcare is a situation in which a basic government-provided healthcare system provides basic care, and a secondary tier of care exists for those who can pay for additional, better quality or faster access. Most countries have both publicly and privately funded healthcare, but the degree to which it creates a quality differential depends on the way the two systems are managed, funded, and regulated.

Some publicly funded universal healthcare systems deliver excellent service and the private system tends to be small and not highly differentiated. In other, typically poorer countries, the public health system is underfunded and overstretched, offering opportunities for private companies to deliver better-quality, albeit more expensive coverage.Chen, Zhang, & Hua. (2015). Analysis of two-tier public service systems under a government subsidy policy. Computers & Industrial Engineering, 90, 146-157.

3.15.1   Canada

Main article: Healthcare in Canada

In Canada, there are private and public healthcare providers with complete patient freedom of choice between which doctors and facilities to use.

The public financing system, unofficially known as Medicare, consists of several different systems managed by each province or territory. The federal government distributes funds to the provinces for healthcare providing the provinces design their systems to meet certain criteria which they all do. Most people receiving care in Canada do not pay for their care. The medical provider gets paid a fixed fee for the care provided. The law bans the medical provider from charging patients to supplement their income from Medicare. Medical care providers can set their own fees that are higher than the Medicare reimbursement fee, but the patient must pay all the cost of care, not just the excess.

About 70% of Canada's healthcare funding is via the public system. Another 30% comes from private funding, divided approximately equally between out-of-pocket funding and private insurance, which may be complementary (meeting costs not covered by the public system such as the cost of prescription medicines, dental treatments and copayments) or supplementary (adding more choice of provider or providing faster access to care)[1] There are, however, financial disincentives that make private medicine for services that are covered by Medicare less economic.

Six of Canada's ten provinces used to ban private insurance for publicly insured services to inhibit queue jumping and so preserve fairness in the health care system. In a complex legal decision in 2005, the Supreme Court of Canada ruled that in some circumstances, such bans can be illegal if the waiting period was unduly long.

Some private hospitals operating while the national healthcare plan was instituted (for example, the Shouldice Hernia Centre in Thornhill, Ontario) continue to operate, but they may not bill additional charges for medical procedures. (The Shouldice Hospital, however, has mandatory additional room charges not covered by public health insurance. That effectively places it in the "upper tier" of a two-tier system. Welfare recipients, for example, cannot be referred there.)

Clinics are usually private operations but may not bill additional charges. Private healthcare may also be supplied, both in uncovered fields and to foreigners.

3.15.2   Denmark

Healthcare in Denmark, although primarily subsidised by the government at the county and the national levels health, is supported by complementary insurance plans to cover elective services not covered by the public system; they also help cover copayments.

3.15.3   France

Healthcare in France is a system of private and public physicians, who largely draw their income from the government. There are public as well as private hospitals.

Patients pay a small copayment for certain aspects of care, but many people choose to cover the costs by taking out supplemental health insurance for which a small premium is payable each year.

Thus, France also has a mixed delivery system with complete patient freedom of supplier choice. There is a two-tier funding arrangement, with compulsory funding of core medical services from taxation, with optional private insurance for the cost of copayments.

3.15.4   Germany

Healthcare in Germany has multiple sickness funds, either publicly owned or not-for-profit mutuals. Membership of a sickness fund is compulsory for everyone except certain people earning an income above a certain level, who opt out of the insurance system altogether. Doctors are usually self-employed, and hospitals may be publicly owned, privately owned or not for profit.

3.15.5   Ireland

Healthcare in the Republic of Ireland is financed mainly by the state. However, all citizens have the option of buying additional private health insurance, provided by four companies. They include VHI, a large publicly owned insurer, operating, like all other insurers, community rating; people are insured at the same basic rate regardless of health status. The other insurers are Glo Healthcare, LAYA and Avivia. Also, much smaller restricted membership companies provide benefits for certain professions, such as police officers.

There are public as well as private hospitals. Private patients are often treated in public hospitals, as all privately insured patients have an entitlement to use the publicly funded system.

3.15.6   Netherlands

Healthcare in the Netherlands is essentially single tier, with all persons accessing a common system of private and public providers with complete freedom of choice between providers. Insurers are all private companies. It is heavily subsidized from tax revenues and heavily regulated, with a common, regulated standard insurance policy coverage set nationwide for all providers and a more flexible top up insurance, which is less regulated and set by each company as it chooses.

Insurers set a standard price for each adult for the year for a given region of the country and must insure all people who apply for insurance at that price regardless of the age or health status of the applicant. An equalization fund, which is essentially a national sickness fund funded from a form of income tax on employers and employees, is used to pay for the health care of all children and to compensate insurers if they have more high risk profile clients than the other insurers.

Thus, Dutch insurers welcome the sick and the elderly because they are fully compensated for the higher-risk profile of these clients. People living in more expensive areas of the country have to pay higher premiums, but the elderly and the sick pay the same premiums as everyone else in that region. Social insurance covers the insurance costs of those with limited incomes, such as the unemployed and the permanently disabled.

3.15.7   Singapore

Healthcare in Singapore uses a true two-tier system for both the provider network and the insurance funds. A government-sponsored and subsidized system of hospitals accepts all patients, with a guaranteed list of services. A parallel system of private hospitals provides services not available in public hospitals or available with extra amenities (such as private rooms and other boutique services).

Singapore uses a universal insurance fund in which all citizens are required to participate, as a baseline. Seniors and certain groups are subsidised in their membership in the universal basic insurance fund.

Optional additional supplementary insurance funds are available for purchase for elective coverage, such as for plastic surgery or for extra amenities in hospital.

3.15.8 Switzerland

Healthcare in Switzerland mandates participation in a national healthcare system for all residents. Public hospitals are subsidised, but there are also private hospitals that provide additional services, such as elective services.

In addition to a national universal insurance fund, optional complementary and supplementary private insurance funds are available for purchase.

3.15.9 United Kingdom

The National Health Service (or NHS) provides universal coverage to all residents of the United Kingdom.

Private healthcare has continued parallel to the NHS, paid for largely by private insurance, and is used by about 8% of the population, generally as an add-on to NHS services and mostly obtained by employer funded insurance schemes. That is a taxable benefit to the employee, the value imputed by the tax authorities as income to the beneficiary. Because NHS services are so comprehensive, there are many areas in which the private sector usually does not compete and private insurers almost always refuse to fund. Childbirth and perinatal services are good examples.

Conversely, there are some areas where the NHS does not offer free treatment (cosmetic surgery for vanity purposes, for example) and so the private sector offers a pay-for-service alternative.

Historically, avoiding waiting lists was the main reason that patients opted out of NHS treatment and into private care. Queues of many months were once common. NHS Consultants, who can run both NHS and private services during their NHS contracts, used to be in charge of waiting lists and had a financial incentive to keep the public waiting list long, to ensure a stream of private income to the private business.

Since the Blair government reforms of the NHS, strict rules apply to waiting lists (see hospital choice in the NHS). That and the allocation of better funding in hospitals both reduced waiting times significantly. Most hospital patients are in fact not admitted from a list at all, and those that do, on average, wait less than 9 weeks. Nobody should wait

more than 18 weeks. The 18 weeks is not dead time because it includes the time taken to book a first appointment, to conduct all the tests, for the doctor and patient to agree on the desired treatment, and to book and execute an operation or commence the treatment regime. A patient not seen in the 18 week period without just cause has the legal right to go private at the NHS's expense.

As a result of these improvements, long waiting times reduced, and the private healthcare sector now sells its surplus capacity to the NHS. Dentistry is an area where many practitioners prefer to work privately (because they can set their own fees). NHS dentistry can then be patchy, and some people may find that private dentistry is the only practical option open to them in their locality.

There has always been a degree of private medicine conducted within NHS hospitals, with private work being done in those hospitals and the patient being accommodated in segregated accommodation. Until recently, few NHS patients were ever treated in private hospitals. In the English NHS, however, there has been greater willingness to outsource some work to the private sector, and so some NHS patients do sometimes gain access to private health care facilities at public expense. The equivalent NHS operations in Wales, Scotland and Northern Ireland do not often fund treatment outside of their own facilities.

Whether the NHS funds treatment in a private hospital is a decision for the local commissioning health authority based on formal service contracts.

3.15.10 United States

Further information: Health care in the United States and Obamacare

The United States has a two-tier health system, but most of the population cannot gain access to the public provision tiers. Healthcare provided directly by the government is limited to military and veteran families and to certain Native American tribes. Certain cities and towns also provide free care directly but only to those who cannot afford to pay. Medicare, Medicaid, and the State Children's Health Insurance Program pay for health care obtained at private facilities but only for the elderly, disabled, and children in poor families. Since enacting the Patient Protection and Affordable Care Act in 2010, Medicaid has been substantially expanded, and federal subsidies are available for low-to middle-income individuals and families to purchase private health insurance.

The debate over healthcare reform in the United States has included a proposal for a public option or Medicare for all, a government-run insurance program, available to all US citizens, to compete with or replace private insurance plans.

3.15.11   See also

- Health in Trinidad and Tobago
- Canadian and American health care systems compared
- Health care compared – tabular comparisons of the US, Canada, and other countries not shown above
- Universal health care

3.15.12   References

[1] *Exploring the 70/30 Split: How Canada's Health Care System Is Financed* (PDF), Canadian Institute for Health Information, 2005, retrieved 2009-05-27

3.16   Vermont health care reform

In 2011, the Vermont state government enacted a law functionally establishing the first state-level single-payer health care system in the United States. Green Mountain Care, established by the passage of H.202, creates a system in the state where Vermonters receive universal health care coverage as well as technological improvements to the existing system.

On December 17, 2014, Vermont Democrats abandoned their plan for universal health care, citing the taxes required of smaller businesses within the state.[1]

3.16.1   Planning

In 2010, the State Legislature passed S 88 (which included provisions from Act 128), which enabled the state of Vermont to establish a commission to study different forms of health care delivery in the state.[2] Dr. William Hsiao, a Harvard University professor of economics who was an advisor during Taiwan's transition to single-payer health care,[3] was enlisted to design three possible options to reform Vermont's health care.[4] Hsaio, along with Steven Kappel and Jonathan Gruber, presented the proposal to the legislature of Vermont on June 21, 2010.[5]

The three options were laid out as follows:

- **Option 1**: As laid out by the requirements of Act 128, the first option would create "a government-administered and publicly financed single-payer health benefit system decoupled from employment which prohibits insurance coverage for the health services

provided by this system and allows for private insurance coverage only of supplemental health services."[5] The proposal considered this option to be the easiest path to single-payer, but was critical of the "complex and inefficient process" of proof of residency needs.[5]

- **Option 2**: As laid out by the requirements of S 88, the second option would create "a public health benefit option administered by state government, which allows individuals to choose between the public option and private insurance coverage and allows for fair and robust competition among public and private plans."[5] The commission noted that this option did not provide universal coverage on its own or the enforcement mechanism in place for any possible mandates put in place to achieve more coverage.[5]

- **Option 3**: Act 128 allowed the commission to design a system that met the various principles outlined in Section 2 of the Act.[2] The commission's design ultimately sought out an "approach to Option 3... by combining three studies to ascertain what type of universal health insurance, what methods of financing, and what type of single payer system is most likely to be politically and practically viable for Vermont."[5]

The commission's proposal ultimately considered the third option to be "the most politically and practically viable single payer system for Vermont," noting that Vermont, "a small state with communitarian values," with its existing network of non-profit hospitals and a medical structure that had shown previous support in state intervention, would be "uniquely poised to pass universal health reform."[5]

3.16.2   Legislation

Following the proposal, Democratic state senator Mark Larson introduced H 202 on February 8, 2011, titled Single-Payer and Unified Health System.[6] The bill passed the House on March 24, 2011, with 94 votes in favor and 49 against.[6][7] The bill then passed the Senate on April 26, 2011, with 21 votes in favor and 9 against.[6][8] The conference report legislation passed the Senate on May 3, 2011 with 21 votes in favor and 9 opposed, and the House on May 4, 2011 with 94 votes in favor and 49 against.[6][9] Governor Peter Shumlin signed the bill on May 26, 2011.[6]

Green Mountain Care

The signing of H. 202 led to the creation of Green Mountain Care, described by Kaiser Health News as "a state-funded-and-managed insurance pool that would provide near-universal coverage to residents with the expectation that it would reduce health care spending."[10] Governor Shumlin, in a blog post at *Huffington Post*, described the plan as "a single payer system" that he believed "will control health care costs, not just by cutting fees to doctors and hospitals, but by fundamentally changing the state's health care system."[11] As of January 2013, Vermont was still working out the role of Green Mountain Care and the responsibilities of the bill, as well as how to fund the program. Dr. Hsiao, for example, had proposed an 11% payroll tax on employers, and the administration was required under Act 48 to provide a financing system in 2013.[12] The state also had to align Green Mountain Care with provisions in the Patient Protection and Affordable Care Act, passed by the United States federal government in 2010, which required the creation of a health care exchange in individual states. To launch fully, Green Mountain Care would have had to gain approval from the federal government to use federal health finances to fund the state program.

As of April 2014, Vermont had yet to craft a bill that would address the $2 billion in extra spending necessary to fund the single-payer system,[13][14] and by the end of the year, the state abandoned their plan for universal health care, citing the taxes required of smaller businesses within the state.[1]

3.16.3 Popular opinion and reactions

Dr. Hsiao, in his proposal, noted that "a two-thirds majority of Vermonters said that all Vermonters should be able to get the health care they need when they need it, regardless of their ability to pay even if this means that they would have to pay higher taxes and higher insurance premiums themselves."[5] The bill was passed in the Vermont legislature on party line votes, with Democrats and Progressives in favor and Republicans against. The bill is considered the first single-payer bill to be passed on the state level, but private insurers can continue to operate in the state. Representative Larson has described Green Mountain Care's provisions as "as close as we can get [to single-payer] at the state level."[15]

According to Leigh Tofferi, the director of government, public and community relations for Blue Cross Blue Shield of Vermont, the lack of initial specifics was causing "anxiety" to many providers. The Vermont Medical Society had no position on the bill or on single-payer in general. David Himmelstein, the founder of Physicians for a National Health Program, a single-payer advocacy group, was critical of the plan due to the ability of private insurers to operate in the state, arguing that the plan "give[s] up a significant part of the administrative savings by doing that," but agreeing that Green Mountain Care "lays the foundation" for single-payer.[15]

In the 2014 gubernatorial election, Governor Shumlin was heavily favored for re-election but only received a plurality of the vote, 46.4%, to Republican Scott Milne's 45.1%. The election was decided by the Vermont General Assembly on January 8, 2015; Shumlin defeated Milne by a vote of 110 to 69.[16] *The Burlington Free Press* ascribed the result, in part, to voters' dissatisfaction with the progress the state had made in instituting single-payer health care.[17]

3.16.4 Aftermath

One of the problems found since the abandonment of the Vermont Health Care initiatives is questionable billing from Jonathan Gruber, who according to CNBC has come into connection because of the contract.[18] According to a Vermont State report filed by Doug Hoffer,[19] an invoice sent by Gruber to Vermont on December 30, 2014 for $40,000 increased the amount of scrutiny on the billing.[20]

3.16.5 References

[1] Governor abandons single-payer health care plan, yahoo.com, December 17, 2014

[2] S 88 Archived October 19, 2013, at the Wayback Machine.: An act relating to health care financing and universal access to health care in Vermont. As passed by House and Senate, 2010.

[3] *New York Times*: Health Care Abroad: Taiwan. November 3, 2009.

[4] Vermont Public Radio: Dr. William Hsiao on health care system reform. January 20, 2011.

[5] The Vermont Option: Achieving Affordable Universal Health Care. Dr. William Hsiao, Steven Kappel, Jonathan Gruber, and a team of health policy analysts, June 21, 2010.

[6] Project VoteSmart: H 202 - SINGLE-PAYER AND UNIFIED HEALTH SYSTEM - KEY VOTE.

[7] H. 202

[8] "Vt. Senate approves single-payer plan". Wcax.com. 2011-04-26. Retrieved 2014-12-29.

[9] H. 202 conference report.

[10] Kaiser Health News: Vermont Edges Toward Single Payer. October 2, 2011.

[11] *Huffington Post*: The Economic Urgency of Health Care Reform. August 5, 2011.

[12] *Vermont Business Magazine*: Health care committee to look at insurance subsidies, financing for single payer, role of Green Mountain Care Board. January 14, 2013.

[13] *Bloomberg*: Vermont's Single-Payer Dream is Taxpayer Nightmare. April 24, 2014.

[14] Vox: Forget Obamacare: Vermont wants to bring single-payer to America. April 9, 2014.

[15] American Medical News: Vermont approves universal health program. May 16, 2011.

[16] Free Press Staff (January 8, 2015). "Shumlin defeats Milne in Legislature governor vote". Retrieved May 31, 2015.

[17] "How a two-term incumbent governor nearly lost". Burlington Free Press. November 6, 2014. Retrieved November 11, 2014.

[18] "Obamacare guru Gruber had 'questionable' billing: Audit". CNBC. February 25, 2015. Retrieved February 27, 2015.

[19] "Gruber contract memo final" (PDF). STATE OF VERMONT OFFICE OF THE STATE AUDITOR. February 23, 2015.

[20] "Report: Gruber May Have Overbilled VT". Local 22. February 23, 2015. Retrieved February 27, 2015.

3.16.6   External links

- Vermont's Health Care Reform Portal

- Green Mountain Care

Chapter 4

Text and image sources, contributors, and licenses

4.1 Text

- **Publicly funded health care** *Source:* https://en.wikipedia.org/wiki/Publicly_funded_health_care?oldid=766961621 *Contributors:* Derek Ross, SimonP, Mintguy, Kemkim, Gabbe, Mic, Paul Benjamin Austin, Minesweeper, G-Man, Popsracer, Charles Matthews, Daniel Quinlan, Selket, Nv8200pa, Pakaran, David.Monniaux, Guppy, TruthBeTold~enwiki, Greaser, Bkalafut, Kowey, Seglea, Diberri, Dmn, TOttenville8, Mboverload, Sievert, Djegan, Formeruser-83, Bobblewik, Edcolins, Jmcnamera, Sam Hocevar, Creidieki, Neutrality, Jcw69, Randwicked, Lacrimosus, Kingal86, Rich Farmbrough, Loganberry, Pak21, Notinasnaid, Xezbeth, Bumhoolery, BenjBot, Solers, Shoujun, Reinyday, Silverback, Pearle, Joolz, John Quiggin, Peregrine1, Bz2, Jrleighton, Dtcdthingy, Instantnood, Dryman, Dan100, Mwparenteau, Bastin, FrancisTyers, Mindmatrix, Sprewell, Spymanut, DrThompson, Pol098, Nklatt, Linkspro, SDC, Deltabeignet, Dpv, Drbogdan, Rjwilmsi, Nightscream, PinchasC, PHenry, Vegaswikian, Ligulem, Fred Bradstadt, Baldwin.jim, Deus777, AED, Tombombadil, RobyWayne, Wavelength, RussBot, Hauskalainen, Anonymous editor, Tony1, Blindjustice, JPK, BrownHornet21, AdBo, Mais oui!, Rathfelder, SmackBot, Srnec, Blackfield, Selizabethr, Chris the speller, Thumperward, DHeyward, JonHarder, RolandR, BlueGoose, LiamInCa, Craig Bolon, Flamingblur, Beetstra, Hu12, Levineps, Walton One, Deetdeet, Imacsam, IntrigueBlue, Argon233, LyptonVillage, Centuriono, Kborer, Aquilosion, Klausness, Joe Schmedley, Yellowdesk, Caesarjbsquitti, Matamoros, Mbhiii, Nbauman, Jorfer, Juliancolton, UnicornTapestry, Philip Trueman, Jethro 82, Sfmammamia, Mangostar, MaynardClark, Freedomwarrior, Ravanacker, Dabomb87, Hordaland, Escape Orbit, Sneyton, ClueBot, SomeGuy11112, Historian 1000, Calwolf, Fishiehelper2, Chemnin, DumZiBoT, Doopdoop, BigK HeX, EastTN, Danielroberts, HexaChord, Addbot, Lifeguard Emeritus, Lightbot, Yobot, Randersonn, AnomieBOT, Goodrule, Ulric1313, Citation bot, Kjerzycke, Nugteren, Prowler08, Eet1, Cosmic Cowboy, Alpha-ZX, LincolnSt, Jade0970, Norcelt, Dcirovic, RickRowden, Jesanj, Sugar-Baby-Love, ClueBot NG, Snotbot, Dr.Shah1996, JustBerry, Drchriswilliams, Monkbot, Augerspectre, Rubbish computer, KasparBot, Bender the Bot, Concus Cretus, ThisIsTemp and Anonymous: 146

- **Single-payer healthcare** *Source:* https://en.wikipedia.org/wiki/Single-payer_healthcare?oldid=766436362 *Contributors:* Gabbe, Ronabop, Darkwind, Kaihsu, Selket, DJ Clayworth, Nv8200pa, Wetman, Catskul, E0N, Andrew Levine, HangingCurve, Karn, Jason Quinn, Edcolins, Pgan002, Neutrality, Paradoxian, Klemen Kocjancic, Gerrit, Picapica, Rich Farmbrough, Mrevan, Jjb, Bender235, Tom, Sentience, Alansohn, Rd232, Dachannien, John Quiggin, Wikidea, Netkinetic, Kenyon, TShilo12, Skeejay, Richard Arthur Norton (1958-), Mindmatrix, Scjessey, DanielZimmerman, Rtdrury, Tynman, Rotten, Rjwilmsi, Vegaswikian, Momothemonster, Ground Zero, AED, Nogburt, Gary Cziko, King of Hearts, Mhking, Arzel, Hauskalainen, Wiki alf, Daniel Simanek, Shepazu, Rathfelder, SmackBot, PiCo, Jerdwyer, Cdogsimmons, Half-Shadow, Evilandi, Chris the speller, WikiFlier, Timneu22, Msr69er, Rrburke, J.R. Hercules, Oanabay04, Kevlar67, Andrew c, CartoonDiablo, Curly Turkey, Ohconfucius, Hmoul, AThing, Ser Amantio di Nicolao, Dreslough, A. Parrot, Astuishin, Kanaman, Barry Deutsch, Levineps, K, Joseph Solis in Australia, Jsorens, CmdrObot, Korrector~enwiki, Bradleee, NaBUru38, DumbBOT, EqualRights, Dary.merckens, Id447, Marek69, Kborer, Bigtimepeace, Alphachimpbot, Lfstevens, The Transhumanist, Smith Jones, Xyz or die, Harelx, WhatamIdoing, Atb129, Cpl Syx, Mjhasley, Textorus, Mbhiii, RockMFR, Brastein, CFCF, Dingdongalistic, Nbauman, Mattnad, JayJasper, Jorfer, Kev8551, Kram0263, Diego, JackWikiSTP, RGarella, Sam Blacketer, Hammersoft, Ewillies, Jeff G., FuzzyCuteness, FitzColinGerald, Anarchangel, Jaredstein, Farcaster, Quantpole, Sfmammamia, Note4nick, Jacksonbliss, Dawn Bard, Luckykaa, Flyer22 Reborn, Toddm7878, Nopetro, KittyKat1001001, Hordaland, Escape Orbit, ImageRemovalBot, MqCorey, Ratemonth, Sfan00 IMG, ClueBot, Napzilla, ImperfectlyInformed, Tony Clothes, Sirald66, Drmies, Mild Bill Hiccup, Historian 1000, Excirial, Kwj2772, Navy II, DumZiBoT, EastTN, Thinkaboutitagain, RJHerrick, Ebender1, Danielroberts, Addbot, Davegre, Jafeluv, Queenmomcat, Lifeguard Emeritus, Strykerhorse, A.torch, Neapolitan Sixth, Chzz, Debresser, Peridon, W0129, Elderlander, Drpickem, Yobot, Legobot II, Darx9url, Randersonn, AnomieBOT, Mclazarus, Piano non troppo, Goodrule, Materialscientist, Citation bot, LilHelpa, Eivindsol, ChildofMidnight, Prowler08, Srich32977, Nickmn, Future2008, Anonymswasawoman, Cosmic Cowboy, Open Road Rider, LincolnSt, Richard Cooke, Wikiwawcu, Sko1221, FrescoBot, Tastybrain, Mookie McGee, DivineAlpha, Citation bot 1, CAdillacride, DrilBot, Tegrat, Abductive, Redjw, Tritest, Aerolin55, Jsharker, CS Sterling, Kstart, Rtaser, The Homosexualist, Statsagogo, Topfacts, Udid2, Limape, Trickymaster, Steveblambert, Rodravss, Trappist the monk, Pangjr, 🌀🌀~enwiki, Boomer73, Captain139, North8000, Callanecc, Chriswaco, Jss331, Skakkle, Phoenix and Winslow, Rwillis12, RjwilmsiBot, TimeClock871, Whywhenwhohow, Ghostofnemo, Tommy2010, Dcirovic, Thecheesykid, Illegitimate Barrister, StickeeRich, Thargor Orlando, NicatronTg, Cobaltcigs, H3llBot, Why Other, Jesanj, RayneVanDunem, Joelglee, Isthisuseful, ClueBot NG, Gareth Griffith-Jones, Somedifferentstuff, Jenova20, Tljeffers, Intlaware, Frietjes, Helpful Pixie Bot, Lowercase sigmabot, BG19bot, Dualus, MusikAnimal, Mark Arsten, UIOschwartz, Polmandc, Dreambeaver,

Thewikibeagles, Attleboro, Cyberbot II, ChrisGualtieri, Khazar2, TylerDurden8823, Dexbot, VictorD7, Epicgenius, Lance Friedman, Neo Poz, DragonoftheWest47, EJM86, EllenCT, NorthBySouthBaranof, HoboMcJoe, Cbrillaz, Thurer, Timcameron, Roccodrift, Monkbot, SpekServices, Abuck10, TJH2018, AHusain3141, Rubbish computer, Abelmolina00, Namaya14, J. Gratrix, Ag987, GreenC bot, Bender the Bot, Pizza Margherita, Clanwars13579, Mcgalace and Anonymous: 287

- **Universal health care** *Source:* https://en.wikipedia.org/wiki/Universal_health_care?oldid=769048904 *Contributors:* The Anome, Rsabbatini, Ixfd64, Mac, Darkwind, Zarius, Selket, DJ Clayworth, Nv8200pa, Jeff8765, E0N, AaronS, Rholton, Ericspenguin, Gidonb, Pretzelpaws, Axeman, Tom harrison, Alison, Gilgamesh~enwiki, Grant65, Gugganij, 159753, Sonjaaa, Beland, Robert Brockway, RayBirks, Neutrality, Greedy-Capitalist, Randwicked, SYSS Mouse, Discospinster, Rich Farmbrough, Bender235, Causa sui, Bobo192, Giraffedata, Zetawoof, Klafubra, Alansohn, Anthony Appleyard, LtNOWIS, TimMorris, Rd232, Wikidea, Fat pig73, Evangeline, Eukesh, MattWade, Snowolf, Wtmitchell, Lev lafayette, Vuo, Versageek, Blaxthos, Saxifrage, Richard Arthur Norton (1958-), Mindmatrix, Rtdrury, Schzmo, Rotten, SDC, Cornince, Graham87, Rjwilmsi, Dr.Gonzo, Koavf, Josiah Rowe, Vegaswikian, Ligulem, Yamamoto Ichiro, VKokielov, Wikiliki, AED, Idaltu, King of Hearts, ChrisChiasson, Mhking, JesseGarrett, Volunteer Marek, Wavelength, Hairy Dude, Hauskalainen, Ansell, Gaius Cornelius, Wimt, SamJohnston, Thane, Mfero, Think Fast, Wiki alf, DJ Bungi, Grafen, Kvn8907, Eric Sellars, Shak, Rjljr2, Nephron, RFBailey, Kortoso, DeadEyeArrow, Wknight94, FF2010, 2over0, Nin10dude, Chase me ladies, I'm the Cavalry, GraemeL, ArielGold, Katieh5584, Tim1965, SmackBot, KnowledgeOfSelf, Ssbohio, Pennywisdom2099, Anastrophe, Wdr1, Rachel Pearce, Chris the speller, Persian Poet Gal, RDBrown, Cattus, HartzR, Timneu22, Renamed user Sloane, Deli nk, Macdonja, Kaid100, TheFeds, Rolypolyman, IMFromKathlene, Otus, Shalom Yechiel, Nlapierre, Jhiner, Addshore, Flyguy649, Roadapathy, Khukri, Nrcprm2026, Crd721, DavidMann, Chopin1810, Folding Chair, Ohconfucius, Hmoul, Jet87, Dave314159, Giovanni33, Mikelr, Jidanni, Loodog, DaveHorne, Mgiganteus1, Aleenf1, CPAScott, MarkSutton, Stwalkerster, Levineps, K, Joseph Solis in Australia, Onathinwhiteline, Igoldste, Blehfu, Courcelles, Dan1679, Restoration, J Milburn, JForget, Causantin, Mineralè, SolnzeUSB, JohnCD, Sir kris, Mystylplx, CWY2190, TVC 15, Merlinus, Wooyi, Argon233, TalkAbout, Karimarie, Valentimd, Corpx, Strongbad1982, Skittleys, DumbBOT, Roger Roger, Thematt523, SpK, Salvor Hardin, Woland37, EnglishEfternamn, CieloEstrellado, Medtopic, Epbr123, N5iln, Revrant, Schmidtr1, Kborer, Aquilosion, Pence, GordonRoss, Philippe, BlytheG, 00666, Klausness, AntiVandal-Bot, Obiwankenobi, Jj137, Gregalton, Gdo01, Zadernet, Alphachimpbot, Cartesian1, ClassicSC, Davewho2, Barek, The Transhumanist, Patxi lurra, Fetchcomms, Ph.eyes, HellaNorCal, Nathanjp, Nmcclana, Dmodlin71, GoodDamon, Achero, Citizen33, Necroforest, KEKPΩΨ, The Myotis, Magioladitis, Bongwarrior, VoABot II, Bill114, Nyttend, Caesarjbsquitti, Esalso, KConWiki, JLMadrigal, Indon, Giggy, Animum, Cgingold, Clygeric, Zagubov, Chivista~enwiki, Blabberhand, Matamoros, Tin Man, Textorus, Nlight2, Paliku, Flowanda, Onaraighl, Rettetast, Metobey, Vox Rationis, Jranotarzt, Mbhiii, J.delanoy, Pharaoh of the Wizards, U C L A Steve, Nbauman, AgainErick, Ian.thomson, Laurusnobilis, Acalamari, Thedeadlypython, Bagelmouseuk, Bunk78, Mikael Häggström, Vineetcoolguy, Wesholing, Marcus1234, Jorfer, All Male Action, Moomoo123, Sleepeeg3, AzureCitizen, Packerfan386, Natl1, Scott Illini, Stnemmoc, Andy Marchbanks, TheNewPhobia, Spellcast, Whizbee, Burlywood, Virginiamarybrennan, Christopher Mann McKay, Aucitypops, X!, VolkovBot, CWii, Nathanaver, Jmrowland, Ryan032, Philip Trueman, Fran Rogers, Rollo44, Cosmic Latte, Pspoutz, Laurauden, Jtellerelsberg, Iliketofrolic666, Dipper3, Maxhaase, Martin451, Wikieditor12, Theklingon, SpecMode, Eubulides, Anonymi2, Caelin 14, Brazier20, Nephosp, Clintville, Falcon8765, Skarz, Sf-mammamia, Buddhi.desilva, Hazel77, FlyingLeopard2014, Callmebc, SPQRobin, DimeCadmium, Tiddly Tom, Deusdies, Dawn Bard, Killamanjaro, Whiteghost.ink, Grundle2600, MaynardClark, Jkingre, Momo san, Lucky Mitch, Nopetro, Freedomwarrior, JSpung, Gmb92, Alethe, Mforg, EnOreg, Oxymoron83, Antonio Lopez, Decoratrix, Faradayplank, Wowjungleman, Avnjay, Lightmouse, Sub619, The-G-Unit-Boss, Alex.muller, Soggypancakes, Sanya3, Pekingu, Gtadoc, C'est moi, Gomeying, Witchkraut, TaerkastUA, Snovak8282, Hordaland, DRTllbrg, Escape Orbit, Kanonkas, Miyokan, VanishedUser sdu9aya9fs787sads, Prettyinpink2121, Imthatboy, Faithlessthewonderboy, Atif.t2, Jonas78~enwiki, ClueBot, SummerWithMorons, Danielspencer91, Snigbrook, Gorillasapiens, The Thing That Should Not Be, Nbwoodyal, Cambrasa, EoGuy, ZippyGoogle, Kentuckyjulie, Sarbruis, Arakunem, Saddhiyama, SomeGuy11112, Myvoicex, Drmies, Mild Bill Hiccup, Baksando, JTBX, Boing! said Zebedee, Nualran, LizardJr8, Historian 1000, Mr. Someguy, Rahilrizvi, Puchiko, Excirial, Gnome de plume, Jusdafax, Monobi, Tylerdmace, Paul82346, Fishiehelper2, Iamthegod2, Sun Creator, Ice Cold Beer, JamieS93, Iohannes Animosus, Redthoreau, Nukeless, Crivera3, Weezey, Mlaffs, MilesAgain, Navy II, Proofer47, Aitias, Versus22, Legid, Dontmentionit, Apatens, DumZiBoT, Doopdoop, Kmcarter, Devpty01, XLinkBot, Dark Mage, EastTN, WikHead, Beach drifter, Noctibus, Catgirl, JCDenton2052, Bennybear, RyanCross, Rslate, Randymcmayhem, Danielroberts, HexaChord, The Squicks, Cunard, King Pickle, Addbot, Taty2007, Manivarma, Hda3ku, Lifeguard Emeritus, DougsTech, Blethering Scot, Ronhjones, CanadianLinuxUser, Mentisock, Ccacsmss, Mjwang24, Dr. Universe, Blaylockjam10, Bwrs, Kandomagoo, Myk60640, Tide rolls, OlEnglish, Tomgilk, Weaseloid, JEN9841, Tackle1625, Yobot, Kyinaire, Granpuff, Insilvis, Tohd8BohaithuGh1, CattOfTheGarage, Legobot II, PeeKoo, THEN WHO WAS PHONE?, Randersonn, Reenem, Gp12, Evaders99, Brit hideaway, IndepAmerican, Laurenlt, Marshall Williams2, Tempodivalse, Raimundo Pastor, AnomieBOT, DemocraticLuntz, Bighungryguy, Tavrian, Neptune5000, Piano non troppo, Innab, Goodrule, Clarinetguy097, Ulric1313, Charlie fong, Citation bot, Teeninvestor, Nifky?, Lil-Helpa, Butthumpinuniversity, ShoreCrab, Capricorn42, Pocketnife43, Prowler08, Orof.brown, Tad Lincoln, Denniscunard94, BritishWatcher, Mustangboy4589, Mikeyc333, Omnipaedista, Mind my edits, Cosmic Cowboy, Alpha-ZX, Open Road Rider, Jtokarsbr, Hotchocolita, LincolnSt, Editor182, Josemanimala, A.amitkumar, Griffinofwales, Sko1221, FrescoBot, Predator1087, Bgriggs, Wreasor, Wikiporch, Cedy 30, HJ Mitchell, Raymond Dundas, Steffv, Citation bot 1, Julacho, Dark Charles, Elockid, Redjw, Winter cake, Tritest, Chatfecter, Ratio101, Philly boy92, Norcelt, Gozer502, Kingnomolos, HonouraryMix, Beao, Wwwmahesh, Full-date unlinking bot, Cre8ivE OnE, Pristino, Kstart, Colonel1234, Floboalexander, Statsagogo, Limape, Abc518, Orenburg1, Rodravss, Jookinj, Masterofthewatch, Lotje, Vrenator, LilyKitty, Danieldis47, Theo10011, Aiken drum, Jeffrd10, Mlnb57, Diannaa, Vanished user aoiowaiuyr894isdik43, Acer567, Ludwiggiozer, Dennis-byron, Mean as custard, Nightbeacon, RjwilmsiBot, Vtstarin, Sproshua, Treyfsu, Myownworst, Mountainscout, John of Reading, NapsterX, User2010II, Immunize, Nations United, RA0808, Minimac's Clone, Index-tan, Tommy2010, MajorTJKong, Wikipelli, Emelddir, Erebunium, Warningsfromthefuture, Australisian, Traimb, H3llBot, Shanekruger, Kilopi, AutoGeek, Jmacwikipedista, Why Other, Jesanj, Ginger Conspiracy, Sugar-Baby-Love, Vulgarian Visigoth, WebDTE, Rhollis7, ClueBot NG, Somedifferentstuff, Catlemur, Djodjo666, Jmoore0905, Widr, Guptan99, Giorgos pkls, BG19bot, Dualus, Frze, Cranmills, Nynetworking, Ricordisamoa, Hostager, Lamin25, Der student 5, Biosthmors, Tutelary, Ikeashiasanders29, Vunhex, Ducknish, Nwellington, Hmainsbot1, SomeFreakOnTheInternet, SucreRouge, Ibn Ridwan, Neo Poz, Drchriswilliams, Stainslav, Enenena, Tschida123, Rosco1950, Blaike parker12345, Tertius51, Emily G. Miller, Kathrynmurray, Narky Blert, Markert23, Kazgarr, Fishingbag, Nøkkenbuer, Tejas Subramaniam, Jolly life, Entranced98, Alphazen1000, Tommain, Digigirl9, SkyWarrior, Bender the Bot, Concus Cretus, Lekkio and Anonymous: 915

- **Health policy** *Source:* https://en.wikipedia.org/wiki/Health_policy?oldid=765145657 *Contributors:* Nv8200pa, Robbot, Jmcnamera, Piotrus, Femto, Orangemarlin, Lev lafayette, Woohookitty, Firefishy, Rjwilmsi, Josiah Rowe, Vegaswikian, Nihiltres, CJLL Wright, Bgwhite, Wavelength, Hauskalainen, Ansell, Vincej, Drgregmartin, RazorICE, Closedmouth, Mais oui!, Rathfelder, SmackBot, Jim62sch, Yamaguchi⯑⯑, Ohnoitsjamie, RDBrown, A. B., Khukri, BullRangifer, DMacks, Vgy7ujm, JoshuaZ, Willy turner, Beetstra, Xiaphias, Swedishpenguin, K, CmdrObot, Future Perfect at Sunrise, Hopping, RXPhd, Bobblehead, Kborer, Mentifisto, Obiwankenobi, Gregalton, Fayenatic london, SiobhanHansa, Rich257, Caesarjbsquitti, WhatamIdoing, Cgingold, DGG, Scottalter, Grook Da Oger, Onaraighl, Antony-22, 2help, Bonadea, Funandtrvl, Signalhead, Hersfold, Rollo44, Phadad, FitzColinGerald, Simonwerner, Doc James, Sfmammamia, Android Mouse Bot, Pattigustafson, Commodore2468, Unbuttered Parsnip, Mild Bill Hiccup, Boing! said Zebedee, Historian 1000, Auntof6, Heartland institue, Arjayay, Navy II, DumZiBoT, Doopdoop, EastTN, Rafnerdj, HarlandQPitt, Danielroberts, Addbot, Keepcalmandcarryon, Raimundo Pastor, Geoffpado, Prowler08, Srich32977, Sift&Winnow, Open Road Rider, LincolnSt, VOR1994, Callanecc, John of Reading, Dcirovic, François duplessis, Jesanj, ChuispastonBot, ClueBot NG, RightWingLies, Guptan99, Wbm1058, Chajacobs, PhnomPencil, Hhand, Safehaven86, Dexbot, Benjaminmasonmeier, Billstevens0929, Everymorning, Health Policy Project, Thewikiguru1, Door Dow Win 345, Sondra.kinsey, KasparBot, GlobalStrategy, Kissmyasthma99, Qzd, Utopianic and Anonymous: 65

- **Health economics** *Source:* https://en.wikipedia.org/wiki/Health_economics?oldid=764439912 *Contributors:* SimonP, DavidLevinson, Michael Hardy, NuclearWinner, Wikid, Taxman, Cutler, Ksheka, Andycjp, APH, Willhsmit, Notinasnaid, Bender235, Violetriga, Femto, Arcadian, Mdd, Complex01, John Quiggin, Kurieeto, PAR, Hubriscantilever, Mokus, RainbowOfLight, Versageek, Woohookitty, Ekem, Wikiklrsc, Rjwilmsi, Kilroy-was-here, AED, YurikBot, Hairy Dude, RussBot, Vincej, Morphh, Drgregmartin, Tony1, Etronic2005, Closedmouth, GraemeL, Rathfelder, SmackBot, Reedy, Hcovitz, RDBrown, MartinPoulter, Timneu22, Jorvik, JonHarder, Khukri, EPM, Mouse Nightshirt, Vanished user 9i39j3, Guroadrunner, Beetstra, Hu12, Iridescent, Cheesy Yeast, Mrdthree, CapitalR, CmdrObot, Argon233, Thomasmeeks, Nmourfield, Skittleys, RXPhd, Dumaka, Jamesbuchanan, Medtopic, Thijs!bot, Hermes Agathos~enwiki, Notmyrealname, Dgies, Obiwankenobi, Fayenatic london, MER-C, Neo-Cavalier, Ph.eyes, Roycm, Globalhealth, WhatamIdoing, M-BMor, Hdynes, Cgingold, Scottalter, Jimtheeconomist, Mikael Häggström, Bonadea, Virginiamarybrennan, Mafs.grp, TXiKiBoT, FitzColinGerald, Qxz, Anna Lincoln, Larklight, Leehach, MaCRoEco, Doc James, EdW UK, Jojalozzo, Pattigustafson, Fratrep, Altzinn, Denisarona, ShelleyAdams, The Thing That Should Not Be, Historian 1000, NICK-NEWTON, Busa428, Dbillig, Doopdoop, Jytdog, EastTN, Ost316, Rslate, Tayste, Addbot, Download, Tide rolls, Swarm, Yobot, Sked123, FeydHuxtable, Raimundo Pastor, AnomieBOT, Mbiama Assogo Roger, Bluerasberry, Citation bot, Chrisampson, Bbarkley, Ncahill, Srich32977, Sift&Winnow, Rxcomms, FrescoBot, Ladwiki, Prakash021, Yulianian, 76student, Bbarkley2, Cgalexander, Luisxx24, Swanb, Bento00, EmausBot, John of Reading, Greath68, Cit helper, Jesanj, Drakedoug, ClueBot NG, Rezabot, Cm1ab, Helpful Pixie Bot, Cait Rico, Takeshi-br, Snow520, Heather Husson, MrBill3, JohanSonn, HO123, Ditzahedva, HoagL, SFK2, ChrisSampson87, Nahedshazly, Ashleyleia, 8digital, Banzai6666, Allthekidsinthestreet, Pattipeeples, Monkbot, Riceissa, L1189960, Martinwolfejr, KasparBot, Alkaturuk, Concus Cretus and Anonymous: 133

- **Public health** *Source:* https://en.wikipedia.org/wiki/Public_health?oldid=768947214 *Contributors:* ClaudineChionh, Olivier, Edward, Infrogmation, Michael Hardy, Kku, Gbleem, Ahoerstemeier, Ronz, Agtx, Andrevan, Greenrd, Freechild, Shizhao, RedWolf, Wereon, Aetheling, Diberri, Mintleaf~enwiki, Zigger, Zmaj~enwiki, Niteowlneils, Jfdwolff, Siroxo, Djegan, Wmahan, Erich gasboy, J3ff, APH, Neutrality, Wyllium, Rich Farmbrough, Notinasnaid, Mjpieters, Pavel Vozenilek, Bender235, El C, Triona, Femto, Jpgordon, Evolauxia, Viriditas, ZayZayEM, Maurreen, Arcadian, La goutte de pluie, Sam Korn, Storm Rider, Danski14, Alansohn, Gargaj, John Quiggin, Howrealisreal, Wouterstomp, Malo, Snowolf, Raymm, JALockhart, Kelly Martin, Peter Hitchmough, MONGO, Rickjpelleg, Graham87, Cuchullain, FreplySpang, Bikeable, Dpr, Rjwilmsi, Ingternet, SMC, Kodami, Sango123, FlaBot, AED, RexNL, TeaDrinker, Liontamer, PhotoSydney, Chwyatt, YurikBot, Pseudomonas, Salsb, Leighblackall, Drgregmartin, Rjensen, Nucleusboy, Ezeu, Zwobot, PanchoS, Nikkimaria, Donald Albury, GraemeL, Rathfelder, Jkpjkp, Hardscarf, Earlmj01, SmackBot, Moeron, Gregmce, Edgar181, Xaosflux, Pzavon, Ohnoitsjamie, Hmains, Paulleake, Dschroder, Silly rabbit, Deli nk, Kevin Ryde, FordPrefect42, Chinawhitecotton, DHN-bot~enwiki, Para, Pencheon, Can't sleep, clown will eat me, Jahiegel, ThatPaige, Snowmanradio, JonHarder, Khukri, Merylholl, Novazed, Vedek Dukat, Stor stark7, Bejnar, JzG, DO11.10, Battlemonk, T g7, Euchiasmus, Lapaz, Pdn30, Tazmaniacs, NongBot~enwiki, Jxb311, Beetstra, Dbo789, Santa Sangre, PRRfan, TastyPoutine, Geologyguy, Hu12, Levineps, Iridescent, Courcelles, Rhetth, Chovain, Bobfrombrockley, Nadyes, Argon233, ShelfSkewed, Cydebot, Soltanski, Mattbartek, Lightofglory, Matrix61312, Mato, Anthonyhcole, Dancter, Aldis90, Medtopic, Epbr123, Marek69, Missvain, Mrmrbeaniepiece, Cyclonenim, Majorly, Fayenatic london, Mack2, Ben Harris-Roxas, Kauczuk, Snali, Murftown, Hydrostatics, The Transhumanist, MegX, Kirrages, Globalhealth, Ben wolff, Hayduke lives, VoABot II, Drabs, Presearch, WhatamIdoing, Cgingold, APHL, Edward321, Valerius Tygart, Pvosta, Yobol, Axlq, Epiding, Keith D, R'n'B, Manticore, J.delanoy, Sinissa, Nev1, CFCF, Boghog, All Is One, Smeto, WiiAlbanyGirl, Cjeffery826, Keithengineer, Dessources, WJBscribe, Janethurley, DASonnenfeld, Funandtrvl, Deor, ABF, Ferrari250, QuackGuru, Seraphim, JhsBot, Sabrinaj, Mlh325, KC Panchal, Davin, Lola Voss, Optigan13, Brianga, Mvleblanc, Doc James, Phad~enwiki, EmxBot, Tarunseem, AngChenrui, Bfpage, Schleef, SieBot, Tkhoffman, Yintan, LeadSongDog, Beppie2006, GlassCobra, Gpinder, Wikibruger, Jsfouche, Pattigustafson, Laurnet9, Reneeholle, Capitalismojo, Denisarona, Dmannsanco, Rahman92a, Sfan00 IMG, ClueBot, Ksherin, Healthwise, Unbuttered Parsnip, Tomas e, Mild Bill Hiccup, Rampera, CounterVandalismBot, Blanchardb, Th17kit, Angkorgo2, Pojoman, Mollyegg, Cphp, Loop 9, Linda Smart, MasterOfHisOwnDomain, XLinkBot, Zackfield100, Delicious carbuncle, Mohsena, NellieBly, Artaxerxes, Courtneylynn45, Zodon, RyanCross, Addbot, Proofreader77, Some jerk on the Internet, Megan marie2008, LaaknorBot, Penrise, West.andrew.g, Aao2107, Lightbot, Hjl7, Luckas-bot, Yobot, Kenny88888, Publichealthier, Public Health Foundation Of India, Raimundo Pastor, AnomieBOT, Nutriveg, Jim1138, Suloshini, Crecy99, Bluerasberry, Citation bot, Nmolina92, ArthurBot, Xqbot, Nugteren, Watertree, Cureden, Capricorn42, PrevMedFellow, Anna Frodesiak, J04n, ⯑⯑⯑⯑, Riotrocket8676, Southmills, GenOrl, JoannaAdcock, Joaquin008, FrescoBot, Kevkiev, Tobby72, Steve Quinn, Austria156, Ιωάννης Καραμήτρος, Citation bot 1, Data-visualization-tools, Knyckis, Sjohn151, ElsevierTim, TennisGrandSlam, Mathiaseu, Sweetpaseo, FoxBot, Jshapi4, TobeBot, Trappist the monk, Vrenator, Ердfeн Карсыбеков, Diannaa, Motibr1~enwiki, Mean as custard, RjwilmsiBot, Bento00, Yeori1317, Fibeewkl, Maneeta89, Ionut Cojocaru, EmausBot, John of Reading, Orphan Wiki, Trilliumz, Funkyjazzz, Socialjustice23, Mjabf, RenamedUser01302013, Waithought, Moswento, Wikipelli, Dcirovic, PhosphateBufferedSaline, Wolfehenson, Jandrewc, H3llBot, Netha Hussain, Erianna, Jesanj, Noodleki, Donner60, Publichealth2010, ChuispastonBot, Spicemix, Wardrubrecht, Noophilic, ClueBot NG, Imansubarkah, Rthandle, Intermittentgardener, Hetz3486, O.Koslowski, MBC2011, Pctan, Guptan99, Ajh93ucla11, MAntonSciortino, Helpful Pixie Bot, BG19bot, Parizellina, Chajacobs, Annakatanna, Lkahnmd, Ibohyd, Leroy e. brown, MrBill3, Klilidiplomus, Jazgonz, Ježofska, BattyBot, Justincheng12345-bot, Lbockhorn, Academīca Orientālis, Chisholmredproject, Aliwal2012, TylerDurden8823, Petardugz, Healthhistory, Graphium, ComfyKem, ChrisSampson87, Elainengai, Jwluk, Dpaes, Shafiq.sims, Biogeographist, Ibn Ridwan, John de Norrona, Mrm7171, MartinPoulter Jisc, Drchriswilliams, Inaaaa, ProfessorHB, Mon3oturf, Dodi 8238, Saeid196721, Drsoumyadeepb, Ryk72, Melcous, Monkbot, Amuseclio, NomvulaWakaBani, EvMsmile, Kal Hamner, Ahm08001, Godsy, 1989, Mll mitch, Ujimix, HelpUsStopSpam, Harsh Patel Scientist, KasparBot, Adam9007, Yugoosaf, Healthyhelp, GlobalStrategy, Medicaljj, Composcompos12, Chadwick1842, Marzbars52, Prevail Health Solutions, Wangela323, Emoriar1, ZackNU, Effie Greathouse, Outaouaisregina, Wikisanchez, KATMAKROFAN, Colinwikipedia, Iambic Pentameter, Nadech007, Thewestwind, FatherTuck, Little Trekker and Anonymous: 362

- **All-payer rate setting** *Source:* https://en.wikipedia.org/wiki/All-payer_rate_setting?oldid=768659501 *Contributors:* BD2412, Rjwilmsi, Bgwhite, Racklever, Lfstevens, AnomieBOT, Hazard-Bot, BG19bot, Biosthmors, Dexbot, PrimeBOT and Anonymous: 3

- **Brian Day** *Source:* https://en.wikipedia.org/wiki/Brian_Day?oldid=765313346 *Contributors:* Bearcat, Kbh3rd, Dave.Dunford, Woohookitty, Alaney2k, Ground Zero, Bgwhite, Wavelength, TransUtopian, Ageless, NeilN, Chris the speller, Khazar, Checkguy, Cydebot, Absentis, JustA-Gal, Demophon, Waacstats, Theroadislong, MetsBot, DerHexer, Canuckle, Quelquechosedautre, NinjaRobotPirate, Ponyo, Capitalismojo, ClueBot, Fagin1800, Arjayay, Navy II, Evertonian47, DumZiBoT, TutterMouse, Tassedethe, Yobot, AnomieBOT, DemocraticLuntz, Everton61, Kelseyboultbee, Everton62, Tritest, Skyerise, Kathleen5454, John of Reading, Iselilja, TehPiratePoo, Verbcatcher, BattyBot, Cwobeel, Malerooster, Ozzie10aaaa, KasparBot, HealthLaw1, Pirbawa, Lifebringer6211, InternetArchiveBot, Danitfischtein, GreenC bot and Anonymous: 22

- **Healthcare reform in the United States** *Source:* https://en.wikipedia.org/wiki/Healthcare_reform_in_the_United_States?oldid=769152385 *Contributors:* Shii, Edward, Lousyd, Bpt, Ronz, Stevenj, Darrell Greenwood, Darkwind, BenKovitz, Deisenbe, Charles Matthews, Whisper-ToMe, Selket, DJ Clayworth, Grendelkhan, JerryFriedman, HaeB, Ancheta Wis, JamesMLane, Stevietheman, Chowbok, Beland, Reagle, Mike Rosoft, Discospinster, Rich Farmbrough, Mrevan, SamEV, Bender235, KarlHallowell, Crust, Longroad, WideArc, Alansohn, Arthena, Rd232, Geo Swan, Sligocki, MattWade, BanyanTree, Mikeo, Fryede, Stuartyeates, Woohookitty, Mindmatrix, Dandv, Wikiklrsc, SCEhardt, Zzyzx11, Dysepsion, Paxsimius, Numbskull816, BD2412, TorArne, Drbogdan, Rjwilmsi, Nneonneo, Yug, SchuminWeb, Ground Zero, Gjudd, Tedder, Bgwhite, Ravenswing, The Rambling Man, Wavelength, Hairy Dude, Arzel, Phantomsteve, Hauskalainen, Pigman, Chris Capoccia, Sasuke Sarutobi, Varnav, NawlinWiki, Rjensen, Slarson, Dhollm, Danlaycock, Wknight94, Mike Serfas, Ehlkej, SmackBot, Prototime, Ikip, Keanu, Kslays, Orser67, Ghosts&empties, Sjrsimac, Chris the speller, Kurykh, Macdonja, JavaJake, Nbarth, ACupOfCoffee, A. B., Emurphy42, Kelvin Case, Threeafterthree, Kingdon, Cybercobra, Lostart, Jeff Wheeler, Fuzzypeg, Pats1, Ohconfucius, Ser Amantio di Nicolao, Soap, JorisvS, Ckatz, JHunterJ, Frontier teg, Hiiiiiiiiiiiiiiiiiiiiii, SQGibbon, PRRfan, Michael J Swassing, Hu12, Quaeler, ThuranX, Levineps, Iridescent, K, Sameboat, Donmac, Synaptic DX, Morgan Wick, CmdrObot, The ed17, TVC 15, Hemlock Martinis, Phatom87, Jac16888, Cydebot, Reywas92, Treybien, Rifleman 82, Dancter, B, EqualRights, Thematt523, Epbr123, N5iln, Aleph-4, Mareoftenebrae, Headbomb, Missvain, Affiray, Universe Man, Notmyrealname, Jimmuldrow, Obiwankenobi, Prolog, Yellowdesk, Erxnmedia, Jabam, Fetchcomms, Connormah, Sarahj2107, Ling.Nut, Crazytonyi, Jatkins, Iploya, KConWiki, Cgingold, Kbs.sidhu, Nat, Dw31415, JaGa, Jodi.a.schneider, Sameerkale, Alikaalex, Racepacket, Tvoz, Charles Edward, Brothejr, Mbhiii, Lilac Soul, RockMFR, CFCF, Nbauman, Richiekim, Extransit, Dave Dial, L'Aquatique, Allreet, Nwbeeson, Jorfer, Flatterworld, Octavabasso, AzureCitizen, Ja 62, Copsi, PFR, Wkurzius, Jeff G., Raggz, Philip Trueman, Jbram 2002, Mkcmkc, Xenophrenic, DaraParsavand, Anna Lincoln, Cmcnicoll, Falcon8765, Farcaster, Sfmammamia, Pklon, AmigoNico, MarkWolf1, Dawn Bard, Discrete, Arbor to SJ, Nopetro, Jdaloner, Lightmouse, Kumioko (renamed), AuburnPilot, Spitfire19, NastalgicCam, Jongleur100, Capitalismojo, ImageRemovalBot, Moorehaus, ClueBot, SummerWithMorons, QueenofBattle, The Thing That Should Not Be, Nbwoodyal, EoGuy, ImperfectlyInformed, Showtime2009, Farras Octara, Historian 1000, Fibrebunny, Wsmith4474, Excirial, Diderot's dreams, DBlade, Sun Creator, Mindstalk, Iamsodeman, NuclearWarfare, Fire 55, Redthoreau, Navy II, Thingg, Liberalcynic, Bubblecuffer, DOR (HK), Elukenich, Apatens, DumZiBoT, Doopdoop, XLinkBot, Ninja247, EastTN, Rreagan007, WikHead, Alexius08, Serge3378, Rslate, The Squicks, Addbot, Jafeluv, DOI bot, Alphaa10, Lifeguard Emeritus, Ronhjones, OBloodyHell, Laurinavicius, Scientus, MrOllie, Bassbonerocks, Mjwang24, Debresser, NittyG, CarTick, Jrgilb, Tassedethe, Kandomagoo, Myk60640, Tide rolls, Pietrow, Zorrobot, JEN9841, GarethH1, Luckas-bot, Yobot, Kartano, Legobot II, ThinkingTwice, Randersonn, Pganas, Maxí, DrFleischman, Lbook52, LaurenIt, AnomieBOT, 264356triv, Rjanag, Innab, Goodrule, Danishroots, Materialscientist, Citation bot, Maison4800, Xqbot, Ingersollian, Wagners46, InpoliticTruth, Prowler08, PrevMedFellow, Srich32977, Mykjoseph, GrouchoBot, Sift&Winnow, Patrickstocks, Cosmic Cowboy, Open Road Rider, LincolnSt, Dreitmen, Noble Spear, Cgersten, Marcgoldwein, Maryhodder, Sko1221, FrescoBot, Mark Renier, Stu.W UK, Whoosit, Weetoddid, Clearcrash1, TheHoger, Citation bot 1, Galmicmi, Klubbit, Pinethicket, I dream of horses, Omerta62, Redjw, Tritest, Chatfecter, John Asfukzenski, Tom.Reding, Calmer Waters, George Orwell III, Fat&Happy, Toonmore, Norcelt, Richard, OrangeReform, Turian, Kstart, Merlion444, Statsagogo, SplintersRSplendid, Vinegaroon, Likwidal, Limape, Trappist the monk, Hellraiser7, Masterofthewatch, MichaelLNorth, NortyNort, Commandr Cody, Adsfasfasdjfasjdfhasdhf, Afhaalchinees~enwiki, Finland 203, Suomi Finland 2009, KirkWayland, Leiko49, Capt. James T. Kirk, Danieldis47, Diannaa, ThinkEnemies, Sammetsfan, Antisoapbox, Dennisbyron, Minimac, Rilixy, Stang5litre, RjwilmsiBot, Khin2718, TimeClock871, Fedorparetsky, Myownworst, Aotthp, Chessofnerd, Whywhenwhohow, Sliceofmiami, John of Reading, Lucien504, HiMyNameIsFrancesca, Omnia mutantur, Dewritech, GoingBatty, Lynnflint, Qrsdogg, Lex Pecunia, Ksspauld, Dcirovic, Nschooley, Oescp, John Shandy`, Zbase4, Bresdd, Phillycodehound, Logicalmaster, Mattybinx, Greath68, Donkeyscommand, Tcrawfo8, MithrandirAgain, Robertmmuniz, Lbrto, Thargor Orlando, Hanagiat, AOC25, Chilibimbambumo, Git2010, Shanekruger, Martonc, Nikkwa, Whitneysmith24, AutoGeek, Sbmeirow, TyA, Fishman0, Jesanj, Ginger Conspiracy, Sugar-Baby-Love, Tbird104, Sven Manguard, MaryD99, Xanchester, ClueBot NG, HeroicXiphos15, Lawnmower145, MelbourneStar, Thomas Keats, Ramillav, 65 fdt 6a, Widr, Helpful Pixie Bot, Tlleap, Proofofthis, Kendage124, Ericaet, Dualus, Nynetworking, Meatsgains, Paulangelluk, Biosthmors, StarryGrandma, ChrisGualtieri, EuroCarGT, Clark Wonderful, Qexigator, Dexbot, Mogism, Markermarker, Cupco, Neo Poz, Lemerson1125, EllenCT, DavidLeighEllis, Classicwiki, Evolution and evolvability, SJ Defender, InterestedInKansas, Beneficii, Monkbot, Rctuason, Black dragon 2014, AHusain3141, Rubbish computer, JJMC89, Bender the Bot, Ckcouzens and Anonymous: 425

- **Medicare (Canada)** *Source:* https://en.wikipedia.org/wiki/Medicare_(Canada)?oldid=769001205 *Contributors:* Dreamyshade, Robert Merkel, Eclecticology, SimonP, Ryguasu, Montrealais, Ewen, Edward, Karada, Radicalsubversiv, Theresa knott, Bueller 007, Boffyflow, The Tom, Yggdrasil, Vanieter, Timc, Maximus Rex, SD6-Agent, Bearcat, RedWolf, TMLutas, Dhodges, Mushroom, Anthony, Jord, Hylaride, Coralys, Steggall, Marcie, Erich gasboy, Quarl, HistoryBA, Thincat, JulieADriver, Creidieki, Neutrality, JamesTeterenko, Freakofnurture, Mark Zinthefer, Discospinster, Rich Farmbrough, Kaisershatner, Mwanner, Spoon!, Shoujun, Spinboy, Pearle, Guy Harris, Sjschen, Samaritan, Dsm iv tr, Wtshymanski, Versageek, Michaelm, TheIguana, Mindmatrix, KrisK, Dah31, SCEhardt, SDC, Siqbal, BD2412, FreplySpang, Rjwilmsi, DeadlyAssassin, Baldwin.jim, AED, McAusten, JYOuyang, Freejerk, Bgwhite, Peter Grey, Albanaco, Wavelength, Briaboru, CambridgeBayWeather, Gcapp1959, Tetsuo, Tony1, Arundel, Zzuuzz, GraemeL, JoanneB, Mais oui!, Canadianism, SmackBot, CarrieD, Chris the speller, Bluebot, Tomfulton, NCurse, Miquonranger03, Antonrojo, Fishhead64, 1sttomars, Cybercobra, Curly Turkey, Fremte, JohnI, Chillychick, Robbie dee, Astuishin, DabMachine, JoeBot, Anger22, Tawkerbot2, IronChris, Deetdeet, P-Chan, CmdrObot, Ruslik0, Argon233, Cydebot, Absentis, NorthernThunder, Gimmetrow, Erich Schmidt, Headbomb, Tellyaddict, Vilje på Hjul, AntiVandalBot, Inks.LWC, Caesarjbsquitti, WLU, CliffC, Airstrom, J.delanoy, UlliD, AlphaFactor, Hoffmansk, RmanB17499, Rularue, Sahyogi, Canking, Biglovinb, Ihubling, Spellcast, Adrian two, WatchAndObserve, MonsterSound, Reginald Perrin, Sfmammamia, Runewiki777, DivaNtrainin, Undisputedvoiceofreason, OMCV, The-G-Unit-Boss, Vice regent, The Four Deuces, ClueBot, Bluenoser73, Fagin1800, The Thing That Should Not Be, ExPatMatt, R2SBD, Trivialist, Wellingdon, Excirial, Dropsoffire, Tfgglobal, NERIC-Security, DumZiBoT, Facts707, Spoonkymonkey, AnnaFrance, Quercus solaris, Lightbot, Yobot, AnomieBOT, Swdandap, Moxy, A.amitkumar, FrescoBot, CircleAdrian, Citation bot 1, Sookevista, Introvert3, Kathleen5454, Rr parker, RjwilmsiBot, Moswento, Dcirovic, Thecheesykid, Zictor23, H3llBot, Seattle, Polisher of Cobwebs, Ego White Tray, HandsomeFella, Sampson T, ClueBot NG, Shivanshu3, Zingplex, Helpful Pixie Bot, Vivpat, Mark Arsten, Brendan.Oz, BattyBot, Cyberbot II, Fosterliberty, Beam-O-Flight, Carlislecum, Jonnycanuck, Tboxler, Supdiop, GreenC bot, Bender the Bot and Anonymous: 190

- **National Health Service** *Source:* https://en.wikipedia.org/wiki/National_Health_Service?oldid=769241960 *Contributors:* The Anome, Michael Hardy, G-Man, Kaihsu, Kierant, Owain, Nmg20, Marcos, Discospinster, Twobells, Alansohn, Rodw, Rwendland, Tainter, Brookie, LoopZilla, Ekem, Pol098, SDC, BD2412, Tim!, Kinu, Jmcc150, GünniX, Whistler, Phantomsteve, Hauskalainen, Rsrikanth05, Rjensen, RFBailey, Jpbowen, Lucasreddinger, DRosenbach, Sandstein, Barryob, Chase me ladies, I'm the Cavalry, Mais oui!, Rathfelder, Tom Morris, Mauls, Aleksmot, Ottawakismet, Thom2002, JaT~enwiki, Mattythewhite, Breadandcheese, DeFacto, Khukri, Kuru, Gnevin, Dl2000, BananaFiend, Iridescent, Richard75, Pi, Bonás, Myasuda, Cydebot, MBRZ48, Sharkli, Scroggie, Optimist on the run, Legis, Epbr123, Salavat, Mentifisto, BenJWoodcroft, Jamie S, 200cake, Responsible?, Snowded, Zagubov, Keith D, R'n'B, Fondls, J.delanoy, JaySherman88, Knight of BAAWA, Rbakker99, Flatterworld, Doomsday28, KylieTastic, Indubitably, Omutumo, Dirkbb, Euryalus, Jauerback, Angusmca, Grundle2600, Markdask, Bentogoa, Mtaylor848, Jza84, ClueBot, Geoffreyrivett, Excirial, Fishiehelper2, D0nnie Dark0 96, JasonAQuest, Knezovjb, DumZiBoT, ברוקולי, XLinkBot, D.M. from Ukraine, Addbot, Catfish61, CanadianLinuxUser, Douglas the Comeback Kid, Proxima Centauri, Chamal N, Favonian, Zorrobot, Frehley, Luckas-bot, Yobot, 2D, Aoso0ck, Raimundo Pastor, AnomieBOT, Petercascio, Justme89, Roadnote, Chromenano, ArthurBot, LilHelpa, Xqbot, Gymnophoria, Doulos Christos, January2009, Verbum Veritas, LincolnSt, Jade0970, DrSearch, Efelante planante Efelante, RedBot, Ecoleg, Smifis, Cnwilliams, Drutton57, Merlinsorca, Ysgol Rhiwabon, RjwilmsiBot, Skamecrazy123, Rayman60, EmausBot, Sir Arthur Williams, Sky4t0k, Parkywiki, Wikipelli, Fæ, Druzhnik, Unreal7, Tolly4bolly, Rcsprinter123, Gsarwa, Matthewrbowker, ClueBot NG, Somedifferentstuff, Widr, Exurbis67, Nationalstudentsurvey, BG19bot, Steve Milburn, Kaltenmeyer, George Ponderevo, Darkness Shines, Compfreak7, Safehaven86, Anbu121, EricEnfermero, BattyBot, YFdyh-bot, Dexbot, Mogism, ChrisSampson87, Ozzie10aaaa, LanternSmirk, Rob984, Melonkelon, Oliknibbs, Ugog Nizdast, Bomph, Drchriswilliams, Amortias, The Original Bob, Wizzjiggy, Nhssos, Crystallizedcarbon, Liance, Papitizer, PriceDL, HymanFam, Absolutelypuremilk, Jason.nlw, User 75649, Zeromonk, Neve-selbert, Blitzernnn, Jenifar87, Bender the Bot, Cadmus90, Stikkyy, Gcgosling, Johnnycb, Sideboard1 and Anonymous: 158

- **PAMI** *Source:* https://en.wikipedia.org/wiki/PAMI?oldid=750093283 *Contributors:* Rathfelder, Fma12, Cydebot, Magioladitis, David Eppstein, Addbot, Sherlock4000, John of Reading, Dewritech, BG19bot, Facucaldo123 and Anonymous: 1

- **Political positions of Dennis Kucinich** *Source:* https://en.wikipedia.org/wiki/Political_positions_of_Dennis_Kucinich?oldid=748537298 *Contributors:* Vsync, Walloon, Tom harrison, Ofus, Jmcnamera, Klemen Kocjancic, Rich Farmbrough, Bender235, Pharos, Echuck215, Paisan30, Woohookitty, Jersyko, GregorB, GoldRingChip, BD2412, Rjwilmsi, Koavf, Ground Zero, TexasAndroid, Buss, Mikeblas, Nikkimaria, Sarefo, Matt Heard, SmackBot, InverseHypercube, Timneu22, JzG, Levineps, Hikui87~enwiki, Gregbard, Cydebot, W.A.C., Timjowers, Zigzig20s, SteveSims, Harelx, Tvoz, R'n'B, Mbhiii, Svetovid, Edward4321, JayJasper, Olegwiki, Foofighter20x, Xenophrenic, Srikipedia, Jocke666, CoolKid1993, Darth Kalwejt, Jdaloner, JL-Bot, History Wizard, Grundyc, EoGuy, Zelogan, Minstrelo, Rodnicholsev, Yobot, DrFleischman, Jim1138, Maximilian Caldwell, Ulric1313, Ingersollian, Purplebackpack89, FrescoBot, Adam9389, Sashay, Shante!, The Homosexualist, Historyfeller, BlueSal, RjwilmsiBot, John of Reading, Dewritech, Blackjackshellac, GoingBatty, Truthsort, Fdr2001, Thargor Orlando, H3llBot, Wikidude10000, Phiclub, Frietjes, Technical 13, BG19bot, ISTB351, Cyberbot II, ChrisGualtieri, Dobie80, ArmbrustBot, GreenC bot and Anonymous: 48

- **Public health insurance option** *Source:* https://en.wikipedia.org/wiki/Public_health_insurance_option?oldid=764238783 *Contributors:* Edward, Iota, Bluejay Young, Jmcnamera, Rich Farmbrough, Viriditas, Alansohn, Wikidea, Bad Graphics Ghost, Rjwilmsi, Mick gold, Ground Zero, Bgwhite, Hauskalainen, Johno95, Rathfelder, SmackBot, C.Fred, Ohnoitsjamie, Chris the speller, Nahum Reduta, RolandR, Will Beback, Gobonobo, K, Cowicide, Wwallacee, Cydebot, Dr.enh, DumbBOT, Zalgo, Magioladitis, Jatkins, KConWiki, Brothejr, Mbhiii, RockMFR, J.delanoy, Nbauman, NewEnglandYankee, Jorfer, Hof1187, Kuni Leml, Atlpedia, Tapalmer99, Thatotherdude, Explicit, ClueBot, Tvol, Gnome de plume, Redthoreau, Pradtke, XLinkBot, EastTN, The Squicks, Proofreader77, Ivanhale, Yobot, AnomieBOT, Bluerasberry, Dvd-junkie, Amaury, Kikodawgzzz, Jonesey95, Σ, Masterofthewatch, Malik El Djebena, Danieldis47, Cellurl, Lammidhania, Leagilly, Yeng-Wang-Yeh, Shawm74, Fieldzee08, Grant Rowland, Neo-wikipedian, BlueSal, RjwilmsiBot, Becritical, Thrind, John of Reading, RenamedUser01302013, Truthsort, Thargor Orlando, Calliostoma, Openstrings, Siparuna, Sugar-Baby-Love, BG19bot, Ariftech, Safehaven86, Cyberbot II, Khazar2, SabinaForest, Iamsorandom, Everymorning, Neo Poz, Blondeguynative, GreenC bot, Bender the Bot and Anonymous: 87

- **Public health system in India** *Source:* https://en.wikipedia.org/wiki/Public_health_system_in_India?oldid=731147818 *Contributors:* Vegaswikian, Shyamsunder, Cydebot, Ekabhishek, The Anomebot2, Mild Bill Hiccup, Arjayay, Yobot, AnomieBOT, Austria156, Bamyers99, Arcandam, Abdulkazad123, Capankajsmilyo and Anonymous: 11

- **Public hospital** *Source:* https://en.wikipedia.org/wiki/Public_hospital?oldid=760001672 *Contributors:* WhisperToMe, Beland, Longhair, Davidruben, Giraffedata, Peter McGinley, Rjwilmsi, Vegaswikian, Sbrools, Wavelength, Welsh, SmackBot, Chris the speller, Dl2000, Synaptic DX, Malleus Fatuorum, Typochimp, Jhw57, Student7, Joseph123454321, The Thing That Should Not Be, Dthomsen8, Addbot, DOI bot, Kyle1278, Alfie66, Luckas-bot, AnomieBOT, Rangasyd, Materialscientist, Citation bot, Likesausages, CompliantDrone, FrescoBot, Mba123, UrbanNerd, ClueBot NG, DorkDoctor, HazelAB, I am One of Many, Tentinator, JustBerry, MoePa, Skr15081997, Monkbot, Prof. Mc, Friar-Tuck1981, Some Gadget Geek, SilverplateDelta and Anonymous: 45

- **Social insurance** *Source:* https://en.wikipedia.org/wiki/Social_insurance?oldid=752117737 *Contributors:* Robbot, DocWatson42, Piotrus, ArnoldReinhold, BD2412, Chobot, Hauskalainen, Neo-Jay, Maksim-bot, Guat6, Beetstra, Iridescent, Thomasmeeks, Cydebot, NorthernThunder, WhatamIdoing, J.delanoy, TXiKiBoT, EuTuga, Vipinhari, Baumfreund-FFM, BotKung, Gamsbart, LizardJr8, Leadwind, DumZiBoT, BRPXQZME, EastTN, Good Olfactory, Addbot, SpBot, Jarble, Blablablob, Gothika, Erud, Mats33, RibotBOT, LilyKitty, Traimb, RayneVanDunem, ClueBot NG, DJL5rice, Solardrum, MerlIwBot, BG19bot, Mogism, Cerabot~enwiki, Lugia2453, KasparBot, DatGuy and Anonymous: 25

- **Socialized medicine** *Source:* https://en.wikipedia.org/wiki/Socialized_medicine?oldid=766131412 *Contributors:* Robert Merkel, The Anome, AlexWasFirst, Galizia, KF, Edward, Pnm, Paul Benjamin Austin, Minesweeper, Ams80, Jll, Charles Matthews, David.Monniaux, Guppy, Bkalafut, Kowey, Seglea, Unfree, Djegan, Steggall, Jmcnamera, Haggis, Chowbok, Pgan002, Beland, Neutrality, Kingal86, Prestonmarkstone, Rich

- **Hospital Insurance and Diagnostic Services Act** *Source:* https://en.wikipedia.org/wiki/Hospital_Insurance_and_Diagnostic_Services_Act? oldid=721233482 *Contributors:* Dreamyshade, Woohookitty, Pol098, Chris the speller, Good Olfactory, Yobot, Gwickwire, ~riley, Curtaintoad and RMD6

- **List of countries by health insurance coverage** *Source:* https://en.wikipedia.org/wiki/List_of_countries_by_health_insurance_coverage? oldid=756738797 *Contributors:* Apatens, Ronhjones and Anonymous: 1

- **List of countries with universal health care** *Source:* https://en.wikipedia.org/wiki/List_of_countries_with_universal_health_care?oldid= 766822965 *Contributors:* Rjwilmsi, GünniX, Bgwhite, Wavelength, Keithonearth, Kintetsubuffalo, Chris the speller, Invenio, Meno25, Obi-wankenobi, Magioladitis, CFCF, DadaNeem, Steel1943, Cnilep, S.Örvarr.S, Whiteghost.ink, Mx. Granger, Ratemonth, Vitilsky, Ottawahitech, SchreiberBike, Apatens, Grayfell, Yobot, Fraggle81, Reenem, AnomieBOT, Materialscientist, LilHelpa, FrescoBot, CaptainFugu, Degen Earth-fast, F3ew, Trappist the monk, RjwilmsiBot, Myownworst, Communitarian35, John of Reading, Communist00, Parkywiki, Winner 42, Dcirovic, K6ka, GermanJoe, ClueBot NG, Somedifferentstuff, ☺☺ȸ, Catlemur, Djodjo666, Widr, BG19bot, Chess, Laom20, Nynetworking, Yasht101, Russellcarden, David.moreno72, Cyberbot II, Sim(ã)o(n), Mogism, Decgal, Lugia2453, Master of Time, Ginsuloft, Czixhc, Drchriswilliams, Feo3dr, Dansallves, Emily G. Miller, Monkbot, SantiLak, Demoniccathandler, Sciophobiaranger, Shafi5001, United Union, 123rwiki, Rubbish computer, AbhiRiksh, Lux-hibou, Robin De Banque, Anahit falack, InternetArchiveBot, Alphazen1000, GreenC bot, Bender the Bot, Fulanito García, Stvgruppetta, FloridaArmy and Anonymous: 65

- **Massachusetts health care reform** *Source:* https://en.wikipedia.org/wiki/Massachusetts_health_care_reform?oldid=766911551 *Contributors:* Edward, Tb, Selket, David.Monniaux, Beland, CaribDigita, Neutrality, Humblefool, D6, Sahasrahla, Chemboss, Richi, Pearle, CoreyEdwards, Polarscribe, Sligocki, Grenavitar, Geraldshields11, Drbreznjev, Stemonitis, Scarykitty, Woohookitty, Xmp, Kosher Fan, Wikiklrsc, GoldRingChip, BD2412, Rjwilmsi, Koavf, Vegaswikian, AED, KarlFrei, Psoreilly, King of Hearts, Wasted Time R, Ravenswing, Wavelength, Bdell555, Rms125a@hotmail.com, Deriobamba, Mardus, Fagles, Sardanaphalus, SmackBot, Holon67, Nil Einne, Hmains, Chris the speller, Jprg1966, Quackslikeaduck, Cybercobra, The PIPE, Kendrick7, Beetstra, Levineps, ChrisCork, CmdrObot, Mcstrother, TVC 15, Argon233, Cydebot, Zgystardst, EqualRights, Dolph Yehudi, Rabin06, Pihp, Yellowdesk, Kigali1, Davew128, MN57798, VoABot II, Yakushima, Appraiser, Cgingold, Olsonist, Tracer9999, MartinBot, U C L A Steve, Scaraway, Mcintosh3102, Mrmuk, Scott Illini, Andy Marchbanks, Hirolovesswords, 88wolfmaster, Dough4872, Dawn Bard, Alexbook, Toddst1, Nopetro, Antonio Lopez, Int21h, FifeOpp08, ImageRemovalBot, Ereq, Midtempo, Krvel07, Supertouch, Jwihbey, Shaliya waya, Ottawahitech, Historian 1000, Edknol, 718 Bot, Mindstalk, NuclearWarfare, Tafdc, Gnickett1, Apatens, DumZiBoT, Ninja247, Bud08, EastTN, Isabelwh, Jafeluv, PantsB, Rayguest, Bcgh345, Download, Anoblecause, JEN9841, Magicpiano, Pwingle, Thw949, DiverDave, AnomieBOT, Sb101, Yachtsman1, Citation bot, LilHelpa, Srich32977, Dark Charles, Jonesey95, Chatfecter, Wellnessgal, FFM784, Entscholar, Dennisbyron, RjwilmsiBot, Myownworst, Nhajivandi, Dricks20815, H3llBot, Kilopi, Pinroot, ClueBot NG, Somedifferentstuff, Nnicitalars, Benneyoboy, Healthcaretime, Doolinnc, Man of Mystery and Magic, BattyBot, Healthcareadvocate, ChrisGualtieri, SD5bot, Khazar2, Masscare, Abstractematics, Davidgblackburn, Everymorning, Cbrillaz, Monkbot, Econbrett, Markensontl, Snoogansnoogans, GreenC bot and Anonymous: 112

- **National health insurance** *Source:* https://en.wikipedia.org/wiki/National_health_insurance?oldid=742520179 *Contributors:* AxelBoldt, Edward, Selket, DJ Clayworth, Nv8200pa, Beland, Neutrality, Picapica, Lacrimosus, Bender235, Jeffrey O. Gustafson, Mindmatrix, Rjwilmsi, Vegaswikian, AED, Hauskalainen, Closedmouth, Rathfelder, SmackBot, Chris the speller, Kevlar67, RolandR, Wwolcott43, Doug Weller, BetacommandBot, Kborer, Obiwankenobi, Bongwarrior, Cgingold, Mbhiii, J.delanoy, Sam Blacketer, Sfmammamia, Historian 1000, Kannie, SchreiberBike, Navy II, Apatens, Lifeguard Emeritus, Counterheg, Yobot, Randersonn, Bugger4stalin, Trash stalinazis, AnomieBOT, Goodrule, Citation bot, Prowler08, Cosmic Cowboy, LincolnSt, Sko1221, Onetrail, Norcelt, Limape, Alex MacIntosh88, RayneVanDunem, Wuerzele, Rb53100 and Anonymous: 36

- **Primary healthcare** *Source:* https://en.wikipedia.org/wiki/Primary_healthcare?oldid=757505278 *Contributors:* Edward, Mac, Mcapdevila, Shiftchange, Rich Farmbrough, PaulHanson, Versageek, Abanima, Mindmatrix, Prashanthns, Mandarax, BD2412, Rjwilmsi, AED, Tedder, Vmenkov, YurikBot, Bhny, Bovineone, Draeco, Jpbowen, San taunk, Htonl, BOT-Superzerocool, Chriswaterguy, Rathfelder, Parvagilla, SmackBot, Chairman S., Wklee, Chinawhitecotton, Khukri, Kavibhalla, Iridescent, Hopsyturvy, Neelix, Cydebot, Jaydenm, Citations, RobDe68, Blathnaid, Zeitlupe, MER-C, Pax:Vobiscum, Rettetast, Brothejr, Kalyan gnp, Naniwako, TXiKiBoT, Bleaney, Eubulides, Ziphon, Sfmammamia, SieBot, Nopetro, Fimbriata, Millstream3, Nancy, TheCatalyst31, ClueBot, Snigbrook, Markneth, Princeattractive, Kofiannansrevenge, Namazu-tron, Danielroberts, Addbot, Yobot, Wlahead, Raimundo Pastor, Eumolpo, Sherry007020, Renamed user 39932kk3, FrescoBot, Citation bot 1, Brasenose, Tintenfischlein, I dream of horses, Serols, RjwilmsiBot, Alph Bot, Bertberry, Becritical, Shanekruger, Tolly4bolly, Stevewetson, Jesanj, Paulkweaver, Cforrester101, DemonicPartyHat, ClueBot NG, Korrawit, Widr, Guptan99, Helpful Pixie Bot, Supotmails, Marcocapelle, Conifer, Mogism, Ellaliao, Amt10, Np5377, Zoyanazni, Rjr-17, Dbmulder, Jomonoe123, Fuzzypillow7, Kca68, Cyclozodiac, Fianaw, Thl9015, Kwx913, RuhNaimi, Ramanjanda, Mololom, Ibn Ridwan, YiFeiBot, Drchriswilliams, BelindaOfalda, Csutric, Monkbot, Ujimix, Harsh Patel Scientist, Sweepy, Bender the Bot, Bh 1902 and Anonymous: 63

- **Rajiv Gandhi Jeevandayee Arogya Yojana** *Source:* https://en.wikipedia.org/wiki/Rajiv_Gandhi_Jeevandayee_Arogya_Yojana?oldid= 752768324 *Contributors:* Yamaguchi図図, Benstown, Niceguyedc, AnomieBOT, FrescoBot, Woodlot, Spirit of Eagle, Capankajsmilyo and AbhiRiksh

- **Rashi Fein** *Source:* https://en.wikipedia.org/wiki/Rashi_Fein?oldid=768817269 *Contributors:* SteveFoerster, Bender235, DePiep, Ground Zero, Patken4, Rathfelder, Cydebot, Connormah, MaynardClark, Tassedethe, Yobot, John of Reading, ClueBot NG, Gothicfilm, Marcocapelle, Spiderjerky, IRMA12345, KasparBot, Bender the Bot and Anonymous: 2

- **Right to health** *Source:* https://en.wikipedia.org/wiki/Right_to_health?oldid=756829399 *Contributors:* Utcursch, Viriditas, Sam Korn, Kurieeto, Toussaint, Prashanthns, Rjwilmsi, SmackBot, Apers0n, Cybercobra, Irn, Eastlaw, DewiMorgan, Fuseau, Maurice Carbonaro, Nefer209, LeaveSleaves, Pierre-Alain Gouanvic, Dodger67, Kaitayun, Drmies, DanielDeibler, Arjayay, Addbot, Dawynn, Lightbot, SasiSasi, Fraggle81, TaBOT-zerem, AnomieBOT, JackieBot, Citation bot, AlasdairEdits, ملهو, Thehelpfulbot, Nickkokay, LilyKitty, Dcirovic, Wikignome0530, ClueBot NG, Shaya88, Fay.farstad, CitationCleanerBot, Jami430, BattyBot, David.moreno72, Lilibeeh, Bdmorrison, Melonkelon, Johncrogers, Gransford, Amolutrankar, Roccodrift, CNMall41, Monkbot, Halal Capone, Bender the Bot and Anonymous: 18

- **Two-tier healthcare** *Source:* https://en.wikipedia.org/wiki/Two-tier_healthcare?oldid=760623265 *Contributors:* SimonP, Montrealais, Edward, Zanimum, SD6-Agent, Bearcat, Saforrest, Zoney, Beland, Randwicked, Qutezuce, John FitzGerald, Rupertslander, Bobo192, Mdkarazim,

Mindmatrix, Lapsed Pacifist, Baldwin.jim, Ground Zero, AED, Nihiltres, Wavelength, Hauskalainen, Aeusoes1, Whobot, Rathfelder, Smack-Bot, Xchbla423, Phuzion, Pewwer42, Afitillidie13, WinBot, YK Times, Canjth, War wizard90, Jmcw37, K.d.stauffer, Dawn Bard, Perspectoff, Yintan, Thesavagenorwegian, Spazure, Hordaland, ClueBot, Historian 1000, PixelBot, WikHead, Addbot, Fluffernutter, Yobot, Legobot II, AnomieBOT, Materialscientist, LincolnSt, Mean as custard, Myownworst, Sugar-Baby-Love, MuhannadDarwish, Jtdla, Khazar2, Comp.arch, ABCABC123123, Melcous and Anonymous: 61

- **Vermont health care reform** *Source:* https://en.wikipedia.org/wiki/Vermont_health_care_reform?oldid=763617936 *Contributors:* Edward, Coemgenus, Ground Zero, Teneriff, JustAGal, JEH, Textorus, Yobot, Guy1890, Liberal92, AnomieBOT, Tiller54, Brucewh, Designate, Myownworst, Josve05a, Thargor Orlando, RayneVanDunem, ClueBot NG, Safehaven86, DallasSchneider, InternetArchiveBot, GreenC bot, Bender the Bot and Anonymous: 14

4.2 Images

- **File:A_coloured_voting_box.svg** *Source:* https://upload.wikimedia.org/wikipedia/en/0/01/A_coloured_voting_box.svg *License:* Cc-by-sa-3.0 *Contributors:* ? *Original artist:* ?

- **File:Ahmed-mater-phcc-aseer.jpg** *Source:* https://upload.wikimedia.org/wikipedia/commons/4/40/Ahmed-mater-phcc-aseer.jpg *License:* CC BY-SA 3.0 *Contributors:* Own work *Original artist:* Info-ahmedmater

- **File:Ambox_current_red.svg** *Source:* https://upload.wikimedia.org/wikipedia/commons/9/98/Ambox_current_red.svg *License:* CC0 *Contributors:* self-made, inspired by Gnome globe current event.svg, using Information icon3.svg and Earth clip art.svg *Original artist:* Vipersnake151, penubag, Tkgd2007 (clock)

- **File:Ambulancias_DYA_Las_Arenas.jpg** *Source:* https://upload.wikimedia.org/wikipedia/commons/0/00/Ambulancias_DYA_Las_Arenas.jpg *License:* CC BY 3.0 *Contributors:* Own work *Original artist:* User:Javierme Javier Mediavilla Ezquibela

- **File:Ambulatorio_del_Norte.JPG** *Source:* https://upload.wikimedia.org/wikipedia/commons/9/96/Ambulatorio_del_Norte.JPG *License:* GFDL *Contributors:* Own work *Original artist:* Bobjgalindo

- **File:Aneurin_Bevan_and_his_wife_Jenny_Lee_in_Corwen_(15368872658).jpg** *Source:* https://upload.wikimedia.org/wikipedia/commons/8/87/Aneurin_Bevan_and_his_wife_Jenny_Lee_in_Corwen_%2815368872658%29.jpg *License:* CC0 *Contributors:* Aneurin Bevan and his wife Jenny Lee in Corwen *Original artist:* Geoff Charles

- **File:Bandera_Castilla-La_Mancha.svg** *Source:* https://upload.wikimedia.org/wikipedia/commons/d/d4/Bandera_Castilla-La_Mancha.svg *License:* Public domain *Contributors:* Dibujada a partir de Image:FlagofCastile.png *Original artist:* Valadrem (http://valadrem.blogspot.com)

- **File:Bandera_de_Castilla_y_León.svg** *Source:* https://upload.wikimedia.org/wikipedia/commons/1/13/Flag_of_Castile_and_Le%C3%B3n.svg *License:* CC BY 3.0 *Contributors:* Own work *Original artist:* **Rastrojo** (D•ES)

- **File:Bandera_de_Navarra.svg** *Source:* https://upload.wikimedia.org/wikipedia/commons/3/36/Bandera_de_Navarra.svg *License:* Public domain *Contributors:* This vector image includes elements that have been taken or adapted from this: <a href='//commons.wikimedia.org/wiki/File:Escudo_de_Navarra_(oficial).svg' class='image'><img alt='Escudo de Navarra (oficial).svg' src='https://upload.wikimedia.org/wikipedia/commons/thumb/4/4b/Escudo_de_Navarra_%28oficial%29.svg/11px-Escudo_de_Navarra_%28oficial%29.svg.png' width='11' height='20' srcset='https://upload.wikimedia.org/wikipedia/commons/thumb/4/4b/Escudo_de_Navarra_%28oficial%29.svg/17px-Escudo_de_Navarra_%28oficial%29.svg.png 1.5x, https://upload.wikimedia.org/wikipedia/commons/thumb/4/4b/Escudo_de_Navarra_%28oficial%29.svg/22px-Escudo_de_Navarra_%28oficial%29.svg.png 2x' data-file-width='550' data-file-height='978' /></a> Escudo de Navarra (oficial).svg (by Miguillen). *Original artist:* Miguillen

- **File:Bandera_de_la_Comunidad_Valenciana_(2x3).svg** *Source:* https://upload.wikimedia.org/wikipedia/commons/1/16/Flag_of_the_Valencian_Community_%282x3%29.svg *License:* Public domain *Contributors:* Own work *Original artist:* Mutxamel

- **File:BenTaubHospitalHoustonTX.JPG** *Source:* https://upload.wikimedia.org/wikipedia/commons/f/fe/BenTaubHospitalHoustonTX.JPG *License:* Public domain *Contributors:* Own work *Original artist:* WhisperToMe

- **File:Budgetary_Impact_of_Health_Reform_Bills.JPG** *Source:* https://upload.wikimedia.org/wikipedia/commons/4/45/Budgetary_Impact_of_Health_Reform_Bills.JPG *License:* CC BY-SA 3.0 *Contributors:* Own work *Original artist:* Marcgoldwein

- **File:Burying_Plague_Victims_of_Tournai.jpg** *Source:* https://upload.wikimedia.org/wikipedia/commons/7/7d/Burying_Plague_Victims_of_Tournai.jpg *License:* Public domain *Contributors:* http://supotnitskiy.ru/stat/stat8.htm *Original artist:* Unknown<a href='https://www.wikidata.org/wiki/Q4233718' title='wikidata:Q4233718'><img alt='wikidata:Q4233718' src='https://upload.wikimedia.org/wikipedia/commons/thumb/f/ff/Wikidata-logo.svg/20px-Wikidata-logo.svg.png' width='20' height='11' srcset='https://upload.wikimedia.org/wikipedia/commons/thumb/f/ff/Wikidata-logo.svg/30px-Wikidata-logo.svg.png 1.5x, https://upload.wikimedia.org/wikipedia/commons/thumb/f/ff/Wikidata-logo.svg/40px-Wikidata-logo.svg.png 2x' data-file-width='1050' data-file-height='590' /></a>

- **File:Calendario_común_de_vacunación_infantil._España_2016.png** *Source:* https://upload.wikimedia.org/wikipedia/commons/b/b3/Calendario_com%C3%BAn_de_vacunaci%C3%B3n_infantil._Espa%C3%B1a_2016.png *License:* Copyrighted free use *Contributors:* Calendario común de vacunación infantil. Calendario recomendado para el año 2016. Consejo Interterritorial del Sistema Nacional de Salud. MSSSI de España. *Original artist:* Ministerio de Sanidad, Servicios Sociales e Igualdad de España.

- **File:Carte_Européenne_d'Assurance_Maladie_France.jpg** *Source:* https://upload.wikimedia.org/wikipedia/commons/2/24/Carte_Europ%C3%A9enne_d%27Assurance_Maladie_France.jpg *License:* CC BY-SA 3.0 *Contributors:* Own work *Original artist:* Zeugma fr (talk) (Antoine FLEURY-GOBERT)

- **File:Centro_salud_Ansoáin3.jpg** *Source:* https://upload.wikimedia.org/wikipedia/commons/9/92/Centro_salud_Anso%C3%A1in3.jpg *License:* CC BY-SA 3.0 *Contributors:* Own work *Original artist:* Miguillen

- **File:Changes_in_Coverage_Health_Care_Bills.png** *Source:* https://upload.wikimedia.org/wikipedia/commons/e/e4/Changes_in_ Coverage_Health_Care_Bills.png *License:* CC BY-SA 3.0 *Contributors:* Own work (Original text: *I (Marcgoldwein (talk)) created this work entirely by myself.*) *Original artist:* Marcgoldwein (talk)

- **File:Charité_(Berlin).jpg** *Source:* https://upload.wikimedia.org/wikipedia/commons/2/29/Charit%C3%A9_%28Berlin%29.jpg *License:* CC BY-SA 4.0 *Contributors:* Own work *Original artist:* Raimond Spekking

- **File:Clinicaprivadaensevilla.JPG** *Source:* https://upload.wikimedia.org/wikipedia/commons/f/fd/Clinicaprivadaensevilla.JPG *License:* GFDL *Contributors:* Own work *Original artist:* Frobles

- **File:Coat_of_arms_of_Massachusetts.svg** *Source:* https://upload.wikimedia.org/wikipedia/commons/5/57/Coat_of_arms_of_ Massachusetts.svg *License:* Public domain *Contributors:*

- Seal_of_Massachusetts.svg *Original artist:* Seal_of_Massachusetts.svg: Adaptation by User:Sagredo

- **File:Commons-logo.svg** *Source:* https://upload.wikimedia.org/wikipedia/en/4/4a/Commons-logo.svg *License:* PD *Contributors:* ? *Original artist:* ?

- **File:Compensation_-_Gross_and_Net_of_Health_Insurance_Premiums.png** *Source:* https://upload.wikimedia.org/wikipedia/commons/ 7/7f/Compensation_-_Gross_and_Net_of_Health_Insurance_Premiums.png *License:* Public domain *Contributors:* White House CEA Report June 2009 *Original artist:* White House Council of Economic Advisors

- **File:Comunidades_autónomas_de_España.svg** *Source:* https://upload.wikimedia.org/wikipedia/commons/b/b4/Comunidades_aut%C3% B3nomas_de_Espa%C3%B1a.svg *License:* CC-BY-SA-3.0 *Contributors:* Basado en Image:Autonomous communities of Spain no names.svg, realizado por Habbit, edited by Nnemo *Original artist:* Rodriguillo, edited by Nnemo

- **File:Connectorroundlogo.png** *Source:* https://upload.wikimedia.org/wikipedia/en/a/a5/Connectorroundlogo.png *License:* Fair use *Contributors:*

  The logo may be obtained from Massachusetts health care reform.

  Original artist: ?

- **File:Crystal_Clear_app_kedit.svg** *Source:* https://upload.wikimedia.org/wikipedia/commons/e/e8/Crystal_Clear_app_kedit.svg *License:* LGPL *Contributors:* Own work *Original artist:* w:User:Tkgd, Everaldo Coelho and YellowIcon

- **File:Delegacionprovincialdesalud.JPG** *Source:* https://upload.wikimedia.org/wikipedia/commons/7/7f/Delegacionprovincialdesalud.JPG *License:* GFDL *Contributors:* Own work *Original artist:* Frobles

- **File:Dennis_Kucinich.jpg** *Source:* https://upload.wikimedia.org/wikipedia/commons/e/ef/Dennis_Kucinich.jpg *License:* Public domain *Contributors:* http://www.gpoaccess.gov/pictorial/109th/oh.html *Original artist:* Unknown<a href='https://www.wikidata.org/wiki/Q4233718' title='wikidata:Q4233718'><img alt='wikidata:Q4233718' src='https://upload.wikimedia.org/wikipedia/commons/thumb/f/ff/Wikidata-logo. svg/20px-Wikidata-logo.svg.png' width='20' height='11' srcset='https://upload.wikimedia.org/wikipedia/commons/thumb/f/ff/Wikidata-logo. svg/30px-Wikidata-logo.svg.png 1.5x, https://upload.wikimedia.org/wikipedia/commons/thumb/f/ff/Wikidata-logo.svg/40px-Wikidata-logo. svg.png 2x' data-file-width='1050' data-file-height='590' /></a>

- **File:Dependencias_hospitalariasdeurgencias.JPG** *Source:* https://upload.wikimedia.org/wikipedia/commons/9/9b/Dependencias_ hospitalariasdeurgencias.JPG *License:* GFDL *Contributors:* Own work *Original artist:* Frobles

- **File:Directors_of_Global_Smallpox_Eradication_Program.jpg** *Source:* https://upload.wikimedia.org/wikipedia/commons/7/77/ Directors_of_Global_Smallpox_Eradication_Program.jpg *License:* Public domain *Contributors:* This media comes from the Centers for Disease Control and Prevention's Public Health Image Library (PHIL), with identification number **#7079**. *Original artist:*

  - Photo Credit:
  - Content Providers(s): CDC

- **File:Dr_Ulhas_Patil_Medical_College_And_Hospital_1.jpg** *Source:* https://upload.wikimedia.org/wikipedia/commons/0/0d/Dr_Ulhas_ Patil_Medical_College_And_Hospital_1.jpg *License:* CC BY-SA 3.0 *Contributors:* Own work *Original artist:* AbhiRiksh

- **File:EHIC_Slovenia.jpg** *Source:* https://upload.wikimedia.org/wikipedia/commons/a/ad/EHIC_Slovenia.jpg *License:* GFDL 1.2 *Contributors:* http://sl.wikipedia.org/wiki/Slika:EUKZZ.jpg *Original artist:* http://sl.wikipedia.org/w/index.php?title=Uporabnik:Andrej5632

- **File:EU_and_EFTA.svg** *Source:* https://upload.wikimedia.org/wikipedia/commons/a/ad/EU_and_EFTA.svg *License:* CC BY-SA 2.5 *Contributors:*

- EU27-2009_EFTA_and_Eastern_Partnership.svg *Original artist:* Europe_countries.svg: Júlio Reis

- **File:Ecard-rückseite-österreich.png** *Source:* https://upload.wikimedia.org/wikipedia/commons/1/1e/Ecard-r%C3%BCckseite-%C3% B6sterreich.png *License:* CC-BY-SA-3.0 *Contributors:* Own work *Original artist:* Griaß-ti (talk)

- **File:Edit-clear.svg** *Source:* https://upload.wikimedia.org/wikipedia/en/f/f2/Edit-clear.svg *License:* Public domain *Contributors:* The *Tango!* Desktop Project. *Original artist:*

  The people from the Tango! project. And according to the meta-data in the file, specifically: "Andreas Nilsson, and Jakub Steiner (although minimally)."

- **File:Elektronische_Gesundheitskarte_Mustermann_RS.svg** *Source:* https://upload.wikimedia.org/wikipedia/commons/2/22/ Elektronische_Gesundheitskarte_Mustermann_RS.svg *License:* Public domain *Contributors:* selbst erstellt nach einer Vorlage des Bundesministeriums für Gesundheit; allgemeine Informationen zur eGK: Die elektronische Gesundheitskarte *Original artist:* Lumu (<a href='//commons.wikimedia.org/wiki/User_talk:Lumu' title='User talk:Lumu'>talk</a>)

- **File:Elena_Arizmendi_Neutral_White_Cross.PNG** *Source:* https://upload.wikimedia.org/wikipedia/commons/c/c8/Elena_ Arizmendi_Neutral_White_Cross.PNG *License:* Public domain *Contributors:* http://www.taringa.net/posts/imagenes/3173865/ Fotos-Antiguas-de-Mexico-2-Politica.html *Original artist:* H Gutierrez

- **File:Flag_of_Switzerland.svg** *Source:* https://upload.wikimedia.org/wikipedia/commons/f/f3/Flag_of_Switzerland.svg *License:* Public domain *Contributors:* PDF Colors Construction sheet *Original artist:* User:Marc Mongenet

  Credits:

- **File:Flag_of_Turkey.svg** *Source:* https://upload.wikimedia.org/wikipedia/commons/b/b4/Flag_of_Turkey.svg *License:* Public domain *Contributors:* Turkish Flag Law (Türk Bayrağı Kanunu), Law nr. 2893 of 22 September 1983. Text (in Turkish) at the website of the Turkish Historical Society (Türk Tarih Kurumu) *Original artist:* David Benbennick (original author)

- **File:Flag_of_the_Balearic_Islands.svg** *Source:* https://upload.wikimedia.org/wikipedia/commons/7/7b/Flag_of_the_Balearic_Islands.svg *License:* CC0 *Contributors:* ? *Original artist:* ?

- **File:Flag_of_the_Basque_Country.svg** *Source:* https://upload.wikimedia.org/wikipedia/commons/2/2d/Flag_of_the_Basque_Country.svg *License:* CC BY-SA 2.5 *Contributors:* own work (modification of the former image at this page) *Original artist:* Daniele Schirmo aka Frankie688

- **File:Flag_of_the_Canary_Islands.svg** *Source:* https://upload.wikimedia.org/wikipedia/commons/b/b0/Flag_of_the_Canary_Islands.svg *License:* Public domain *Contributors:* ? *Original artist:* ?

- **File:Flag_of_the_Community_of_Madrid.svg** *Source:* https://upload.wikimedia.org/wikipedia/commons/9/9c/Flag_of_the_Community_of_Madrid.svg *License:* CC0 *Contributors:* ? *Original artist:* ?

- **File:Flag_of_the_Czech_Republic.svg** *Source:* https://upload.wikimedia.org/wikipedia/commons/c/cb/Flag_of_the_Czech_Republic.svg *License:* Public domain *Contributors:*

  - -xfi-'s file
  - -xfi-'s code
  - Zirland's codes of colors

  Original artist:
  (of code): SVG version by cs:-xfi-.

- **File:Flag_of_the_Netherlands.svg** *Source:* https://upload.wikimedia.org/wikipedia/commons/2/20/Flag_of_the_Netherlands.svg *License:* Public domain *Contributors:* Own work *Original artist:* Zscout370

- **File:Flag_of_the_Region_of_Murcia.svg** *Source:* https://upload.wikimedia.org/wikipedia/commons/a/a5/Flag_of_the_Region_of_Murcia.svg *License:* CC0 *Contributors:* ? *Original artist:* ?

- **File:Flag_of_the_United_Kingdom.svg** *Source:* https://upload.wikimedia.org/wikipedia/en/a/ae/Flag_of_the_United_Kingdom.svg *License:* PD *Contributors:* ? *Original artist:* ?

- **File:Flag_of_the_United_States.svg** *Source:* https://upload.wikimedia.org/wikipedia/en/a/a4/Flag_of_the_United_States.svg *License:* PD *Contributors:* ? *Original artist:* ?

- **File:Folder_Hexagonal_Icon.svg** *Source:* https://upload.wikimedia.org/wikipedia/en/4/48/Folder_Hexagonal_Icon.svg *License:* Cc-by-sa-3.0 *Contributors:* ? *Original artist:* ?

- **File:Gross_Costs_of_Health_Coverage.png** *Source:* https://upload.wikimedia.org/wikipedia/commons/5/51/Gross_Costs_of_Health_Coverage.png *License:* CC BY-SA 3.0 *Contributors:* Own work (Original text: *I (Marcgoldwein (talk)) created this work entirely by myself.*) *Original artist:* Marcgoldwein (talk)

- **File:HealthEconPlumbing.gif** *Source:* https://upload.wikimedia.org/wikipedia/en/3/37/HealthEconPlumbing.gif *License:* PD *Contributors:* ? *Original artist:* ?

- **File:Health_Care_Spending_in_Switzerland_Per_Capita,_1998_to_2008.JPG** *Source:* https://upload.wikimedia.org/wikipedia/commons/2/20/Health_Care_Spending_in_Switzerland_Per_Capita%2C_1998_to_2008.JPG *License:* Public domain *Contributors:* Own work *Original artist:* Sugar-Baby-Love

- **File:Hemodialysismachine.jpg** *Source:* https://upload.wikimedia.org/wikipedia/commons/f/fc/Hemodialysismachine.jpg *License:* CC-BY-SA-3.0 *Contributors:* ? *Original artist:* ?

- **File:Hospital_Torrecárdenas_2.JPG** *Source:* https://upload.wikimedia.org/wikipedia/commons/2/2f/Hospital_Torrec%C3%A1rdenas_2.JPG *License:* GFDL *Contributors:* Own work *Original artist:* Schumi4ever

- **File:Hospital_Valdecilla.PNG** *Source:* https://upload.wikimedia.org/wikipedia/commons/7/79/Hospital_Valdecilla.PNG *License:* Public domain *Contributors:* Own work *Original artist:* Desmondrx

- **File:Hospitalinfantilesevilla.JPG** *Source:* https://upload.wikimedia.org/wikipedia/commons/f/f7/Hospitalinfantilesevilla.JPG *License:* GFDL *Contributors:* Own work *Original artist:* Frobles

- **File:Hscportallogo.png** *Source:* https://upload.wikimedia.org/wikipedia/en/7/78/Hscportallogo.png *License:* Fair use *Contributors:* http://www.hscni.net *Original artist:* ?

- **File:Image_of_Triangle_Shirtwaist_Factory_fire_on_March_25_-_1911.jpg** *Source:* https://upload.wikimedia.org/wikipedia/commons/8/87/Image_of_Triangle_Shirtwaist_Factory_fire_on_March_25_-_1911.jpg *License:* Public domain *Contributors:* http://www.ilr.cornell.edu/trianglefire/primary/photosIllustrations/slideshow.html?image_id=746&sec_id=3#screen *Original artist:* Unknown<a href='https://www.wikidata.org/wiki/Q4233718' title='wikidata:Q4233718'><img alt='wikidata:Q4233718' src='https://upload.wikimedia.org/wikipedia/commons/thumb/f/ff/Wikidata-logo.svg/20px-Wikidata-logo.svg.png' width='20' height='11' srcset='https://upload.wikimedia.org/wikipedia/commons/thumb/f/ff/Wikidata-logo.svg/30px-Wikidata-logo.svg.png 1.5x, https://upload.wikimedia.org/wikipedia/commons/thumb/f/ff/Wikidata-logo.svg/40px-Wikidata-logo.svg.png 2x' data-file-width='1050' data-file-height='590' /></a>

- **File:Israeli_Health_Care_Spending_as_a_Percentage_of_GDP.jpg** *Source:* https://upload.wikimedia.org/wikipedia/commons/8/86/ Israeli_Health_Care_Spending_as_a_Percentage_of_GDP.jpg *License:* Public domain *Contributors:* Own work (Original text: *I (Sugar-Baby-Love (talk)) created this work entirely by myself.*) *Original artist:* Sugar-Baby-Love (talk)

- **File:Kinderarzt.jpg** *Source:* https://upload.wikimedia.org/wikipedia/commons/a/a6/Kinderarzt.jpg *License:* Public domain *Contributors:* german wikipedia, original source was http://www.defense.gov/photos/Aug2004/040818-A-1300H-053.html (not available) *Original artist:* Sgt. Vernell Hall, U.S. Army

- **File:Laprascopy-Roentgen.jpg** *Source:* https://upload.wikimedia.org/wikipedia/commons/c/c7/Laprascopy-Roentgen.jpg *License:* Public domain *Contributors:* Medical x-ray (flouroscopy) *Original artist:* HenrikP

- **File:Lester_B._Pearson_with_a_pencil.jpg** *Source:* https://upload.wikimedia.org/wikipedia/commons/a/a1/Lester_B._Pearson_with_a_ pencil.jpg *License:* Public domain *Contributors:* This image is available from Library and Archives Canada under the reproduction reference number **e002505448** and under the MIKAN ID number 3607934
  Original artist: Toronto Star

- **File:Life_expectancy_vs_healthcare_spending.jpg** *Source:* https://upload.wikimedia.org/wikipedia/commons/d/d6/Life_expectancy_vs_ healthcare_spending.jpg *License:* CC BY-SA 4.0 *Contributors:* OurWorldInData.org *Original artist:* Max Roser

- **File:Lock-green.svg** *Source:* https://upload.wikimedia.org/wikipedia/commons/6/65/Lock-green.svg *License:* CC0 *Contributors:* en:File: Free-to-read_lock_75.svg *Original artist:* User:Trappist the monk

- **File:Logo_SERGAS.png** *Source:* https://upload.wikimedia.org/wikipedia/commons/3/3d/Logo_SERGAS.png *License:* Public domain *Contributors:* Orde de 17 do abril de 2007 pola que se establecen o símbolo, o logotipo e o manual de identidade corporativa do Servizo Galego de Saúde DOG_20070511_NUM_091.PDF page 21 *Original artist:* Xunta de Galicia

- **File:Logo_pami.png** *Source:* https://upload.wikimedia.org/wikipedia/commons/f/f1/Logo_pami.png *License:* CC BY 2.5 *Contributors:* http: //www.pami.org.ar/ *Original artist:* PAMI INSSJP

- **File:Logotipo_del_SERMAS_(RPS_10-03-2012).png** *Source:* https://upload.wikimedia.org/wikipedia/commons/d/d5/Logotipo_del_ SERMAS_%28RPS_10-03-2012%29.png *License:* Public domain *Contributors:* Own work *Original artist:* Raimundo Pastor

- **File:Logotipo_del_Servicio_Andaluz_de_Salud.svg** *Source:* https://upload.wikimedia.org/wikipedia/commons/8/8a/Logotipo_del_ Servicio_Andaluz_de_Salud.svg *License:* CC BY-SA 4.0 *Contributors:* Own work *Original artist:* NACLE

- **File:MRT_Myanmar.jpg** *Source:* https://upload.wikimedia.org/wikipedia/en/9/9a/MRT_Myanmar.jpg *License:* CC-BY-SA-3.0 *Contributors:* ? *Original artist:* ?

- **File:Mammogram.jpg** *Source:* https://upload.wikimedia.org/wikipedia/commons/d/dd/Mammogram.jpg *License:* Public domain *Contributors:*

- http://www.cancer.gov/cancertopics/pdq/screening/breast/Patient/page3 *Original artist:* National Cancer Institute

- **File:Maple_Leaf_(from_roundel).svg** *Source:* https://upload.wikimedia.org/wikipedia/commons/f/fc/Maple_Leaf_%28from_roundel%29. svg *License:* CC-BY-SA-3.0 *Contributors:*

- Roundel_of_the_Royal_Canadian_Air_Force_(1946-1965).svg *Original artist:* Roundel_of_the_Royal_Canadian_Air_Force_(1946-1965).svg: F l a n k e r

- **File:MedCorpsBC.gif** *Source:* https://upload.wikimedia.org/wikipedia/commons/e/e2/MedCorpsBC.gif *License:* Public domain *Contributors:* ? *Original artist:* ?

- **File:Medicare_and_Medicaid_GDP_Chart.png** *Source:* https://upload.wikimedia.org/wikipedia/commons/b/b3/Medicare_and_Medicaid_ GDP_Chart.png *License:* Public domain *Contributors:* http://www.cbo.gov/ftpdocs/93xx/doc9317/05-29-NASI_Speech.pdf *Original artist:* CBO and farcaster

- **File:Medicare_brand.svg** *Source:* https://upload.wikimedia.org/wikipedia/commons/c/cd/Medicare_brand.svg *License:* Public domain *Contributors:* http://www.medicareaustralia.gov.au/public/migrants/files/1856-21-medicare-enrolment-children-adopted-from-overseas.pdf *Original artist:* Uploader.

- **File:Medicare_spending_per_capita.png** *Source:* https://upload.wikimedia.org/wikipedia/commons/f/fd/Medicare_spending_per_capita. png *License:* Public domain *Contributors:* White House CEA Report June 2009 *Original artist:* This is a work of the United States Federal Government, copied with a new header

- **File:Ms._magazine_Cover_-_Spring_2010.jpg** *Source:* https://upload.wikimedia.org/wikipedia/commons/e/e7/Ms._magazine_Cover_-_ Spring_2010.jpg *License:* CC BY-SA 4.0 *Contributors:* Ms. magazine *Original artist:* Liberty Media for Women, LLC

- **File:NHS.svg** *Source:* https://upload.wikimedia.org/wikipedia/commons/7/73/NHS.svg *License:* Public domain *Contributors:* :en:Image:NHS.svg *Original artist:* Unknown<a href='https://www.wikidata.org/wiki/Q4233718' title='wikidata:Q4233718'><img alt='wikidata:Q4233718' src='https://upload.wikimedia.org/wikipedia/commons/thumb/f/ff/Wikidata-logo.svg/20px-Wikidata-logo.svg.png' width='20' height='11' srcset='https://upload.wikimedia.org/wikipedia/commons/thumb/f/ff/Wikidata-logo.svg/30px-Wikidata-logo.svg.png 1.5x, https://upload.wikimedia.org/wikipedia/commons/thumb/f/ff/Wikidata-logo.svg/40px-Wikidata-logo.svg.png 2x' data-file-width='1050' data-file-height='590' /></a>

- **File:NHS_Scotland.svg** *Source:* https://upload.wikimedia.org/wikipedia/commons/9/9a/NHS_Scotland.svg *License:* Public domain *Contributors:* http://www.scot.nhs.uk/wp-content/uploads/2016/02/cropped-NHS_Logo_ds.png *Original artist:* NHS Scotland

- **File:NHS_logo_in_Wales.png** *Source:* https://upload.wikimedia.org/wikipedia/en/8/84/NHS_logo_in_Wales.png *License:* Fair use *Contributors:*
  The logo may be obtained from NHS Wales.
  Original artist: ?

- **File:Snow-cholera-map-1.jpg** *Source:* https://upload.wikimedia.org/wikipedia/commons/2/27/Snow-cholera-map-1.jpg *License:* Public domain *Contributors:*
(This image was originally from en.wikipedia; description page is/was here.)
Original artist: John Snow

- **File:Tarjetasanitariaindividual.JPG** *Source:* https://upload.wikimedia.org/wikipedia/commons/a/a8/Tarjetasanitariaindividual.JPG *License:* GFDL *Contributors:* Own work *Original artist:* Frobles

- **File:The_cow_pock.jpg** *Source:* https://upload.wikimedia.org/wikipedia/commons/d/d6/The_cow_pock.jpg *License:* Public domain *Contributors:* Library of Congress, Prints & Photographs Division, LC-USZC4-3147 (color film copy transparency), archival TIFF version (4 MB), converted to JPEG with the GIMP 2.4.5, image quality 88. *Original artist:* James Gillray

- **File:The_hospital_ship_USNS_Mercy_(T-AH_19)_June_6,_2012,_in_Manado,_Indonesia,_during_Pacific_Partnership_2012_ 120606-N-CW427-402.jpg** *Source:* https://upload.wikimedia.org/wikipedia/commons/6/6a/The_hospital_ship_USNS_Mercy_%28T-AH_ 19%29_June_6%2C_2012%2C_in_Manado%2C_Indonesia%2C_during_Pacific_Partnership_2012_120606-N-CW427-402.jpg *License:* Public domain *Contributors:* http://www.defenseimagery.mil/imageRetrieve.action?guid=93697b964dff8134cfcb199873f2e6f41fb4b97f&t=2 *Original artist:* MC3 Clay M. Whaley

- **File:Torrelodones._Centro_de_Salud_y_Canto_del_Pico.jpg** *Source:* https://upload.wikimedia.org/wikipedia/commons/f/ff/ Torrelodones._Centro_de_Salud_y_Canto_del_Pico.jpg *License:* CC-BY-SA-3.0 *Contributors:* Own work *Original artist:* Paconi

- **File:Total_health_expenditure_per_capita,_US_Dollars_PPP.png** *Source:* https://upload.wikimedia.org/wikipedia/commons/8/80/Total_ health_expenditure_per_capita%2C_US_Dollars_PPP.png *License:* Public domain *Contributors:* I (Sugar-Baby-Love (talk)) created this work by myself, using tools from the free charting site chartgo.com along with public OECD information as mentioned above. *Original artist:* Sugar-Baby-Love (talk)

- **File:U.S._Insurance_Contributions_(1990_to_2010).jpg** *Source:* https://upload.wikimedia.org/wikipedia/commons/b/b4/U.S._Insurance_ Contributions_%281990_to_2010%29.jpg *License:* Public domain *Contributors:* Own work (Original text: *I (Sugar-Baby-Love (talk)) created this work entirely by myself.*) *Original artist:* Sugar-Baby-Love (talk)

- **File:U.S._Uninsured_and_Uninsured_Rate_(1987_to_2008).JPG** *Source:* https://upload.wikimedia.org/wikipedia/commons/4/4d/U.S. _Uninsured_and_Uninsured_Rate_%281987_to_2008%29.JPG *License:* Public domain *Contributors:* "Income, Poverty, and Health Insurance Coverage in the United States: 2008", United States Department of Commerce: United States Census Bureau, Page 22, released through the U.S. Government Printing Office in Washington in 2009. A version is avilable online here. *Original artist:* The report was composed by Carmen DeNavas-Walt, Bernadette D. Proctor, and Jessica C. Smith.

- **File:Unbalanced_scales.svg** *Source:* https://upload.wikimedia.org/wikipedia/commons/f/fe/Unbalanced_scales.svg *License:* Public domain *Contributors:* ? *Original artist:* ?

- **File:Universal_health_care.svg** *Source:* https://upload.wikimedia.org/wikipedia/commons/2/25/Universal_health_care.svg *License:* CC BY-SA 3.0 *Contributors:* This file was derived from: BlankMap-World6.svg
Original artist: NuclearVacuum, Obi-wan Kenobi, Apatens

- **File:Visiting_Nurse_Service_of_New_York_Logo.jpg** *Source:* https://upload.wikimedia.org/wikipedia/en/6/6c/Visiting_Nurse_Service_ of_New_York_Logo.jpg *License:* Fair use *Contributors:* The Visiting Nurse Service of New York *Original artist:* ?

- **File:Vista_Login_Manager_Cropped.svg** *Source:* https://upload.wikimedia.org/wikipedia/commons/1/15/Vista_Login_Manager_Cropped. svg *License:* GPL *Contributors:* Image:Vista-Login Manager2.png, from [1] *Original artist:* Sa-Ki at DeviantArt, traced by User:Stannered

- **File:Wiki_letter_w.svg** *Source:* https://upload.wikimedia.org/wikipedia/en/6/6c/Wiki_letter_w.svg *License:* Cc-by-sa-3.0 *Contributors:* ? *Original artist:* ?

- **File:Wiki_letter_w_cropped.svg** *Source:* https://upload.wikimedia.org/wikipedia/commons/1/1c/Wiki_letter_w_cropped.svg *License:* CC-BY-SA-3.0 *Contributors:* This file was derived from Wiki letter w.svg: <a href='//commons.wikimedia.org/wiki/File:Wiki_letter_w.svg' class='image'><img alt='Wiki letter w.svg' src='https://upload.wikimedia.org/wikipedia/commons/thumb/6/6c/Wiki_letter_w.svg/50px-Wiki_ letter_w.svg.png' width='50' height='50' srcset='https://upload.wikimedia.org/wikipedia/commons/thumb/6/6c/Wiki_letter_w.svg/75px-Wiki_ letter_w.svg.png 1.5x, https://upload.wikimedia.org/wikipedia/commons/thumb/6/6c/Wiki_letter_w.svg/100px-Wiki_letter_w.svg.png 2x' data-file-width='44' data-file-height='44' /></a>
Original artist: Derivative work by Thumperward

- **File:Wikisource-logo.svg** *Source:* https://upload.wikimedia.org/wikipedia/commons/4/4c/Wikisource-logo.svg *License:* CC BY-SA 3.0 *Contributors:* Rei-artur *Original artist:* Nicholas Moreau

- **File:Wikiversity-logo.svg** *Source:* https://upload.wikimedia.org/wikipedia/commons/9/91/Wikiversity-logo.svg *License:* CC BY-SA 3.0 *Contributors:* Snorky (optimized and cleaned up by verdy_p) *Original artist:* Snorky (optimized and cleaned up by verdy_p)

- **File:Wikivoyage-Logo-v3-icon.svg** *Source:* https://upload.wikimedia.org/wikipedia/commons/d/dd/Wikivoyage-Logo-v3-icon.svg *License:* CC BY-SA 3.0 *Contributors:* Own work *Original artist:* AleXXw

- **File:World_Health_Organisation_building_from_west.jpg** *Source:* https://upload.wikimedia.org/wikipedia/commons/6/6e/ World_Health_Organisation_building_from_west.jpg *License:* GFDL *Contributors:* Own work *Original artist:* Yann (<a href='//commons.wikimedia.org/wiki/User_talk:Yann' title='User talk:Yann'>talk</a>)

4.3 Content license

- Creative Commons Attribution-Share Alike 3.0